MEDICATION SAFETY
Dispensing Drugs Without Error

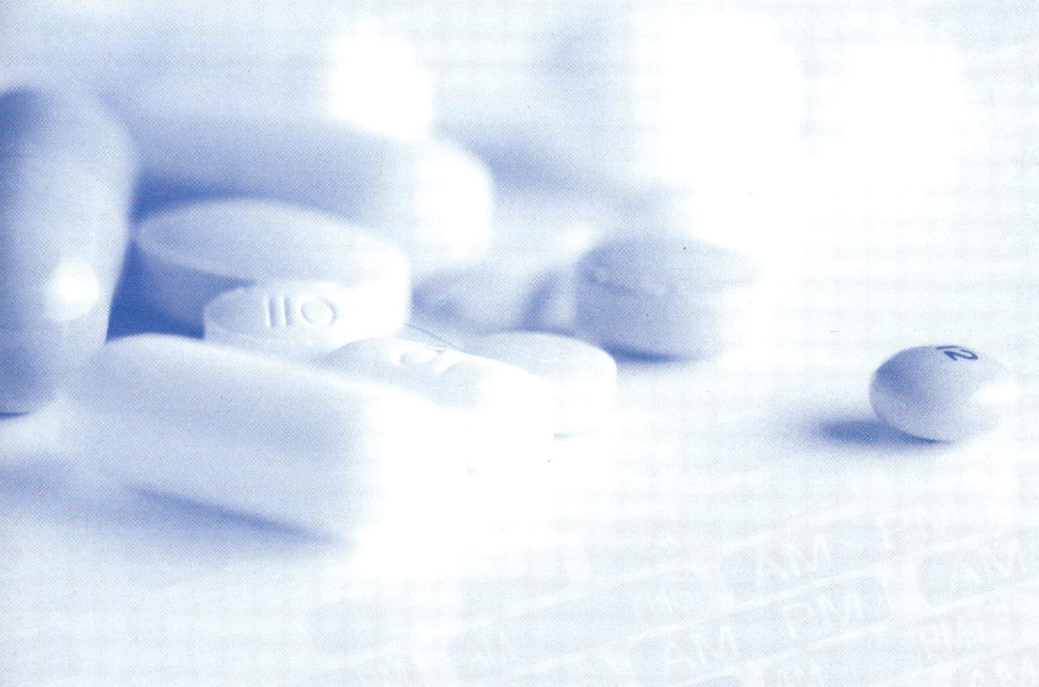

MEDICATION SAFETY
Dispensing Drugs Without Error

KENNETH R. BAKER, BS Pharm, JD

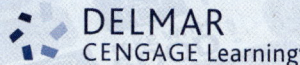
DELMAR
CENGAGE Learning

Australia • Brazil • Japan • Korea • Mexico • Singapore • Spain • United Kingdom • United States

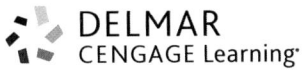

Medication Safety: Dispensing Drugs Without Error
Kenneth R. Baker, BS Pharm, JD

Vice President, Careers & Computing:
Dave Garza

Director of Learning Solutions:
Matthew Kane

Senior Acquisitions Editor: Tari Broderick

Managing Editor: Marah Bellegarde

Product Manager: Natalie Pashoukos

Editorial Assistant: Nicole Manikas

Vice President, Marketing: Jennifer Baker

Marketing Director: Wendy Mapstone

Associate Marketing Manager:
Jonathan Sheehan

Senior Production Director:
Wendy A. Troeger

Production Manager: Andrew Crouth

Content Project Manager: Allyson Bozeth

Senior Art Director: Jack Pendleton

© 2013 Delmar, Cengage Learning

ALL RIGHTS RESERVED. No part of this work covered by the copyright herein may be reproduced, transmitted, stored or used in any form or by any means graphic, electronic, or mechanical, including but not limited to photocopying, recording, scanning, digitizing, taping, Web distribution, information networks, or information storage and retrieval systems, except as permitted under Section 107 or 108 of the 1976 United States Copyright Act, or applicable copyright law of another jurisdiction, without the prior written permission of the publisher.

> For permission to use material from this text or product,
> submit all requests online at **www.cengage.com/permissions**
> Further permissions questions can be e-mailed to
> **permissionrequest@cengage.com**

International Edition:

ISBN-13: 978-1-1332-8446-8
ISBN-10: 1-1332-8446-9

Cengage Learning International Offices

Asia
www.cengageasia.com
tel: (65) 6410 1200

Brazil
www.cengage.com.br
tel: (55) 11 3665 9900

Latin America
www.cengage.com.mx
tel: (52) 55 1500 6000

Australia/New Zealand
www.cengage.com.au
tel: (61) 3 9685 4711

India
www.cengage.co.in
tel: (91) 11 4364 1111

UK/Europe/Middle East/Africa
www.cengage.co.uk
tel: (44) 0 1264 332 424

**Represented in Canada by
Nelson Education, Ltd.**
www.nelson.com
tel: (416) 752 9100 / (800) 668 0671

Cengage Learning is a leading provider of customized learning solutions with office locations around the globe, including Singapore, the United Kingdom, Australia, Mexico, Brazil, and Japan. Locate your local office at:
www.cengage.com/global

For product information and free companion resources:
www.cengage.com/international

Visit your local office: **www.cengage.com/global**

Printed in the United States of America
1 2 3 4 5 6 7 16 15 14 13 12

Dedication

To my wife, partner, supporter,
and friend
Kay Baker, RN

To my sons:
Stephen Baker
Jason Baker

To my grandchildren:
Logan
Alexandra
Zachary
Hannah
Jordan
Drew
Aaron

Preface

Purpose

This book is specifically written for pharmacy technicians as a guide to reducing medication errors. While introducing the theory behind continuous quality improvement (CQI), the focus of this book is on real, day-to-day, practical applications of the CQI workflow in pharmacy. The emphasis is on the role of pharmacy technicians as a driving force in serving patients, including their responsibility for delivering the right drug with the right directions to the right patient.

This book recognizes, however, that pharmacy technicians' duties go beyond dispensing. Portions of the text explore ways in which pharmacy technicians can assist pharmacists to fully carry out their ever-increasing duties in the areas of counseling and prospective drug review.

Technicians who are students today may someday be pharmacy trainers and managers. With this in mind, there are chapters on training, monitoring, and constructing quality pharmacy systems.

Mission: A Note from the Author

Having studied and worked in the field of medication errors and continuous quality improvement for over 25 years, I have become convinced that the keys to reducing medication errors in pharmacy are well-trained and educated pharmacy technicians. Pharmacists and members of management are important, but it is the trained and educated pharmacy technician who will make a CQI system work.

The fulfillment of pharmacy's obligation to "First, do no harm," depends upon the commitment of those pharmacy technicians who are on the front line of patient service. The roles of the pharmacist are changing. Those important new roles can be fully achieved only if pharmacy technicians are trained in the art and science of pharmacy dispensing in a way that minimizes medication errors.

I wrote this book because medication errors can and must be reduced and because pharmacy technicians are critical to achieving that goal. I have designed CQI systems for pharmacy chains and independent pharmacies.[1] After giving countless lectures, writing scores of articles, and spending hours teaching about designing and implementing CQI workflow systems, I have been frustrated by the

---

[1] These programs were codesigned with David Brushwood, noted in the "Acknowledgments" section. Without the help of David and the pharmacies also noted in the "Acknowledgments," these programs would not have been possible.

lack of textbooks designed to train technicians in the practical issues of reducing medication errors.

There are many books that discuss theories of quality. Many are great. I use them, quote from them, and have authored chapters[2] in some, but they are not designed for training technicians. This book discusses day-to-day issues in quality such as the use of best practices and how, where, and why steps should be placed in the pharmacy's workflow to reduce medication errors. From my years as a trial lawyer, I particularly thought it was important that the lessons be illustrated by stories, court cases, professional liability claims, and hypothetical situations in a way that students would be able to relate to the matters discussed. Stories can make abstract ideas come alive to a jury and to a class of students.

I envisioned a book about quality in pharmacy that could be used not only in a course dedicated to teaching quality, but also in the dispensing laboratory and a pharmacy-operations class. I hope this text will help students understand, design, and implement a workflow based upon total quality management (TQM) and CQI principles aimed at minimizing medication errors.

Structure and Organization

The book focuses on the pharmacy technician's role in day-to-day pharmacy operations as they relate to reducing medication errors. Throughout, the text is illustrated by real, pharmacy-liability cases and claims to help readers relate to the dangers of medication errors and how attention to pharmacy processes can prevent them.

Edwards Deming's philosophy of quality management, process workflow, and monitoring using statistical control is woven through the text combining theory with the day-to-day application of CQI. Along with the role of the pharmacy technician, the book discusses the emerging roles of pharmacists, with an emphasis on ways in which technicians can assist pharmacists in protecting and educating their patients.

This book discusses how to identify where errors could occur and how to guard against them. The chapters on workflow provide concrete examples of a CQI pharmacy workflow and discuss why each step is necessary. Two important topics in pharmacy CQI are monitoring and training. Pharmacy technicians should understand why and how to monitor the pharmacy's CQI system so that medication error-reduction programs are able to constantly improve.

---

[2] Chapters written by me are listed in "About the Author" in this preface.

Pharmacy-technician students today will be the future trainers and pharmacy managers. One chapter focuses on the importance and techniques used in training members of the pharmacy staff to implement and use the CQI program.

The final chapter discusses how the patient can be brought into and made a part of the pharmacy's quality system. The patient often provides the last chance to prevent a medication error. Included is a discussion of the pharmacy staff's role in helping patients avoid medication errors caused by prescribers and even by the patients themselves.

SPECIAL AIDS AND FEATURES

Throughout the text, the student will find illustrations and drawings designed to help understand the concepts described. These visual and other aids are presented in various ways to provide context and aid comprehension: stories, hypotheticals, court cases, and facts from insurance company claims. In addition, the book provides the following special aids and features:

1. **OBJECTIVES** are given at the beginning of each chapter to enable the instructor and students to know what information they can expect from the material.

2. An **OUTLINE** of each chapter provides the students with the subject matter and method of organization of the material discussed.

3. **KEY TERMS** in each chapter precede the text and are highlighted when first used in the chapter. These key terms provide a context for phrases and words with which the students may be unfamiliar.

4. **STUDIES, GRAPHS, AND CHARTS** relating to professional liability claims are used throughout the text. Many of these claims are provided through the courtesy of Pharmacists Mutual Insurance Company, the leader in pharmacy malpractice insurance. These provide a real-world setting for the topic being discussed.

5. **FORMS AND TOOLS** are presented that are designed as aids for pharmacy technicians when working with pharmacists or analyzing an error. An example is a counseling algorithm identifying especially vulnerable patients for the pharmacist counseling or drug review consideration. These forms and tools provide concepts students may use later in their careers to design their own forms and tools to enhance their pharmacy practice.

6. **PRESCRIPTIONS AND DRAWINGS** illustrating best practices or training techniques described in the text are used to enhance the text. Pharmacy technicians may be called upon to improve quality workflows in the future. This material is presented to help the students understand how techniques are used and why they work.

7. A detailed **QUALITY-ASSURANCE WORKFLOW** with specific steps and best practices is included. The workflow presented is not intended as a process to be followed, but to provoke thought and understanding for when the students may in their careers be called upon to design or redesign a system of CQI workflow.

8. **QUALITY NOTES** provide additional comments and information on topics in a particular chapter. These notes are to provoke thought and point the students to additional subjects related to the specific material.

9. **RxERCISES** are presented as part of each chapter. Instructors may use these as assignments or as the basis of a conversation, argument, or debate. They are "think" pieces allowing the students to become part of the topic being discussed.

10. **Links and Citations** are provided throughout the book and at the end of each chapter. It is hoped students will follow one or two of these references for more in-depth information on the subjects cited.

ADDITIONAL TEACHING AND LEARNING RESOURCES

Instructor Companion Site

(ISBN 978-1-1115-3947-4)

An Instructor Companion Site is available that includes the Instructor Resources.

To access the Instructor Companion site, go to http://login.cengage.com

- *If you have a Cengage SSO account:* Sign in with your e-mail address and password.

- *If you do not have a Cengage SSO account:* Click "Create My Account" and follow the prompts.

Instructor's Manual

The instructor's manual includes answers to the review questions contained within the textbook. The review questions are designed to assess the student's accomplishment of the chapter objectives and may be useful as a homework assignment or simply as a self-assessment tool.

PowerPoint® Presentations

More than 400 PowerPoint slides are designed to aid instructors in planning their class presentations. If a student misses a class, a printout of the slides for a lecture provides a helpful review page. Instructors should feel free to add their own slides for additional topics introduced to the class.

Computerized Test Bank in ExamView®

The test bank includes approximately 400 test questions. These include multiple-choice, matching, and short-answer questions. Users can add their own questions. This software allows the user to create tests in less than 5 minutes, with the ability to print them out in a variety of layouts. It also has electronic "take-home testing" (put test on disk) and Internet-based testing capabilities.

ACKNOWLEDGMENTS

There are too many people and companies who have helped me in writing this book and gathering information to list all. Without the following, however, I could not have conceived of or presented the ideas and information contained in this book.

Pharmacists Mutual Insurance Company and the following individuals who have built and sustained this important part of the profession of pharmacy:

Edward Yorty, FCAS, MAAA, President

Ed Berg, CPA, CPCU, ARe, MBA, President (retired)

Kirk Hayes, CPCU, President (retired)

Don McGuire, BS Pharm, JD, Senior Vice President, Risk Management, General Counsel

Frank Gartland, BS Pharm, JD, formerly Vice President and General Counsel

(Pharmacists Mutual and its subsidiary, PMC Quality Commitment, Inc., provided several graphs, charts, and examples used in this book.)

Renaud Cook Drury Mesaros, PA, and the attorneys and staff who have provided encouragement and assistance while I wrote this book. In particular a special thanks to Bill Drury, Steve Mesaros, David McDowell, Mike Wolver, Carol Romano, Margie McCarthy, and Charlie Hover, along with all the other excellent attorneys and staff who have made Renaud Cook Drury Mesaros, PA, one of the finest law firms in the state of Arizona.

The following individuals to whom I must give special recognition:

David Brushwood, who taught me much of what I know in this area and who worked with me to develop (invent) Pharmacy Quality Commitment®

Mike Cohen and Donna Horn of ISMP, who shared with me much of their knowledge, experience, and wisdom in how to reduce medication errors

The following institutions that helped me refine my understandings and ideas:

American Society for Pharmacy Law

University of Iowa, College of Pharmacy

University of Florida, College of Pharmacy

Midwestern University, College of Pharmacy, Glendale Campus

Hy-Vee Pharmacies, Kmart Corporation, and Eckert Drugs, which allowed me to design and/or implement, along with Dave Brushwood, CQI systems that they put into practice

NASPA and the 50 state pharmacy associations in the nation that provide the Pharmacy Quality Commitment® quality-assurance and monitoring programs to pharmacies across the United States

Countless colleges of pharmacy and professors who allowed me to lecture to their students and thereby hone, and often modify, my messages of quality assurance and CQI programs to reduce medication errors

Reviewers

Alaric Barber, RPhT, CPhT, MBA
Pharmacy Technician Consultant/Instructor
Corinthian Colleges, Inc.
Santa Ana, CA

Lezlie Cohn-Oswald, CPhT
Clinical Pharmacy Technician
Professional Standards Board Chair–VHA
Pharmacy Technician Externship Associate Program Director–VASLCHCS
Salt Lake City, UT

Katie McGlothlen, MHA, CPhT
Pharmacy Technician Program Director
Brookline College
Phoenix, AZ

Lorraine C. Zentz, CPhT, PhD
Author/Instructor
Cengage Learning/Ed2Go
Mesa, CO

About the Author

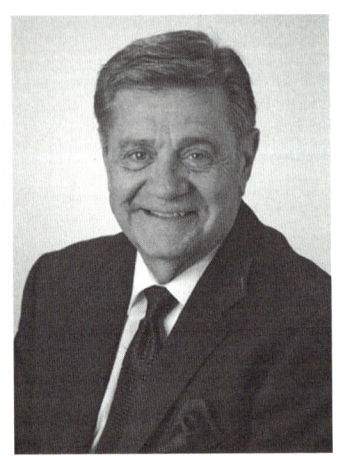

Ken Baker is a pharmacist and an attorney. He practices law, of counsel, with the Phoenix, Arizona, law firm of Renaud Cook Drury Mesaros, PA. Ken also consults on subjects ranging from pharmacy law, pharmacy compounding, insurance, risk management, reducing medication errors, and quality-assurance systems. His clients include Pharmacists Mutual Insurance Company and PMC Quality Commitment, Inc.

In addition to consulting and law practice, Ken teaches as adjunct faculty at Midwestern University College of Pharmacy in Glendale, Arizona, where he teaches courses in Ethical Decision Making and Risk Management / Patient Safety. He is also adjunct assistant professor for the University of Florida, where he teaches three courses (State Regulations; Enterprise Risk Management; and Pharmaceutical Crimes) in the Masters of Pharmacy Internet program. Previously, Mr. Baker taught Pharmacy Law and Ethics at the University of Iowa.

Following graduation from Purdue University, School of Pharmacy, Ken practiced pharmacy prior to returning to law school. He worked in independent and chain pharmacies and managed a chain pharmacy in Indianapolis, Indiana. Upon graduation from Indiana University School of Law, Indianapolis (cum laude), Ken entered law practice in Lebanon, Indiana, where he practiced general trial law, including service as a deputy prosecuting attorney for Boone County, Indiana.

Ken practiced law for several years before joining Pharmacists Mutual Insurance Co. where he was senior vice president and general counsel as well as executive vice president of PMC Quality Commitment, Inc., a Pharmacists Mutual subsidiary. Ken served for two years as the executive director of the Pharmacy Compounding Accreditation Board in Washington, DC.

Ken Baker is past president of the American Society for Pharmacy Law and the Iowa Pharmacy Foundation. His publications and presentations include:

Articles and Speeches: Ken speaks widely and writes various articles in the fields of risk management, pharmacy law, pharmacist liability, compounding, and medication errors.

Rx School, Continuing Education: Bimonthly online CE for pharmacists and technicians

Law Review: The OBRA-90 Mandate and Its Developing Impact on the Pharmacist's Standard of Care, *Drake Law Review* (Vol. 44, No. 3)

Book Chapters:

- Risk Management, in *Quality and Safety in Pharmacy Practice*, Terri L. Warholak and David P. Nau, Eds. New York: McGraw-Hill, 2010

- Fundamentals of Insurance, in *Pharmacy Management, Leadership, Marketing, and Finance* (scheduled for second edition), Marie A. Chisholm-Burns, Allison Vaillancourt, and Marvin Shepherd, Eds. Burlington, MA: Jones and Bartlett, 2011

- Managing Risks—The Basics, in *Pharmacy Management, Leadership, Marketing, and Finance* (scheduled for second edition), Marie A. Chisholm-Burns, Allison Vaillancourt, and Marvin Shepherd, Eds. Burlington, MA: Jones and Bartlett, 2011

- Principles of Professional Liability Insurance for Pharmacists, in *Pharmacy Law Desk Reference*, Delbert D. Konnor, Ed. Philadelphia, PA: Haworth Press, 2007

- Documentation in Pharmacy Practice, in *Pharmacy Practice Manual*, 2nd ed., Larry E. Boh, Ed. Lippincott, Williams and Wilkins, 2001

Drug Topics: Bimonthly column, print and digital eds., *Pharmacy Law*

Textbook: Baker, K. R., *Medication Safety: Dispensing Drugs without Error*. Delmar, NY: Delmar Cengage Learning. (Anticipated publication date: March 2012)

For more information and samples of articles, see www.kenbakerconsulting.com

Table of Contents

Dedication v

Preface vi

Acknowledgments x

Chapter 1: The Theory of Quality 1

Chapter 2: The Role of the Pharmacy Technician
               in Reducing Medication Errors 25

Chapter 3: Role of the Pharmacist 52

Chapter 4: Prescription Workflow 77

Chapter 5: Identify the Risks 104

Chapter 6: Best Practices and Other Tools 138

Chapter 7: Refining the Workflow 169

Chapter 8: Training for Quality 191

Chapter 9: Monitoring and Learning from Mistakes 220

Chapter 10: The Role of the Patient in Preventing Medication Errors 251

Glossary 270

Index 279

CHAPTER 1

The Theory of Quality
A Pharmacy Imperative

OBJECTIVES

Upon completion of this chapter, the reader should be able to:

1. Explain the need for a quality system in the practice of pharmacy.
2. Understand the role of paradigms in medication errors.
3. Describe the extent of the medication-error problem in community pharmacy.
4. Discuss the importance of the Institute of Medicine (IOM) reports on quality in health care.
5. Describe an error as the term is used in pharmacy.
6. Explain the importance of Edwards Deming in the field of quality.
7. Discuss statistical controls in the implementation of a quality system.
8. List ways in which collecting information regarding near-misses can improve a quality system in a pharmacy.
9. Explain the importance of management in implementing a quality plan.
10. Discuss the role of Japan in the development of quality in the United States.

KEY TERMS

Adverse drug event: Any incident in which the use of a medication (drug or biologic) at any dose, a medical device, or a special nutritional product (for example, dietary supplement, infant formula, medical food) may have resulted in an adverse outcome in a patient. (See http://www.jointcommission.org/sentinelevents/se_glossary.htm)

Adverse event: An injury related to medical management, in contrast to complications of disease. Medical management includes all aspects of care, including diagnosis and treatment, failure to diagnose or treat, and the systems and equipment used to deliver care. Adverse events may be preventable or nonpreventable. (See http://www.who.int/patientsafety/events/05/Reporting_Guidelines.pdf)

Ambulatory: A health care facility that services patients who are not in a hospital, nursing home, or otherwise institutionalized. An outpatient pharmacy located in a hospital and retail or community pharmacies are both examples of ambulatory pharmacies.

Best practice: Best practices are techniques used in the pharmacy profession as a way of stopping or catching mistakes before they reach a patient. They are called "best practices" because they have proven effective in use. An example of a best practice is a **national drug code (NDC)** check during which the number on the manufacturer's bottle is checked against the NDC number printed on the pharmacy receipt.

Community pharmacy: Formerly referred to as a *drugstore* or *retail pharmacy*, the community pharmacy is usually located in commercial areas and serves the general public. It may be an independent pharmacy or a unit of a chain pharmacy.

Continuous quality improvement (CQI): Developed from the writings and teachings of Dr. Edwards Deming, CQI is the name often used in pharmacy for a systematic plan to reduce medication errors by identifying the risks, developing a plan, implementing and training staff in the use of the plan, and monitoring the results with the concept of using that information to further improve the workings of the plan.

Cubic centimeter (cc): A unit of measure often used in medicine. One cc is approximately equivalent to one milliliter (mL). A standard teaspoon is considered to be about 5 cc or 5 mL. A dosage of 5 cc measured in a marked cup or syringe is a more accurate dose than "1 teaspoonful" because teaspoons may vary in size.

Errors: Also referred to as *preventable adverse medical events*, errors are mistakes made anywhere in health care. In pharmacy, an error is usually considered to be a mistake that reaches a patient.

Mechanical error: In the Pharmacists Mutual Insurance Company Claims Study, a mechanical error is defined as *wrong drug*, *wrong strength of drug*, or *wrong directions*. Mechanical errors account for over 80 percent of all claims in the study.

Medical error: Includes all errors throughout the medical professions. The Institute of Medicine, in a summary of its publication, *To Err is Human: Building a Safer Health System*, wrote:

> Medical errors can be defined as the failure of a planned action to be completed as intended or the use of a wrong plan to achieve an aim. Among the problems that commonly occur during the course of providing health care are **adverse drug events** and improper transfusions, surgical injuries and wrong-site surgery, suicides, restraint-related injuries or death, falls, burns, pressure ulcers, and mistaken patient identities. High error rates with serious consequences are most likely to occur in intensive-care units, operating rooms, and emergency departments.

(See http://www.iom.edu/~/media/Files/Report Files/1999/To-Err-is-Human/To Err is Human 1999 report brief.pdf)

Medication error: The standard definition provided by the National Coordinating Council for Medication Error Reporting and Prevention is:

> A medication error is any preventable event that may cause or lead to inappropriate medication use or patient harm while the medication is in the control of the health care professional, patient, or consumer. Such events may be related to professional practice, health care products, procedures, and systems (including prescribing; order communication; product labeling, packaging, and nomenclature; compounding; dispensing; distribution; administration; education; monitoring; and use).

(See: http://www.nccmerp.org/aboutMedErrors.html)
> A medication error is any error occurring in the medication use process. It may be in prescribing, dispensing, or administering a drug. It may also include the overuse or underuse of medication. It includes a mechanical error, a drug review error, or a counseling error.

National drug code (NDC): Each drug manufactured in the United States under the authority of the Food and Drug Administration (FDA) is given a unique number code. The code is divided into three segments that identify the manufacturer (four or five digits), the product or drug (three or four digits), and the size of the package (one or two digits). Because the number is also in the pharmacy's computer and printed on each pharmacy receipt, it can be checked against the NDC number on the manufacturer's bottle.

Near-misses: In pharmacy, a mistake that does not reach the patient, or is caught before it does, is often called a "near-miss." In order to be considered a near-miss, the mistake must have moved from the process or step where it was made to the next step or process. For example, if a mistake is made when typing the information for the label into the computer but is caught before it leaves the computer station, it does not meet the definition of a near-miss.

Paradigm: A common set of patterns or forms that experience has taught us to expect. A paradigm is the lens through which we see the things around us. They help us make quick decisions. A typical paradigm is that high-quality items cost more than low-quality items. While many times paradigms are true and can be useful in helping us recognize patterns, some paradigms are not correct and may lead to mistakes in judgment.

QID (qid): A Latin abbreviation for "four times a day." Prescriptions are often written using such older style of abbreviations. Other common Latin abbreviations are QD (qd) (every day), BID (bid) (twice a day), and TID (tid) (three times a day).

Quality-related event (QRE): "Quality-related event" is a name given to a shorthand method used to describe the total of all errors and near-misses. In some instances it is used to describe only errors, but actually it refers to both.

Total quality management (TQM): TQM was the original name given to the systematic process of management and quality improvement by Dr. Edwards Deming.

Workflow: Pharmacy quality systems are arranged as a series of processes that begin at one end of the prescription-dispensing area and move to the other end. Workflows are usually designed as a straight-line flow with some deviation for special processes.

OUTLINE

- **The Theory of Quality**
- **Introduction to Quality in Pharmacy**
  - The Institute of Medicine Report
- **The Father of CQI: Story of W. Edwards Deming**
  - Background and Concepts
  - Applying the Principles to Pharmacy
  - Paradigms
    - *The Case of the Wrong Shortcut*
- Applying Quality Concepts to the Practice of Pharmacy
- **Statistical Control**
- **Why Quality Is Important**
- **Efficiency—A Side Effect of Quality**
  - *The Case of the Near-Miss*
- **The Risk-Management Process**
- **Summary**

RxErcise 1-A   A Study of Theory

This first chapter is designed to give a background for the study of **continuous quality improvement (CQI)** and the reduction of **medication errors**. If you do not understand all parts of the theory, do not worry. You need not be an expert in the theory in order to reduce the risk of errors in the pharmacy.

After reading this chapter:

- Discuss why quality is important.
- Explore what the history of quality systems can teach about management in relation to quality.

While discussing these topics, consider that a few years from now you may be a part of management. For now, studying theory can be useful in recognizing what should be expected from those throughout the pharmacy.

Important: In this first chapter, relax; enjoy the stories and the theories. What we discuss here will become clearer as we get into the more practical applications of the quality processes associated with the role of the pharmacy technician.

INTRODUCTION TO QUALITY IN PHARMACY

Every year, three million potentially serious or even deadly prescription errors are dispensed by community pharmacies in the United States. That was the conclusion of a study conducted by Auburn University College of Pharmacy.[1] The results of this study were the subject of an article concerning quality in American drugstores that appeared in the *Wall Street Journal* in January 2004.[2] Quoting the Auburn study, which found an overall error rate in community pharmacies of 1.8 percent, the *Wall Street Journal* headline shouted, "A Typical Pharmacy Filling 250 Prescriptions Daily Makes an Average of Four Mistakes." Using a widely accepted estimation that community pharmacies fill over three billion prescriptions each year, the Auburn study calculated that each year there are over 50 million errors at the community level of pharmacy practice. Of these, the study reported, only 4 percent were judged to be capable of causing serious injury or even death.

When patients present their prescriptions to the drugstore in their neighborhood, or when the physician sends a drug order to the hospital pharmacy, the expectation is that the medication order will be filled correctly. Pharmacists and pharmacy technicians all make the same pledge—First, I will do no harm. Of all the jobs performed each day in a pharmacy, filling each prescription correctly must be considered paramount. If quality is imperative in any field, it certainly must be considered such in the practice of pharmacy.

Quality is more than just reminding ourselves to be careful or deciding we are going to double-check every time. Quality is more than a list of pharmacy **best practices**, such as using **national drug code (NDC)** checks and "echoing back" every telephoned prescription. Quality is a plan. With a plan, medication errors can be prevented.

No plan is perfect. No matter how good its quality-assurance plan is, a pharmacy will never eliminate all errors. But a good plan can reduce the number and frequency of errors and make prevention more likely. Without a plan, error prevention is very much a measure of luck.

The Institute of Medicine Reports

In 1999 the Institute of Medicine (IOM), as part of an ongoing study on the quality of health care in the United States, released a report on the larger problem of medical errors. The conclusion of the study was explosive to both the health care community and to society generally. This initial report, *To Err is Human: Building a Safer Health System*,[3] was followed by several additional reports. Of particular import to pharmacy was the Quality Chasm Series, including *Crossing the Quality Chasm: A New Health System for the 21st Century; Patient Safety, Achieving a New Standard for Care; and Preventing Medication Errors.*[4]

The IOM reported that medical errors are one of the leading causes of death in the United States. Extrapolating the results from two studies conducted in different parts of the country, the IOM estimated that between 44,000 and 98,000 deaths occur each year as a result of medical errors in hospitals in the United States. The IOM made the gravity of the situation clear: "Even when using the lower estimate, deaths due to medical errors exceed the number attributable to the eighth-leading cause of death. More people die in a given year as a result of medical errors than from motor vehicle accidents (43,458), breast cancer (42,297), or AIDS (16,516)."[5]

The IOM estimates that more than 6,000 people die each year from medication errors alone.⁶ Not all of the incidences originate from pharmacies or from the pharmacy profession. Some may be the result of physician or nursing mistakes; some may even be the result of patient errors. Many, however, are preventable. In hospitals alone, "two out of every 100 admissions experience a preventable **adverse drug event**, resulting in average increased hospital costs of $4,700 per admission or about $2.8 million annually for a 700-bed teaching hospital."⁷ Note the use of the word "preventable" in that statistic.

In addition to exploring the problems associated with medical errors (or, as the IOM referred to them, "preventable adverse medical events"), it provides suggestions. Many of the recommendations require government actions. However, pharmacies need not wait for governments to act. Recommendation 4.1 provides, with only slight modification, a good set of goals that pharmacies can adopt immediately:

1. Set a goal for patient-safety improvement each month.
2. Track progress in meeting this goal.
3. Issue an annual report on patient safety to management, staff, and even patients.

Without setting goals, real progress will be difficult. We in pharmacy can learn much from the IOM's Quality Chasm Series, especially the importance of studying quality systems and fully implementing a continuous quality improvement (CQI) plan in every pharmacy. Merely having a CQI plan, however, is not sufficient. Staff must be trained, goals must be measured, and compliance must be enforced.

*Preventing Medication Errors,*⁸ the fourth book in the IOM Quality Chasm Series, notes that not all medication errors are **mechanical** (wrong drug, wrong strength, or wrong directions) mistakes made in the pharmacy. The IOM reviewed several studies in **ambulatory** clinics and found that medication errors came from many sources. Among those cited were:⁹

- of the prescriptions examined, 21 percent contained at least one writing error;
- in one clinic's hemodialysis unit, 97.7 percent of the patients were subject to at least one prescribing error;
- in an ambulatory chemotherapy unit, 3 percent of the doses administered contained an error;
- in one clinic, 15 percent of prescription refills were missing from the patient's record;

- in a study of community pharmacies, 12.4 percent of telephoned prescriptions contained an error;
- examining dispensing samples, one study found that 17 percent of the labels referred to enclosed prescribing information that was absent.

The IOM also reviewed reports of errors in hospitals, nursing homes, and even pediatric hospitals, and cited problems of overutilization and underutilization with over-the-counter drugs. The editors also looked at the costs associated with these medication errors, citing a United States General Accounting Office (GAO) report finding that preventable medication errors in one nursing home cost "$340,942 over a 2-year period."[10]

It is not surprising, then, that the IOM report *Preventing Medication Errors* concluded that more needs to be done. The cost in terms of money, suffering, and unnecessary pain dictates that everyone in health care should do what they can to prevent the next medication error from reaching a patient. The only proven way to do that is through a systematic program of continuous quality improvement.

Quality Note 1-A   Institute of Medicine Reports

The IOM report *To Err is Human: Building a Safer Health System* is available on the Internet and can be read free. http://www.nap.edu/readingroom Search for *To Err is Human*.

All four of the quality reports can be found in the National Academies Press (NAP) reading room.

THE FATHER OF CQI: STORY OF W. EDWARDS DEMING

In 1979 William Conway, an executive with the Nashua Corporation, noted that Japanese manufacturers could produce copying machines at a higher level of quality and at lower costs than their American competitors. He sent a team of engineers to Japan to study their method of manufacturing and to learn their secrets. What Conway discovered was that the "Japanese system" was actually an American plan of quality and management.[11]

Conway also learned that by implementing this American plan, the Japanese were able to increase their efficiency, leading to increased profit margins and decreased selling prices for their products. The overall result was higher quality, lower prices, and greater sales, which gave the Japanese a competitive edge over the rest of the world, including the United States.

Conway's engineers also learned that American manufacturers had rejected this same plan in favor of the older style of management that had been the standard in the United States for decades. This **total quality management (TQM)** plan introduced continuous quality improvement into the manufacturing process. TQM, by its nature, led to a continuous cycle of increased efficiency, greater profits, lower prices, and further competitive advantage.

Conway learned it was an American mathematician, Edwards Deming, PhD, invited to Japan following World War II, who introduced the plan to them. Conway hired him as a consultant to his Nashua Corporation.

Conway's discovery was duplicated by NBC, which in 1980 aired a documentary entitled "If Japan Can . . . Why Can't We?"[12] Many American companies began embracing Deming's management and quality ideas, including Ford Motor Company, which hired him as a consultant in 1981 and credited him as being an important element in reversing Ford's losses and introducing a profitability that within five years exceeded that of General Motors (GM). By using Deming's teachings, Ford increased the quality of its automobiles. As a result, sales increased and profits continued to surpass its American competitors into the next decade. Today, many companies worldwide utilize the Deming philosophy of quality management. Almost all continuous quality improvement (CQI) systems used in American pharmacy today can trace their origins back to Edwards Deming and his system of total quality management (TQM).[13]

Background and Concepts

It is important to understand the background and concepts of this American plan for quality. Start with Edwards Deming, the man who was instrumental in the renewed success of the Nashua Corporation and Ford Motor Company.

Born in Sioux City, Iowa, in 1900, Deming obtained his PhD from Yale University in mathematics in 1928. Much of his early work was in statistics for the United States Department of Agriculture and the Census Bureau, as well as with Bell Laboratories. He was later a professor at New York University and Columbia University, where he was a member of the faculty into his nineties. Throughout his career he felt that his particular management philosophy, along with statistical process control, were keys to quality improvement.

Following the end of World War II, Deming was invited to Japan, where he introduced his concepts of management and quality to Japanese manufacturing companies. At the time Edwards Deming arrived in Japan, its manufacturers were known as producers of substandard, low-quality goods. Thirty years later, using the principles taught by this American mathematician, Japanese manufactures led the world in quality, efficiency, and competitive pricing. If this was a Japanese miracle, the head magician was an American. Today, the most sought-after prize for quality among Japanese manufacturers is the Deming Prize, named after Edwards Deming.

Between 1979 and 1982, Ford Motor Company lost $3 billion. Ford had a problem and in 1981, it hired Dr. Deming as a consultant. By 1982 the company started a comeback and by 1986 was the most profitable American auto company; its earnings exceeded GM for the first time since the 1920s. The Ford chairman credited the teachings of Edwards Deming for much of the dramatic turnaround.[14]

What surprised Ford when it hired Deming to teach quality was that most of his teachings were on a method and philosophy of management. The key to quality was not harder work, but better management and higher expectations. Most of the problems with quality, Deming said, can be traced to the actions of management.[15] Management and statistical control lead to continuous improvement of the process that results in lower variability of the product. This low variability is an important part of the definition of quality.

Quality starts with management and its acceptance of Deming's 14 management principles.[16] These principles were originally written with manufacturers in mind, but they can be readily adapted to today's pharmacy practice. The 14 principles laid out by Deming are:

1. Create constancy of purpose towards improving products and services, allocating resources to provide for long-range needs rather than short-term profitability.

2. Adopt the new philosophy for economic stability by refusing to allow commonly accepted levels of delays, mistakes, defective materials, and defective workmanship.

3. Cease dependence on mass inspection by requiring statistical evidence of built-in quality.

4. Reduce the number of suppliers for the same item by eliminating those that do not qualify with statistical evidence of quality; end the practice of awarding business solely on the basis of price.

5. Search continually for problems in the system to constantly improve processes.

6. Institute modem methods of training to make better use of all employees.

7. Focus supervision on helping people do a better job; ensure that immediate action is taken on reports of defects, maintenance requirements, poor tools, inadequate operating definitions, or other conditions detrimental to quality.

8. Encourage effective, two-way communication and other means to drive out fear throughout the organization and help people work more productively.

9. Break down barriers between departments by encouraging problem solving through teamwork, combining the efforts of people from different areas such as research, design, sales, and production.

10. Eliminate use of numerical goals, posters, and slogans for the work force that ask for new levels of productivity without providing methods.

11. Use statistical methods for continuing improvement of quality and productivity, and eliminate work standards that prescribe numerical quotas.

12. Remove all barriers that inhibit the worker's right to pride of workmanship.

13. Institute a vigorous program of education and retraining to keep up with changes in materials, methods, product design, and machinery.

14. Clearly define top management's permanent commitment to quality and productivity and its obligation to implement all of these principles.

Applying the Principles to Pharmacy

Consider these points as they might be applied to pharmacy management. For example, under the first principle, a consistent method of filling prescriptions should be established that works the same when one patient is waiting or when several people are waiting. One small pharmacy chain had instructed its pharmacists and technicians in techniques that were to be used to work faster when the number of people in line exceeded a particular number. After studying Deming, this pharmacy's manual was changed. The new instructions emphasized the need to care for each patient, regardless of how busy the pharmacy was. The pharmacy found that working faster was counterproductive because customer satisfaction decreased and there was a concern that errors could increase. Concentrate, the new manual said, on caring for each patient and on filling one prescription at a time. Focus, not on short-term problems, but on long-term success and profits, by doing the job right the first time and delivering the correct prescription each time. This principle also teaches that each technician and pharmacist in the pharmacy prescription-filling workflow uses the same procedures and best practices to produce uniform workflow for each prescription.

Under the second principle, neither management nor staff any longer accepts that there will be a certain number of errors and **near-misses**. Each near-miss causes delays and rework. They are not acceptable. When a near-miss occurs, it is treated with the same gravity as an error that reaches a patient. If the pharmacy can reduce the number of near-misses, each of which could lead to errors, fewer errors would follow automatically. Likewise, glitches in software, defects in equipment, and late deliveries by suppliers are no longer acceptable.

The third principle needs to be modified for pharmacy practice. To Deming, mass inspections were inefficient and unproductive. Deming taught increased quality could be obtained through statistical control. As we will see later, statistical control is important in pharmacy in discovering vulnerabilities in the process of prescription filling. However, pharmacy is not like a manufacturing process. To avoid the risk of injury if even one mistake is allowed to reach a patient, pharmacy must also have a process of 100 percent inspection of each prescription. This is discussed later and is an exception to Deming's teachings that we must make in pharmacy.

The fourth principle means that management does not buy from suppliers who cannot consistently provide quality products and service, even if the price is less. Five and six indicate that everyone in the pharmacy strives to constantly improve both processes and employees through training. Under principles seven, eight, and nine, management focuses on its employees by effectively listening to what these workers have to say. Management must encourage communications.

Principle ten reminds us that slogans alone do nothing to improve quality or work habits. People do not make fewer errors because they are told to do so. Employees must be given the tools and methods to succeed. Management cannot set artificial numerical quotas and expect that magically the goals will be met. Methods, principle eleven tells us, must be designed to help the employee meet reasonable expectations.

There must be a constant guard against any barriers that may interfere with an employee's ability to succeed, says principle twelve. One barrier is lack of knowledge and training, as is pointed out in number thirteen. Finally, under fourteen, management must not only have a clear commitment to quality, but it must also communicate this commitment to all, including employees and customers. In pharmacy, this means telling patients that the pharmacy and staff are dedicated to caring for them. "We do not accept mistakes, and neither should you," is the message.

Deming believed teamwork is important in delivering a quality product. This means management and employees must work together under a set of realistic rules. When management adopts

Deming's principles, it does not mean the work will be easier or that all time pressures will dissolve. It does not mean that there will not be times when the pharmacy has less staff than may be desirable. It does mean that everyone works together in a system of efficient two-way communication, all part of a team working toward a common, realistic goal.

Paradigms

Not only does management need to think about its responsibilities, but everyone in the pharmacy needs to challenge their own paradigms. A **paradigm** is a set of rules or a theory that guides our way of thinking about things. It is the lens through which we see the world.

We all know that in a deck of cards the ace of diamonds is red. If we are shown a red ace of diamonds or a black ace of spades, we recognize them immediately without conscious thought.

We do not need to think about it. It matches our paradigm—in our world, all aces of diamonds are red. But what if one was not? If we are shown a black ace of diamonds or a black ace of hearts, it would take our brains time to correctly identify them. If we were shown a black ace of hearts and then it was quickly put away, we would probably identify it as an ace of spades. Paradigms allow us to make quick decisions. They can also cause us to make errors. In pharmacy we also have paradigms.

The Case of the Wrong Shortcut

A young mother brought a new prescription for her 3-month-old baby into the pharmacy and handed it to the pharmacy technician. The pharmacy technician made sure the prescription contained all of the needed information and began preparing the label by typing the baby's name, the name of the prescribed drug, and directions into the pharmacy computer. The directions on the prescription were written: "Give 3 cc QID," which translates to "Give 3 **cubic centimeters (cc)** four times a day." Three cc is a little more than a half teaspoonful. The manufacturer's bottle was designed to be dispensed with the medication and came supplied with a dropper marked with a 3 cc and a 6 cc measurement.

The pharmacy technician made a mistake. While typing the directions into the computer, she used a shorthand method built into the software that allowed most directions to be entered quickly with a minimum of keystrokes. Using this shortcut, she typed "g 3 qid", which resulted in a label being printed that read "Give 3 teaspoonsful four times daily." A teaspoonful is commonly understood to be 5 cc. Three teaspoonsful were therefore 15 cc or a dose equal to five times that prescribed.

The pharmacy technician who filled the prescription and the pharmacist who checked it both said later that they checked the label and the prescription and did not notice the mistake in the directions. How is that possible? How can an experienced pharmacy technician and pharmacist both miss such an obvious error? The answer may be that their paradigms overruled what their eyes saw.

It is not unusual for a pharmacy to fill 100–200 prescriptions in an eight-hour shift. Technicians and pharmacists will check many prescriptions each day. Almost every time they do, the label is correct. From the Auburn University study of medication errors, a technician and pharmacist may be expected to see 99 correct prescription labels for every 100 prescriptions checked. Statistically, even the one mistake that may be mixed into those 100 prescription labels will probably not be clinically important. Some may have a name spelled wrong or the permitted number of refills incorrectly stated. The paradigm in their mind is that this label is going to be right. The mind sees what it expects to see—a correct label. Understanding the paradigm is a large step in overcoming this problem. Look again at Figure 1-1. The fact that the black card is an ace of diamonds is easier to spot when you realize it may be there.

Most prescriptions are filled correctly without any mistake. Most mistakes are caught before they leave the pharmacy's control. In the example of the baby given 3 teaspoonsful instead of 3 cc, ask yourself again how a trained and experienced pharmacy technician and a pharmacist could have both missed such a glaring mistake in the label. It took at least three mistakes to allow this erroneous label to reach the patient. We occasionally miss mistakes because most prescriptions we check are correct. A quality program is designed to catch the unusual, the outlier. The good news is that only one of the mistakes needs to be caught to prevent an error.

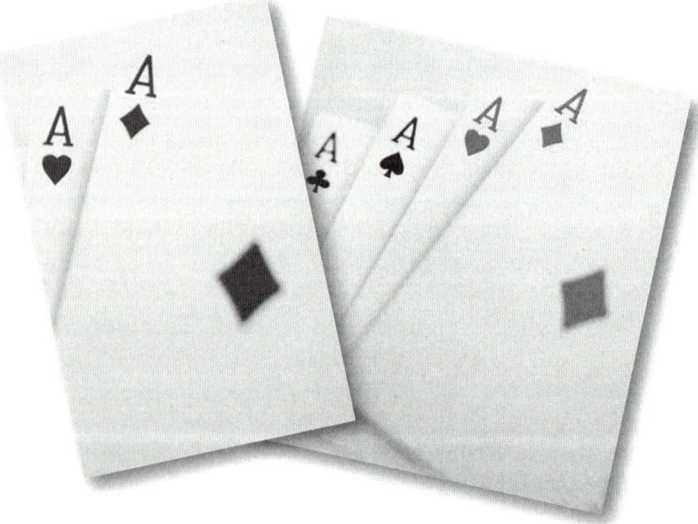

Figure 1-1
Paradigm—Ace of Diamonds
© Cengage Learning 2013

Applying Quality Concepts to the Practice of Pharmacy

A study of Deming's teachings shows that quality does not happen consistently because we will it or because we try hard. The Deming philosophy of constantly increasing quality involves a plan. This plan works in pharmacy as well as in the manufacture of copying machines or automobiles. In addition to making better copiers and cars, this plan can also be used to reduce the number of prescription errors reaching patients.

The first step toward quality is to identify the most common problems. In order to reduce the incidences of patients receiving the wrong drug, or the wrong strength of a prescribed drug, or a prescription with a label containing the wrong directions, we need to know what mistakes are made most often. In addition, we need to know where in the prescription-filling process mistakes are most likely to occur. We need this information because we need to know where to start and which problems are most critical.

Once we know where and what mistakes are most likely to occur, we can implement a plan to reduce these mistakes or to catch them before they reach the patient. To make the plan work we must standardize the process. If the plan involves using the pharmacy best practice of performing an NDC check, it is done at a particular point in the process where we decide it would be most effective. Then we train every person who fills a prescription in our pharmacy to perform the NDC check at the same step in the process. Not only does this standardize our process, it standardizes our training and increases efficiency. It also increases the likelihood that the selected best practice will be done for every prescription.

A plan is effective only if everyone who uses the plan is trained in its use. Ford executives were surprised when Deming, who was hired to increase quality, spent most of his time talking to them not about quality, but about how to manage. The role of management is to provide training and tools to those who do the actual work. Deming told Ford executives that posters and slogans do not work—training does. Lack of training leads to poor performance. Deming said, "Remove all barriers that inhibit the worker's right to pride of workmanship." Workers cannot have pride in what they do if they are not properly trained. The workers are ultimately responsible for quality; management is responsible for allowing the workers to succeed. In order to increase quality, the frontline pharmacists and technicians must be trained to use a planned, standardized workflow.

Once a plan is in effect, we need to know whether it is working and then we can begin thinking about how to further improve it. Deming was a mathematician. What he taught the Japanese, the Nashua Corporation, Ford Motors, and hundreds of other companies was that in order to have a successful quality system, they needed to collect data. In order to know if a pharmacy's plan is working, we need to collect information on each of our mistakes, near-misses, and errors. These errors and near-misses are collectively known as **quality-related events (QREs)**. Once collected, the information should be put in a format that will allow the pharmacy to view it in an illustrative format such as a chart or graph. The information can then be analyzed to determine where improvements can be made.

In pharmacy this means we need to record every mistake or QRE that is made, whether it reaches a patient or was discovered and corrected before the prescription was delivered to the patient. From this data we can learn where, when, what, and how mistakes are made in our pharmacy. At that point, we can adjust the workflow so that even fewer of these mistakes reach the patient. Statistics allow us to continuously increase quality by constantly correcting whatever weaknesses remain in our system.

The plan for prescription quality begins with a commitment by management. It ends when every technician and every pharmacist serving patients attains perfection—in other words, *quality improvement never ends*. With a plan, the goal is that every day the number of mistakes will be slightly lower than the day before and then even lower the next day and the next and the next.

STATISTICAL CONTROL

A basic concept of Deming's theories of quality is statistical control of the system, which he as a mathematician believed to be the secret to constantly improving quality. Statistical control provides a measurement to answer the question: How are we doing? In pharmacy practice this is a way of determining how many prescriptions were filled correctly.

To perform this measurement, the pharmacy must have accurate information. This means the staff must record each mistake or quality-related event (QRE). At the end of each month, the number of mistakes is compared with the number of prescriptions filled. The comparison then provides a percentage QRE rate. The pharmacy can compare this number with the QRE rate for the preceding month. In Figure 1-2, the percentage of QREs (mistakes) made decreased each month as a percentage of prescriptions filled. This is what the pharmacy hopes to see each month. This should be one of the pharmacy's goals.

In addition to knowing how many mistakes were made, a "success rate" can be measured by comparing the number of mistakes that were caught before they reached a patient compared with the number of errors that did reach a patient. Figure 1-3 (Success Rate) shows that in January the pharmacy had 47 QREs. Of these the

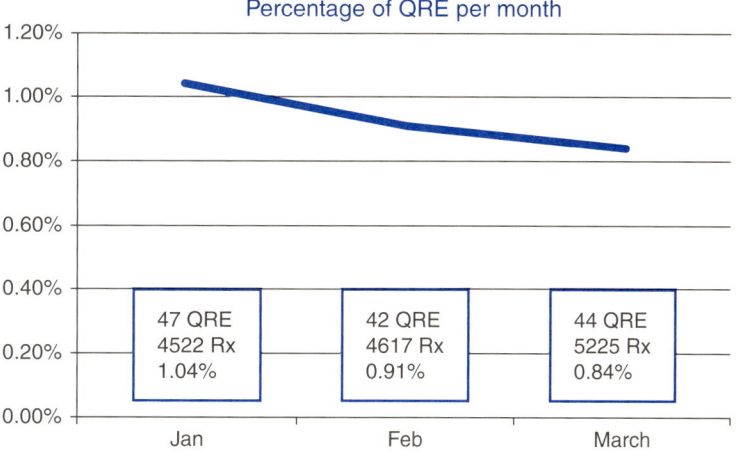

Figure 1-2 QRE Rate
Percentage of QRE per month
© Cengage Learning 2013

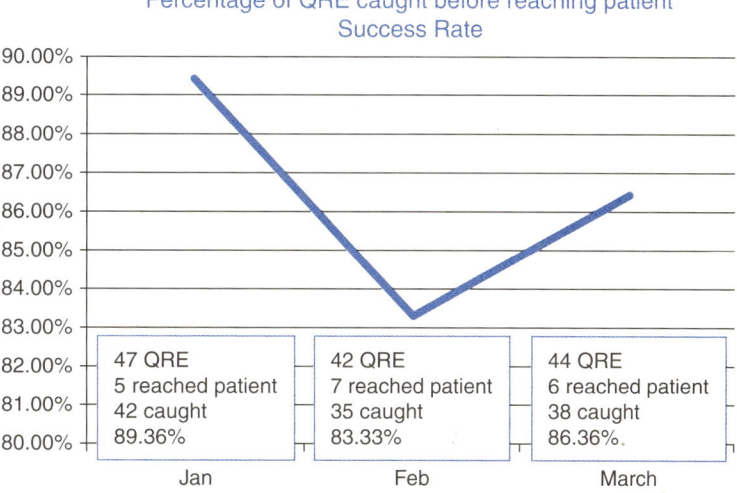

Figure 1-3 Success Rate
Percentage of QRE caught before reaching patient
© Cengage Learning 2013

pharmacy caught 42 before they reached a patient, meaning that five did reach patients and became errors. This success rate means that 89.4 percent of the QREs made that month were caught before they reached a patient. The following month, however, the success rate decreased to 83.3 percent, but came back to 86.4 percent in March. This information can also be used to tell how many errors the pharmacy had compared with the number of prescriptions filled (see Figure 1-4, Error Rate).

16 Medication Safety: Dispensing Drugs Without Error

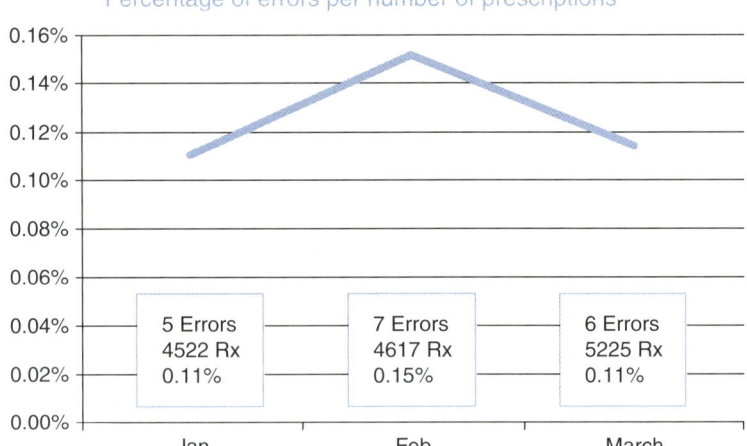

Figure 1-4 Error Rate
Percentage of errors per number of prescriptions
© *Cengage Learning 2013*

> **RxErcise 1-B   *Analyzing the Error Rate***
>
> Examine Figure 1-4, Error Rate. This is a report from your pharmacy for the first quarter of the year. The pharmacist-in-charge has asked you to analyze this chart and interpret the results for the rest of the staff. What do you tell them? Include in your report why the information is important and how the pharmacy can use it to improve quality.

When we collect information on all of the pharmacy's near-misses and errors, it would take little additional time to note where each mistake was made and where it was caught. Armed with this data, we can determine where in our workflow mistakes are most likely to happen and where they can be caught. This information points to the vulnerabilities within our system and allows us to make corrections before mistakes happen and thus before any errors occur. As we continue to note throughout this book, the best way to prevent errors is to prevent the mistakes (QREs) that lead to them.

In this chapter we have looked at a few of the graphs that we can use to constantly improve our system and our workflow. Later, in Chapter 9, we will look more closely at how we might collect and use information, data, and statistics.

Why Quality Is Important

The first job of every pharmacist and pharmacy technician can be stated in the medical maxim: First, do no harm. The essence of this duty is first to fill each prescription accurately as written. While this does not sum up the total commitment of pharmacists and technicians in a quality pharmacy, it is the first area on which pharmacy personnel must concentrate. Above all, a pharmacy should be able to deliver the correct medication to the correct patient with the correct directions for use.

Most professional liability claims against pharmacies, pharmacists, and pharmacy technicians involve filling a prescription with the wrong drug, wrong strength of the drug, or the wrong directions on the label. These filling errors are usually referred to as **mechanical errors**. A study of claims against pharmacies, pharmacists, and pharmacy technicians received by Pharmacists Mutual Insurance Company since 1989 shows that over 85 percent of all claims are for a mechanical error (see Figure 1-5, Pharmacists Mutual Insurance Company Claims Study[17]).

The presence of an insurance liability claim usually indicates that a patient was seriously injured by the pharmacy error. The patient must take time to initiate a claim and claims are paid only if there is some damage. With a professional pharmacy liability claim, the damages are usually a physical injury caused by the error.[18] We will look at sections of this study in more detail in later chapters.

Quality is important in pharmacy because protecting the patient from harm is at the core of the profession. Most prescriptions are filled correctly. Patients expect perfection when they bring a prescription to the pharmacy and when they receive medication in the hospital. All other jobs of a pharmacy technician and a pharmacist are secondary to delivering the prescription correctly, including a pharmacist's drug review and patient counseling. If a pharmacy does not institute a quality program for its professional services, it cannot serve its patients in the long run.

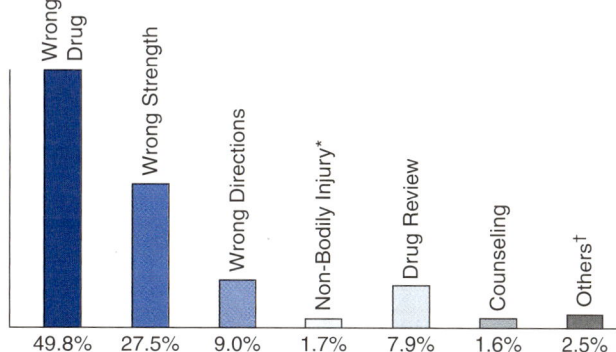

*Non-bodily injury includes release of confidential information; libel, slander, false arrest. Most of these claims were for unauthorized release of confidential information, i.e. a HIPAA violation.
†Others is a group of claims that are each typically less than 1%. The include illegal acts, safety cap violations, compounding claims.

Figure 1-5 Pharmacists Mutual Claims Study
Pharmacists Mutual Claims Study 2010
1989 through 2009
© Cengage Learning 2013

EFFICIENCY—A SIDE EFFECT OF QUALITY

There is a side effect of introducing a quality program into a pharmacy. As the Japanese, the Nashua Corporation, and Ford Motor Company found when they instituted total quality management (TQM), the system became more efficient. That resulted in lower costs and higher profits.

A district manager for a pharmacy chain made the statement he feared that 20 percent of the prescriptions filled in the pharmacies under his control contained some mistake.[19] He went on to say that most of these were near-misses and did not result in an error that reached a patient. He felt from this that his system was working fairly well. A pharmacist working for another chain agreed with the 20 percent near-miss number.[20]

Examine that estimate of 20 percent near-misses among all prescriptions filled. Ask the question: Is this system efficient? By *efficient* we mean the system is cost-effective as opposed to being wasteful in terms of time and money. If this system is inefficient, it requires improvement. If the pharmacy technician is required to fill the same prescription twice, it would appear to be wasteful of the technician's time. An inefficient system will eventually lead to errors. RxErcise 1-C explores these problems.

RxErcise 1-C   An Inefficient System

The pharmacy-chain district manager referred to above may have been exaggerating the percentage, but he should have been concerned that a large number of prescriptions contained a near-miss. Presume the district manager was wrong by a factor of 10, and only 2 percent of the filled prescriptions contained a near-miss. In his district, assume there are 100 pharmacies. (There are actually many more.) Next, assume that his 100 pharmacies each fill 1000 prescriptions a week. (They actually fill, on average, many more.) In his district:

How many prescriptions are miss-filled each week?

How many prescriptions are miss-filled each year?

For each near-miss, someone must discover the problem and then correct the prescription before delivering it to the patient.

Estimate the average number of staff minutes it would take to correct each prescription. Multiply that number by the number of miss-filled prescriptions in a week and then in a year.

If you could institute a quality program in each of the pharmacies in this region, how much time would be saved if you cut the number of near-misses in half?

It would be fun to also estimate how much money the chain could save in this one region.

Time is money. In RxErcise 1-C you are asked to estimate the number of minutes lost in a group of 100 pharmacies. Using simple math, you can expand the number of minutes lost in hours and in days. The importance of this can be seen from the following example.

The Case of the Near-Miss

When a pharmacy technician entered the prescription information into the pharmacy computer, she should have entered "penicillin 250 mg." She made a mistake and instead entered "penicillin 500 mg." The technician at the computer did not notice her error, nor did the technician filling the prescription. Reading off the typed label, the filling technician filled the prescription with penicillin 500 mg. When the pharmacist was checking the prescription, she did notice the mistake and returned the entire receipt, label, and prescription containing 32 tablets of penicillin 500 mg to the technician at the computer system. The technician corrected the entry into the computer, printed a new receipt and label, and passed all of this along with the bottle containing penicillin 500 mg to the filling technician. The filling technician returned the 500 mg penicillin tablets to the correct stock bottle and threw away the prescription bottle with the wrong label affixed. She then pulled the correct drug from the shelf and filled the prescription correctly. She then placed the corrected information in the pharmacist check area where the pharmacist again checked the prescription, this time finding it correct. The old incorrect receipt was destroyed.

Each time a prescription is corrected it must be refilled, at least partly, for free. The pharmacy was unable to collect more money for this prescription that took almost twice the time of a prescription that contained no mistakes. Time was spent for which no profit was generated.

If in RxErcise 1-C you were able to cut the number of mistakes to one per 100, rather than two per 100, you would save the pharmacy money and time. Greater profits, or higher gross margins, allow for greater investment and higher wages. More importantly, if near-misses can be prevented, there would be no errors reaching patients. It is worth repeating: the best way to prevent errors is to prevent the mistakes in the first place or, failing that, to have a system to reduce the risk of a mistake reaching a patient.

THE RISK-MANAGEMENT PROCESS

The risk-management or quality-assurance process can best be described as a continuous circle and can be represented as a four- or five-step cycle. For the purposes of this discussion, the five-step model explains the system best (see Figure 1-6). The first step is to identify where a mistake may be made. (We will explore this in more depth in Chapter 5.) Basically, it means looking at the pharmacy's workflow and answering the question: Where and how could mistakes be made that could result in an error if not caught?

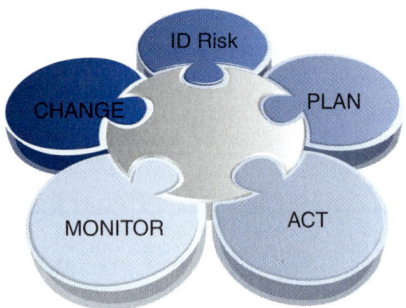

Figure 1-6 Risk-Management Process
© Cengage Learning 2013

The second step is deciding on a technique or best practice to address the risk. If a risk-management technique is chosen, the problem may be managed by putting a plan into effect that will reduce the risk of the mistake happening or increase the likelihood of catching the mistake before it reaches the patient. If a risk-avoidance technique is chosen, the pharmacy may decide not to engage in a certain action—for example, not to compound sterile eye drops or IV solutions. Another technique for dealing with risks is to finance the risk by purchasing enough insurance to cover a claim if the risk should materialize. In this book, we will deal primarily with the technique of managing the risk by instituting a good CQI program.

Best practice is a method of catching or avoiding a mistake by using a practice that has proven effective in the past—for example, checking each filled prescription three times before it is considered finished.

Step three is to make a workflow plan using the technique or best practice selected and putting the plan into effect by training the staff to use the workflow the way it is designed. This may be first instituted on a small scale and then, if successful, throughout the pharmacy.

When the plan is in effect, the results must be monitored. This is step four in the risk-management process. Monitoring will help to answer the question: How well does the plan we put into action work in reducing mistakes? If the system is not perfect (it never is), changes must be made, which is step five. Then the circle is closed by having the entire process start over by identifying where risks of mistakes are possible in the new system.

SUMMARY

In the practice of pharmacy, whether it is hospital or community, the reduction of medication errors begins with management instituting Deming's 14 principles along with a system of continuous quality improvement. Once management has made this commitment, it is up to the pharmacists and pharmacy technicians who are on the front line to make the CQI plan work. Making it work begins with the understanding of the various roles played by each member of the staff in reducing medication errors and even the role that can be played by the patient. A nonpunitive culture will help staff embrace CQI, so that reporting errors is a safe and even rewarding practice in the quest of safer pharmacies.

In this book we will look at the role of the pharmacy technician, the role of the pharmacist, and the various steps in putting a CQI plan into effect. We will look at the importance of training, developing quality habits, and the importance of the pharmacy technician throughout the workflow. We will also review how the pharmacy can be certain its plan is working and how it can use statistics and information about each error to continuously improve its process of filling a prescription.

REVIEW QUESTIONS

1. In the Auburn University study, the authors observed the filling of prescriptions in what type of pharmacies?

    A. Community

    B. Hospital

    C. Nursing home

    D. All of the above

2. What percentage error rate did the Auburn University study find?

    A. 3.1%

    B. 5.0%

    C. 1.8%

    D. 12%

3. The first IOM report in the Quality Chasm Series was published in 1999 and was entitled:

    A. *Preventing Medication Errors*

    B. *To Err is Human*

C. *Quality is Free*

D. *Crossing the Quality Chasm*

4. The IOM reported that _____ were one of the leading causes of death in the United States.

   A. Medication errors

   B. Medical errors

   C. Errors in community pharmacies

   D. Workers' deaths in the workplace

5. A good set of goals for a pharmacy to adopt that are adapted from the IOM report would include:

   A. Set a goal for patient-safety improvement each month.

   B. Track progress in meeting these goals.

   C. Issue an annual report on patient safety.

   D. All of the above

6. One of the first United States companies to hire Edwards Deming to help it institute a quality plan was _____.

   A. The Nashua Corporation

   B. General Motors

   C. Walgreens Pharmacy

   D. Sears, Roebuck and Company

7. Deming's quality program was called:

   A. CQI

   B. TQM

   C. ABC

   D. JDP

8. What is described as one side effect of instituting an effective quality program?

   A. Increased efficiency

   B. Increased cost

   C. Lowered work load

   D. None of the above

9. What is the term used to describe a set of rules or a theory that guides our way of thinking about things?

   A. Mechanical thought

   B. Guided thought

   C. Paradigm

   D. Quick recovery

10. A term that can be used to collectively describe both near-misses and errors is _____.

    A. Quality-related events

    B. Medication errors

    C. Preventable adverse medical events

    D. Patient-qualified events

Endnotes

[1] Flynn, E. A., Barker, K. N., and Carnahan, B. J., National observational study of prescription-dispensing accuracy and safety in 50 pharmacies, *JAPhA*, Vol. 43, No. 2, March/April 2003, pp. 191–200.

[2] A typical pharmacy filling 250 prescriptions daily makes an average of four mistakes, *Wall Street Journal*, January 15, 2004.

[3] Kohn, L. T., Corrigan, J. M., and Donaldson, M. S., Eds., 2000. *To Err is Human: Building a Safer Health System*. Washington, DC: National Academy Press.

[4] The Institute of Medicine has published many reports in the area of quality in health care. See the IOM website at http://www.iom.edu/Reports.aspx?page=1&Series={4EC47331-CA08-4A25-80E6-D4CEB54A485C}

[5] Ibid. at 1.

[6] Ibid. at 2.

[7] Ibid. at 2.

[8] Aspden, P., Wolcott, J. A., Bootman, J. L., and Cronenwett, L. R., Eds., 2007. *Preventing Medication Errors: Building a Safer Health System*. Washington, DC: National Academy Press.

[9] Ibid., p. 112.

[10] Ibid., p. 131.

[11] Gelina, R. J., *Continuous Quality Improvement*, Center for Continuous Quality Improvement, Iowa State University Research Park, 1993.

[12] For more information on the NBC White Paper, see http://www.managementwisdom.com/ifjapcanwhyc.html

[13] Gelina, R. J., *Continuous Quality Improvement*, Center for Continuous Quality Improvement, Iowa State University Research Park, 1993.

[14] For the story of Deming's work with Ford Motor Company, see The Vector Study website: http://www.vectorstudy.com/management_gurus/edwards_deming.htm Also see the discussion at Wikipedia, W. Edwards Deming, http://en.wikipedia.org/wiki/W._Edwards_Deming

[15] Deming E. W., 1986. *Out of the Crisis*. Cambridge, MA: MIT Press.

[16] Ibid.

[17] The latest published Pharmacists Mutual Claims Study is available at the company's website: http://www.phmic.com/phmc/services/RM/profliab/claimsstudy/Pages/TheStoryBehindthePharmacistsMutualClaimStudy.aspx Accessed, August 2, 2010. I found the following on Nov 12, 2011: http://www.phmic.com/phmc/services/RM/profliab/claimsstudy/Pages/TheStoryBehindthePharmacistsMutualClaimsStudy.aspx

[18] Interview with Don McGuire, BS Pharm, JD, General Counsel, Pharmacists Mutual Insurance Company and head of the company's pharmacy professional liability claims department, August 2, 2010 (telephone).

[19] Conversation with Ken Baker, author, August 2009. Identity and all identifying information withheld for privacy concerns.

[20] Conversation with Ken Baker, author, November 2010. Identity and all identifying information withheld for privacy concerns.

CHAPTER 2

The Role of the Pharmacy Technician in Reducing Medication Errors

OBJECTIVES

Upon completion of this chapter, the reader should be able to:

1. Explain the role of pharmacy technicians in systems of quality.
2. List the elements of a basic quality workflow in a pharmacy.
3. Describe the role of the pharmacy technician in receiving a prescription in the pharmacy.
4. Discuss the role of the pharmacy technician in training quality processes.
5. Describe a best practice.
6. Explain the importance of quality for the pharmacy technician in organizing the pharmacy.
7. Discuss duties a pharmacy technician can assume that can reduce the risk of medication errors.
8. List ways in which the pharmacy technician assists the pharmacist as part of the team in the workflow.
9. Explain the importance of "pharmacist only questions."
10. Explain how information collected by a pharmacy technician is necessary for the pharmacist in performing a drug review.

KEY TERMS

American Pharmacists Association (APhA): Formed in 1852, the APhA is the oldest national association representing pharmacists and pharmacy technicians in the United States. See http://www.pharmacist.com

American Society of Health-System Pharmacists (ASHP): Originally called the American Society of Hospital Pharmacists, ASHP was formed as a part of the APhA. Today, ASHP is a strong national association representing hospital pharmacists and pharmacy technicians. See http://www.ashp.org

Controlled substance: While all prescription drugs are controlled by federal and state laws, drugs that have been determined to be addictive have been designated as "controlled substances." Primarily these are narcotics, pain medications, and mood altering drugs such as some stimulants and tranquilizers. They are divided into five schedules, depending on their nature, from Schedule I, considered most addictive with no medical value, to Schedule V, least additive and in some states available without a prescription if sold by a pharmacist to a customer with proper identification. See the Drug Enforcement Administration (DEA) website for drugs in each schedule: http://www.deadiversion.usdoj.gov/schedules/index.html

Drug review, prospective drug review, drug utilization review (DUR): Pharmacists are trained to review prescriptions to ensure patient safety. Medications need to be appropriate for the specific patient, taking into consideration patient age, gender, disease states, drug sensitivities, and allergies. In addition, pharmacists review drug-drug interactions, drug-food interactions, drug–disease state interactions, drug duplications, and patient compliance with prescribed doses and regimens. Also, pharmacists should spend time making sure patients understand their medications. Due to OBRA-90, states are required to have standards for retrospective drug-utilization review and may require prospective drug-utilization review. The Joint Commission standards also mandate prospective drug-utilization review in most settings.

Errors: Also referred to as "preventable adverse drug events." A working definition of errors in pharmacy is mistakes made in the pharmacy that reach a patient. A more complete definition of error from the National Coordinating Council for Medication Error Reporting and Prevention (NCC MERP) is discussed in Chapter 10.

Food and Drug Administration (FDA): A consumer protection agency of the federal government, the FDA regulates the safety and quality of drugs, food, cosmetics, and devices. It was created by the 1906 Pure Food and Drugs Act. See http://www.fda.gov

Herbals: Herbals are medicines usually made or derived directly from plant sources. For most purposes, herbals are not regulated by the FDA as are drugs. They can interfere and interact with drugs in the body. For an overview on herbals, visit Wikipedia: http://en.wikipedia.org/wiki/Herbal

Institute for Safe Medication Practices (ISMP): ISMP is a not-for-profit organization dedicated to making the delivery of drugs in health care safer. It describes itself as a "nonprofit organization devoted entirely to medication error prevention and safe medication use." See http://www.ismp.org

Interactions: Occasionally, drugs can have an effect when used in combination with other drugs, herbals, or even food in ways that can be dangerous. There can be drug-drug (including herbals) interactions or drug-food interactions or drug–disease state interactions. Many of these drug interactions are known and these interactions are among the items pharmacists will screen for when they perform a drug review or DUR.

Mechanical errors: In the Pharmacists Mutual Insurance Company Claims Study, a mechanical error is defined as "wrong drug, wrong strength of drug, or wrong directions." (To look at the study, go to http://www.phmic.com and click on "Services" in the bar at the top and then on "Professional Liability Risk Management" in the menu on the left.) Mechanical errors exceed 80 percent of all claims in the study (click on "Mechanical Errors" in the same menu).

Med-guides: Medication guides are described by the FDA as "paper handouts that come with many prescription medicines. The guides address issues that are specific to particular drugs and drug classes, and they contain FDA-approved information that can help patients avoid serious adverse events." The FDA requires that med-guides be given with certain drugs, currently about 100. See http://www.fda.gov/Drugs/DrugSafety/UCM085729

National Alliance for State Pharmacy Associations (NASPA): NASPA is an association representing all state pharmacy associations in the United States. It features a continuous quality improvement program called Pharmacy Quality Commitment®. See http://www.naspa.us

Near-miss: A pharmacy mistake that does not reach the patient is often called a near-miss. See QRE.

Omnibus Budget Reconciliation Act-90 (OBRA-90) Regulation: In 1990 the federal government passed the Omnibus Budget Reconciliation Act that required, as a small part of the legislation, states to require pharmacists to perform drug reviews, counsel patients, and maintain a patient profile on some patients. By 1993, the states, through their pharmacy practice acts or board of pharmacy regulations, had broadened these requirements.

Over-the-counter medications: Medications that do not require a prescription are referred to as over-the-counter drugs.

Patient profile: By law or regulations, pharmacies are required to maintain a limited amount of information about each patient. These are referred to as "patient profiles" and may include other drugs the patient is taking in addition to general information such as the address and phone numbers. Disease state may be included in some of these patient profiles.

pH: A measurement of acidity, ranging from 1 (most acidic), to 14 (most basic). A pH of 7 is considered neutral, neither acid nor base.

Quality-related events (QRE): A name given to a shorthand method used to describe the total of all errors and near-misses. In some instances it is used to describe only errors, but originally it referred to both.

Rx Only drugs: Originally called "prescription" or "legend drugs." *Rx Only* is the new label given to medications that may not be dispensed except upon an order by a prescriber.

Workflow: Pharmacy-quality systems are arranged as a series of processes that begin at one end of the prescription-dispensing area and move to the other end. They are usually designed as a straight-line flow.

OUTLINE

The Pharmacy Technician Role in Quality Systems
   Pharmacy Technicians—First in the Workflow
   New Division of Labor

Implementing a Quality System
   How Many Errors Do Pharmacies Make?

Recognizing "Pharmacist Only Questions"
   The Case of Heidi Happel
   Sam's Case

Organizer-in-Chief: Make Necessary Information Available

The Pharmacy Technician and the Prescription Workflow
  Receiving the Prescription/Drug Order
  The Case of the 4-Year-Old Child with Pink Eye
  Particularly Vulnerable Patients
  The Address and Phone Number
  The Case of Jimmy's Impatience
  The Telephone Order
  Computer Entry and Preparing the Label
  The Case of Sr., Jr., and the III
  Filling the Prescription/Drug Order
  Preparing for the Pharmacist's Quality Check
  Preparing for Pharmacist's DUR and Counseling
  Delivery to the Floor or the Patient
When Something Goes Wrong
Using Error and Near-Miss Information
Quality Information
Training Others
Participating in Peer Review
Following the Law
Summary

The Pharmacy Technician Role in Quality Systems

In order to reduce the number of medication errors, a quality-assurance system must be a part of any pharmacy's daily workflow. While quality is always a team effort, it must be emphasized that a quality-assurance system will not work if the pharmacy technician is not part of the system. The role of the technician is critical.

In Chapter 1, we described the risk-management or quality-assurance process as a five-step continuous circle (see Figure 1-6).

1. Identify where a mistake may be made.
2. Choose techniques or best practices to reduce, eliminate, or manage the risks; design a plan using those techniques and best practices to define the pharmacy's workflow.
3. Act by putting the plan into effect and training the staff.
4. Monitor the new system.
5. Make changes where necessary.

Pharmacy technicians are in a position to find potential problems in the workflow, particularly in the areas that are their primary responsibility. Recognizing potential problems, they can suggest possible solutions and recommend best practices that can prevent or catch mistakes. Monitoring the system in which they are working, they can recognize when implemented solutions did or did not work. Training of new employees may be entrusted to technicians.

Pharmacy Technicians—First in the Workflow

The pharmacy technician acts in many areas within the dispensing process, often occupying the first position in the workflow.

This gives the technician opportunities to affect quality, especially where he or she may be the main person responsible for:

- receiving the prescription (state law may require a pharmacist to receive new, telephoned prescription orders);
- entering the information into the computer;
- preparing the label and receipt;
- retrieving the correct drug from stock;
- counting, pouring, mixing the prescribed drug;
- placing the drug in an appropriate dispensing container;
- affixing the label to the container holding the drug;
- attaching the label, including auxiliary labels, to the container;
- assembling patient-information material to accompany the finished prescription;
- collecting the finished prescription, patient information, and receipt to be forwarded to the pharmacist;
- reviewing all items and forwarding them to the pharmacist for quality check, drug review, and counseling;
- delivering (depending upon the workflow design) the completed prescription to the patient.

The quality system usually begins when the medication order arrives in the pharmacy either by telephone, by fax, by electronic entry into the computer system, or by a patient at the intake desk. This is the first step in the workflow in filling a prescription correctly with the right drug in the right strength for the right patient and with the right directions. The role of the technician is to receive the order and deliver it to the pharmacist.

In the past, the roles in pharmacy were considerably different. Until relatively recently, pharmacists received the prescriptions, typed the labels, pulled the drugs from the shelves, filled the order, and placed the label on the bottle. If a technician was involved at all, it was to deliver the finished prescription to the patient and collect the money due.

This old method was not very efficient, but in those days it did not matter because the volume was low (a busy pharmacy might fill 100 prescriptions a day). One person could perform a drug review, look for allergies, contraindications, conflicts, overuse and underuse while filling the prescription. The pharmacy technician served as a clerk or perhaps a secretary. If the volume of prescriptions became too heavy, the high gross margin earned on each prescription allowed the pharmacy to hire more pharmacists.

New Division of Labor

By the 1980s the economics of community pharmacy had changed due to competition, third parties, and higher pharmacists' wages. Added to that, laws changed and courts began to require greater legal responsibilities such as direct patient contact through counseling and more drug reviews. The pharmacist could no longer spend time on the mechanical functions of prescription dispensing. Hospital pharmacies began using more auxiliary personnel in expanded roles earlier than community pharmacies.

The question became: Where is the pharmacist's education and expertise most needed or legally required? Generally speaking, the technician can perform, with supervision, most steps required from receiving the prescription through completion of the mechanical filling process.[1] There are legal exceptions such as taking a new telephoned prescription, and there must be a full quality check at the end of the filling process by a pharmacist. While the pharmacist oversees the dispensing of **Rx Only drugs**, it is increasingly the pharmacy technician who prepares the prescriptions. This new division of labor leaves the pharmacist free to concentrate on the clinical aspects that require his or her unique professional talents.

State or federal law requires the supervision or participation of a pharmacist at many points in the process. Three questions must be answered before employing a technician for a particular task.

- Is there a reason for using a pharmacist for that job?
- Can this task be accomplished by a trained technician who does not have the pharmacist's education and experience?
- Does the law allow a pharmacy technician to do the job?

When a patient presents a prescription at the intake desk of an ambulatory pharmacy, a technician reviews the prescription, collects all required information, enters the order in the computer, and prepares a label. Then, the prescription, label, and receipt go to a filling or assembly area where a pharmacy technician pulls the drug from the shelf, counts, weighs or measures the correct quantity, affixes the label to the bottle into which the contents are poured. The finished prescription is placed in line to be checked by a pharmacist, whose knowledge and skill are needed to complete the dispensing function. Pharmacy technicians should check with the law in their state for any exceptions to the rule that each prescription must be checked by a pharmacist before it can be dispensed. In some states a drug order in a hospital can be checked by another technician (known as "tech-check-tech") who has been specially trained and certified. While some states allow a "tech-check-tech" process, it is usually only in accordance with strict rules and usually only in a hospital. The standard rule in most states is and remains that a pharmacist must review the completed prescription order. By placing pharmacists at the end of the mechanical process they are freed to spend more time on clinical pharmacy functions.

> **Quality Note 2-A   A Technician in Charge of the Quality System**
>
> The common wisdom used to be that each pharmacy had to have a pharmacist in charge of the pharmacy's quality system. The emerging thought is that what is critical is that a responsible, trained individual be placed in charge of the system. In larger pharmacies, the individual may be in charge of a team that will work to ensure compliance with the quality program.
>
> While a pharmacist can best understand some of the clinical challenges needed to improve the overall workflow, a technician may be well suited to supervise the mechanical and training aspects of the quality system.
>
> Certain qualities are needed such as respect for everyone in the pharmacy, commitment to making quality key in the system, understanding of the pharmacy's system, and the realization of the importance of the need for a system. In addition, this person must be a teacher and have authority to insist on compliance by the entire staff.

IMPLEMENTING A QUALITY SYSTEM

Management must provide pharmacy staff with the tools needed to succeed. One of those tools is a continuous quality improvement (CQI) system.

Most mechanical mistakes are made during the computer entry and filling (assembly) parts of the workflow process, which are under the control of the pharmacy technician. So it is the technician who is in the best position to stop mistakes before they become errors.

How Many Errors Do Pharmacies Make?

In the Auburn University College of Pharmacy study of 50 community pharmacies we briefly looked at in Chapter 1, it was found that between July 2000 and April 2001, of the 4,481 prescriptions filled in those pharmacies, there were 77 errors—it should be noted that the observers in this study intervened so that no patient actually received the incorrect prescription—and 74 near-misses (mistakes that were caught by pharmacy staff before reaching a patient). Of the 77 errors observed:

- 51 involved a mistake in the labeling,
- 6 were the wrong drug, and

- 8 were the wrong strength of the drug;
- 65 of 77 errors were in the part of the workflow the technician controls.

> **RxErcise 2-A The Importance of Minor Errors**
>
> In the study by Auburn University, 9 of the 77 observed errors involved dispensing the wrong quantity of the drug prescribed, such as putting 29 tablets in a bottle that was supposed to contain 30 tablets. Discuss why, although such mistakes may seem minor, they represent an important measurement of the pharmacy's quality system.

A reasonable conclusion that can be drawn from that study is that pharmacy technicians are in a good position to reduce a majority of medication errors. While it is management's responsibility to provide the quality-assurance program, the pharmacy technician is in the best position to implement it. The pharmacists must assist the technicians by working with them to introduce and organize the overall workflow. The people who can best bring a system to life are those who are closest to the action.

Recognizing "Pharmacist Only Questions"

There are some tasks that should be considered as "pharmacist only" because pharmacists have the required clinical education and training. In some cases the law will specify that only a pharmacist may perform a certain task such as counseling. In Arizona, for example, the board of pharmacy regulation on counseling reads:

R4-23-402. Pharmacist, Graduate Intern, and Pharmacy Intern

A. ....

B. Only **a pharmacist, graduate intern, or pharmacy intern shall provide oral consultation** about a prescription medication to a patient or patient's caregiver in an outpatient setting, including a patient discharged from a hospital.

There are other times when the pharmacy will have a rule restricting who is to perform a particular function. This is not necessarily because only a pharmacist can do these functions, but because the functions are sufficiently important that the pharmacy must limit the number of persons who can handle them. These jobs will usually be done only by the highest professional person on duty at the time, for example, dealing with an unhappy pharmacy customer.

There are also certain questions that are to be directed to the pharmacist, called "pharmacist only questions." If, for example, a patient calls and says, "My prescription is a different color this time," it is a call that should be referred to the pharmacist on duty. Consider the case of Heidi Happel and the questions that were asked by her husband when he was in the pharmacy and the question by Heidi when she later called the pharmacy.

The Case of Heidi Happel

Heidi Happel suffered from severe menstrual pain.[2] Because Heidi was allergic to aspirin, acetaminophen, and ibuprofen, she asked her doctor to prescribe something on prescription that would relieve the cramping. Her doctor prescribed Toradol® (ketorolac), an anti-inflammatory drug that is usually very effective for menstrual pain. Her doctor knew of the patient's allergies, but he did not know that Toradol was contraindicated in a patient who was allergic to aspirin.

Heidi's husband presented the prescription to the pharmacy and was asked if Heidi suffered from any allergies. He answered yes and listed the drugs to which she was allergic. All three of the drugs were already in the computer in Heidi's profile and each was marked as "allergic." According to court testimony in this case, the pharmacy technicians were trained to ask about allergies whenever a new prescription was presented. The prescription was filled correctly and her husband took it home and gave it to Heidi.

About 4:00 p.m., Heidi took the first dose of the Toradol. Within less than an hour, she began having problems breathing and called the pharmacy to ask if the medicine could be affecting her allergy. She was told "No." In actuality, Heidi was suffering from the beginning stages of anaphylactic shock. She later contacted a pharmacist friend who told her there was a cross sensitivity between Toradol and aspirin allergy. He told her to go to the emergency room. She was able to get to the emergency room in time to prevent a worse outcome.

Although the physician did not know, the pharmacist who filled the original prescription was aware that Toradol is contraindicated in patients allergic to aspirin. The pharmacist testified later that had she known the patient was allergic to aspirin, she would not have filled the prescription without calling the doctor.

The court ruled the pharmacist had knowledge of the information in the pharmacy's computer system and that the pharmacy was liable for the incorrect information given to Heidi when she called and asked questions. While it was never discovered who Heidi talked to and who gave her the incorrect information, it appeared it was one of the pharmacy's technicians.

Any question or statement indicating a patient has a question about his or her medicine or may be having a possible adverse reaction to medication is a "pharmacist only question." These must be referred to a pharmacist immediately.

RxErcise 2-B   How Many Errors?

From the short description of the Heidi Happel aspirin-Toradol allergy case, list how many errors you feel were committed by (1) a pharmacy technician or (2) the pharmacist in this case. Note: Assume there was only one pharmacist on duty that day.

CHAPTER 2 • The Role of the Pharmacy Technician in Reducing Medication Errors

Consider Sam's case that took place in an independent pharmacy in a small town in the Midwest. The pharmacist involved owned the pharmacy. Even though the pharmacy had a rule of "pharmacist only questions," mistakes still occurred.

Sam's Case

Sam, almost 80 years old, had been suffering from epilepsy for several years and for the last few years had been successfully treated with a prescription of ¼ grain phenobarbital,[3] a **controlled substance** requiring a new prescription every six months. One morning Sam's physician called in a new prescription for a 100-day supply, which was filled and picked up by Sam later that day.

A couple of hours later, Sam's wife called to say the tablets "did not look the same." She was assured they were correct, and Sam took them for almost three months before it was discovered that the prescription had been erroneously filled with 1 grain phenobarbital. Sam had taken a fourfold overdose for all of those months because a mistake was made in filling the prescription. When given a chance to correct the error before any harm was done, a second mistake was made by not directing the question to the pharmacist. Any question or conversation with a patient that contains a phrase even remotely like "These don't look right" is a "pharmacist only question." It is the technician's duty to make sure these questions are directed to the pharmacist on duty.

Because the pharmacy designates something as a "pharmacist only question," that does not guarantee that any potential problem or error will be prevented. In the example of Sam's phenobarbital, the pharmacy had a "pharmacist only question" policy and when Sam's wife called in, the telephone was given to the pharmacist. In that case the second mistake was made by the pharmacist.

Quality Note 2-B   *Sam's Phenobarbital Rx—How many mistakes to make an error?*

When discussing Sam's ¼ grain phenobarbital prescription that was mistakenly filled with 1 grain tablets, the failure to discover the error when the wife called in was described as the second error. In actuality, it was at least the fifth error involving that prescription that day.

As a new prescription, the information was entered into the computer system as a new prescription and a new number was assigned to it. The pharmacy technician who entered the prescription had done her job correctly.

When a second technician filled the prescription, she grabbed the wrong bottle from the shelf—the 1 grain phenobarbital instead of the ¼ grain (mistake 1). After filling the prescription, the filling technician was to recheck her work. She either failed to recheck or missed the fact that the prescription had been filled with the wrong strength tablet (mistake 2).

After the prescription was filled, it was moved to a pharmacist quality-check area where the pharmacist is required to recheck every item of the prescription. The pharmacist either failed to check the prescription or failed to catch the error (mistake 3).

(Continues)

> **Quality Note 2-B   Sam's Phenobarbital Rx—How many mistakes to make an error? (Continued)**
>
> Although in this particular state the pharmacist was only required to "offer to counsel" patients on new prescriptions—under this state's laws this was considered a new prescription even though Sam had received the same drug several times—the pharmacy policy was to counsel on each new prescription. It was also the pharmacy's procedure to do a "show and tell" counseling, which is not required by law, where the pharmacist would open the sack and take the lid off the bottle during counseling. Either the pharmacist did not counsel or failed to notice the change in tablet size (mistake 4). The pharmacist then missed the fact that a mistake had been made when Sam's wife called in later in the day (mistake 5).
>
> The first the pharmacy knew an error had been made was almost three months after the events occurred. The mistake was finally caught by a nurse at the nursing home where Sam had been committed because it was noticed his mental faculties were becoming impaired. Everyone presumed this was because of age, but when Sam was changed back to ¼ grain phenobarbital, he was back to his old self and was released from the nursing home.

ORGANIZER-IN-CHIEF: MAKE NECESSARY INFORMATION AVAILABLE

When the job is to get the prescription right, everyone has a job to do. The pharmacy technician is the organizer-in-chief, organizing all the necessary information and making sure each person in the prescription workflow has it. The pharmacy technician needs to know what data is available from what source and how it can best be used; for example, in a hospital some of the information may later used by a nurse on the floor. Some of the organizational jobs the pharmacy technician can perform to make sure data is received, stored, and used are:

- Collect information from the patient or caregiver while receiving the prescription or drug order to be used by the pharmacist in performing a prospective drug review
- Pass the information on to the computer entry area
- Enter the collected information into the computer and update the **patient profile**
- Retrieve facts stored in the computer to be used later in the workflow
    - making sure any allergy or drug-incompatibility information is available and known to the pharmacist overseeing the drug review—may be known as **drug utilization review (DUR)**

- noting for the pharmacist in a community pharmacy when counseling is performed other medications the patient is or has recently been taking
- Assemble or place auxiliary labels on the bottle in addition to the prescription label when appropriate
- In a hospital, enter billing information; this may be done automatically, but the pharmacy technician needs to understand and check information
- In a community pharmacy, place receipt and patient-information leaflets with the correct prescriptions
- In a community pharmacy, determine which prescriptions require an FDA med-guide to accompany the prescription and pull or print them so they will be available for delivery to the patient (see Quality Note 2-C for a discussion of FDA med-guides)

Depending on the pharmacy, other information may be collected that may be useful someplace during the workflow. A pharmacy technician should know what information may be needed and make sure it is in place when it is needed.

The Pharmacy Technician and the Prescription Workflow

Receiving the Prescription/Drug Order

If the pharmacy technician is to be the "organizer-in-chief," the job of organizing begins at the start of the workflow. Prior to dispensing any prescription, a pharmacist is expected to perform a **prospective drug review (DUR)** either pursuant to hospital protocol or under the **OBRA-90 regulation** in every state. In Chapter 3 we will take a closer look at the pharmacist's jobs, including the DUR.

A pharmacist cannot adequately perform a DUR unless she or he has all of the information needed, including other medications the patient is taking, all allergies to medications the patient may have, the age of the patient, and other information normally in the patient profile. In a hospital, the pharmacist may have direct access to this information. In a community pharmacy environment, however, the pharmacist will rely more on the pharmacy technician to collect and organize the data.

Patient information is not static. It may not change for years and then may change several times over the next few months. In the earlier example of Heidi Happel, who was allergic to aspirin, it was the policy of the pharmacy to ask about allergies each time a new prescription was received. It would be inefficient for the pharmacist to personally ask this question of each patient with a new prescription. A trained pharmacy technician can easily collect this information and then make sure it is added to the patient computerized profile.

All pharmacies should have a policy to ask about allergies with each new prescription. Most collect it from each new patient, and many ask with each new prescription. However, that is not the end of the information that should be collected by the technician who is trained to ask several other questions. The data is passed to the computer entry station where the patient profile is updated when the new prescription is entered as part of the dispensing process.

The new prescription is then passed on through the rest of the workflow. The information should be documented so it stands out. In addition to allergy information, the receiving technician should ask for or confirm information including:

- Date of birth
- Current address and phone number, including a cell number
- Other medications the patient is taking or has recently taken, including OTC and herbals
- Unusual dosages—any medication taken other than orally or taken more than two at a time
- Legibility of the prescription, particularly if it is hand-written
- Identity of the prescriber, particularly if there is more than one prescriber identified on the prescription blank

RxErcise 2-C   Information Collected

Review the list of items the pharmacy technician is collecting and documenting on the new prescription. For each, discuss why the information is helpful in preventing medication errors and give an example of how it might prove useful.

The Case of the 4-Year-Old Child with Pink Eye

According to Pharmacists Mutual Insurance Company, one of the most common professional pharmacy liability claims is an otic (for the ear) preparation mistakenly used to fill a prescription written for ophthalmic (for the eye) drops. Consider the following claim from Pharmacists Mutual files (names changed to protect privacy).

Mrs. Baxter's 4-year-old son was up all night with an eye infection. She was able to get him into the pediatrician's office as soon as they opened the next day. The child was diagnosed with conjunctivitis, commonly known as "pink eye." The physician prescribed an ophthalmic drop. This drug also comes in an otic form for use in the ear. Both formulations are sterile, but the one for the eye has a neutral **pH** of 7.0, which is the same pH as the eye. If a liquid with a lower pH (more acidic) or a higher pH (more basic) is used in the eye, it will cause a great deal of pain. For example, when companies market a "no-tear" shampoo, they make it at a pH of 7, so there is no pain if it should get into the eye when it is used. Most otic preparations are in the pH range of 2 to 5 (see Figure 2-1, pH Scale).[4]

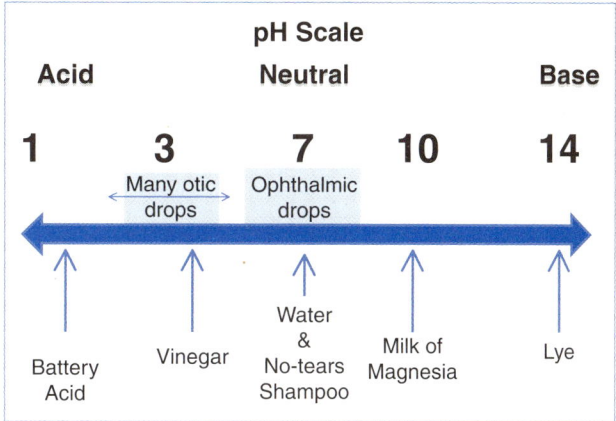

Figure 2-1 pH Scale
© Cengage Learning 2013

Mrs. Baxter brought her child's prescription to the pharmacy as soon as she got out of the physician's office. The label was prepared correctly, but when the bottle was pulled off the shelf, the otic formulation was used by mistake. No one noticed until Mrs. Baxter got home and placed one drop in her son's eye. The little boy screamed in pain. She took him to the emergency room and it was discovered that the pain was caused by the misfilled prescription. The pain was only temporary and there was no lasting damage.

While everyone who had an otic drop placed into their eye would be in pain, when the patient is a child the mistake is more of a problem. Not only is a parent less likely to be forgiving when his or her child is involved in an error, but, more importantly, a child is more sensitive to pain and injury. A lesson here is that while all medication errors should be avoided, it is particularly important when the patient is more vulnerable, such as a child or an older adult.

Particularly Vulnerable Patients

When filling a prescription for a patient under 6 years old or over 60 years old, everyone in the pharmacy should be alerted that this is a particularly vulnerable patient, and should take a couple of extra seconds to check one more time.

This takes us back to the earlier discussion of receiving a new prescription and gathering data where the technician verifies the date of birth of the patient and writes this on the prescription. If the date of birth shows the person is less than 6 years of age or greater than 60, the technician writes the age of the patient in large letters and with another color pen, such as red. As the prescription proceeds through the workflow, each technician and pharmacist is alerted to the fact that this prescription is for a particularly vulnerable patient. Figure 2-2 illustrates a prescription that includes the "Under 6 / Over 60" documentation.

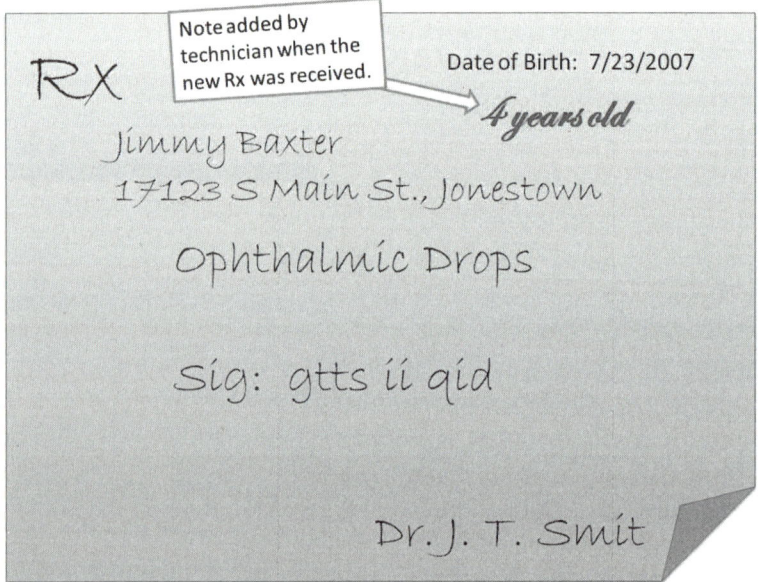

Figure 2-2 under 6, over 60
© Cengage Learning 2013

The Address and Phone Number

Other information that needs to be on each prescription includes the patient's address and telephone number. In RxErcise 2-C, you are asked to state why each piece of information would be helpful in preventing medication errors and to give an example of how each might prove useful. Let us look at one answer that may have been given for one of these items of information—the address and phone number.

Pharmacies may or may not have this information, which often changes and must be updated. It is a part of the patient identification system. In one medical clinic, every time a patient is escorted into a room or area, the staff is trained to ask the patient to verbally repeat their date of birth. This is done to ensure this is the correct patient.

By law, the address is required to be on the prescription for a controlled substance. In addition, the address and the phone number are identifiers. Just as the medical clinic used the birth date as a way of being sure they had the right patient in tow, the pharmacy can use one or both bits of information to be certain they have the correct patient or patient record. A better practice is for two unique identifiers to be used for each patient.

When the pharmacy technician puts the information into the computer, it should be double-checked to be certain this is the correct patient. There can be several patients with the same name, although usually not with the same address or phone number. Collecting the address and phone number on each prescription provides a double check at the computer station and at the other end of the workflow to be certain that the prescription is being given to the correct patient. Consider the case of Jimmy.

The Case of Jimmy's Impatience

Jimmy was 16 years old and went directly to the drugstore from his physician's office.[5] He had a new prescription for allergy medication that he handed in to the pharmacy technician along with his insurance card that showed this was to be charged to Medicaid. Customarily, when a prescription was filled, the insurance card would be handed back in the prescription bag with the filled prescription. Jimmy waited, with the impatience of a typical 16-year-old boy, while several customers in front of him had their prescriptions filled and delivered back.

Finally, a pharmacy clerk held a prescription bag and announced the name "Harold Brown," at which time Jimmy immediately held up his hand, stepped forward, and took the prescription bag. Probably because Jimmy had a Medicaid card, he did not think about paying for the prescription or looking at the receipt. No one else seemed to notice that he did not pay for the prescription in his hand.

Jimmy went home and handed the prescription bag to his mother who opened the bag, took one capsule out of the bottle, and watched as he took it. By the time the mistake was discovered the next day, Jimmy had taken three of the capsules from Harold Brown's prescription.

When Jimmy's mother was asked later whether she had read the prescription label, which was clearly labeled for Harold Brown, she admitted that she looked at the directions but never noticed the name. When Jimmy was asked why he held up his hand when the clerk called out the name of "Harold Brown," he had no answer. Following this incident, the pharmacy started a procedure requiring the patient to give his or her address before a prescription is delivered. In some pharmacies the phone number, rather than the address, is used to identify that the prescription is being picked up for the correct patient. There are other reasons for collecting the address and phone number on each prescription. The pharmacy may need to contact the patient or a member of the patient's family. In the example of Jimmy and Harold Brown's prescription, the mistake was discovered when Harold Brown came in the pharmacy the next morning to pick up his prescription. A search of "Will-Call" showed that Jimmy's prescription had never been picked up, although the clerk remembered giving it to him. The pharmacy had Jimmy's mother's phone number in the file and was able to contact her before Jimmy took more doses.

The Telephone Order

Many orders for medication enter the pharmacy by telephone, fax, or an electronic communication directly into the pharmacy's computer. Each pharmacy will have procedures for handling each of these communication methods. State law usually limits a pharmacy technician's ability to accept a new order over the telephone, although most refill information will be part of the technician's tasks. It is important that each technician know which of these duties can be performed under state laws and under the rules of their practice site.

Computer Entry and Preparing the Label

When a prescription or drug order arrives at the pharmacy, it is just a set of instructions that the pharmacy must enter into a format that can be used by the patient or the nurse. The technician enters the information into the computer and prints the label. The computer is the pharmacy's electronic record-keeping system.

The technician ensures the information is correct and up to date—addresses and phone numbers, new allergies information, drugs taken that are not in the pharmacy's system, drugs taken that do not require a prescription—all must be updated in the computer **patient profile**. Many **Rx only drugs** will interact with **herbals** and **over-the-counter (OTC) medications**. To perform a **drug review**, the pharmacist must be aware of all of this information. Unless herbals and OTC medications are in the computer, the interaction software cannot alert the pharmacist to potential **interactions** or warnings.

When the technician is entering information and prescription data into the computer, there may be a notice generated by the computer software of an allergy, possible overdose, or interaction. When this occurs the technician must see that the pharmacist is made aware of the warning. How this is done will depend on the computer system, the software, and pharmacy policies or procedures. Review the case of Heidi Happel. The pharmacist had all of the pharmaceutical and clinical knowledge she needed regarding the cross allergies. What she did not know was that the computer contained information that Heidi was allergic to aspirin. The problem was not lack of knowledge; the problem was getting the information to where it could have saved the patient a trip to the hospital.

There are several ways technicians can be sure relevant information is available to the pharmacist. One pharmacy has a second computer screen in the pharmacist's final check area. If a warning comes up on the technician's screen during entry, a note can be placed with the label to alert the pharmacist to use the second computer terminal to bring up the patient profile and review the warnings.

One pharmacy that does not have a second computer uses a second printer that prints all warnings and a patient profile. These accompany the prescription and the bottle of the drug to the pharmacist's final check area. Most pharmacy-software programs are set so that a pharmacist is required to come to the computer entry station when a warning appears. Only a pharmacist is supposed to override such a warning. A similar system was in place at the pharmacy Heidi used, but it failed because someone other than the pharmacist apparently overrode the warning on the screen. Every technician needs to know how his or her system for getting information to the pharmacist works and to make sure a warning will get to where it is needed. Most computer systems now have the capability to track who overrides what warnings.

One of the most common mistakes leading to medication errors is entering incorrect directions into the computer. For example, a community pharmacy, while testing a CQI system it had implemented, collected data on every near-miss for 30 days. In the first month, it found 39 percent of all prescriptions entered involved incorrect directions being inputted into the computer. Most of these were caught and corrected before reaching the patient. Similar results have been reported from other pharmacies.[6]

The Case of Sr., Jr., and the III

It is not just the directions that must be entered correctly. A middle-aged man died when he was given his father's heart medication. Three men by the same name resided in the same house and had their prescriptions filled at the same pharmacy. The only difference was the suffix at the end of the names. The oldest male in the household, the grandfather, was senior. Carl, Jr. was his middle-aged son and father to the youngest. The youngest was Carl, III. Several prescriptions for the family were filled on the day of the error. One new prescription was for the grandfather, but the technician used the name on the second line which was "Jr." The prescription was filled with Jr.'s name on it. Carl, Jr. took it without noticing.

An additional problem arises when an error is made during the original fill. Any part of the information incorrectly entered may be refilled incorrectly in the future. Because this problem is so common, some pharmacies require that the original prescription be reviewed at the first refill. Other systems have been developed which scan the original prescription so that the image of the hard copy appears with every refill for a required review.

Filling the Prescription/Drug Order

After the information is entered into the computer, the label and the prescription order usually go to an area where the prescription is filled. Selecting the correct drug, placing the correct label on the bottle, and assembling all needed information with the finished prescription are some of the most important jobs of a pharmacy technician. If filling the drug order means preparing the total parenteral nutrition (TPN) solution or mixing an IV, the technician must be particularly vigilant. All items used in preparing a compounded product must be carefully set out to allow the pharmacist to check all the material both before and after mixing. Each system will have check procedures to avoid errors in this part of the process.

Preparing for the Pharmacist's Quality Check

As noted earlier, a process of "tech check tech" is becoming an accepted practice in hospital settings, and in some states required by law. In the majority of pharmacy settings, whether by practice or by law, a pharmacist must check each prescription for accuracy before it is delivered to a patient. The final check is an extremely important part of every pharmacy's quality-assurance system.

Pharmacies with the ability to record errors and near-misses routinely document when and in which process near-misses are caught. They have found that the majority of all near-misses are caught at the pharmacist's quality checkpoint in the workflow.[7] Near-misses are also caught by technicians at other points and most mistakes are intercepted before they leave the pharmacy. While those facts are positive, they also signal that too many mistakes get through the system and reach a patient.[8] The ideal pharmacy practice would have zero errors reach a patient. One way to accomplish that ideal would be for pharmacy technicians to allow no near-misses to reach the pharmacist's final quality check area.

Preparing for Pharmacist's DUR and Counseling

When we discussed the filling process, we explored some of the information the pharmacist needs to perform an effective drug utilization review (DUR) and counseling. A DUR consists of the pharmacist checking the patient's profile for disease states, allergies, and other drugs the patient is taking that could cause a problem or interaction with the prescribed new drug. In addition, the pharmacist will check for any prescriber error such as when a prescribed amount appears out of the normal range. In such a case, the pharmacist may decide to call the physician and inquire as to whether there is a reason for the atypical dose.

The pharmacist can best do this if a pharmacy technician has prepared the scene. The pharmacist must know about patient allergies and other drugs the patient is taking. Ideally, pharmacists would like to know what disease states (e.g., high blood pressure or diabetes) the patient suffers from and how compliant the patient has been in taking medications. In many ways, the pharmacy's policies and procedures will dictate what information is available and how the technicians collect it, and direct how and what information is presented to the pharmacists. Having the correct information available at the right place may be a matter of life and death.

Delivery to the Floor or the Patient

In a community pharmacy, the filled prescription is usually handed directly to the patient, often by the technician who also collects payment, and, if counseling is needed or recommended, directs the patient to an area with some degree of privacy. In some pharmacies, delivery is done by the pharmacist at the time of counseling. In mail-order pharmacies, the finished prescription is delivered to the mail room or fulfillment center where it is shipped to the patient.

In a hospital, the medication may be delivered directly to the nursing station or loaded into a mechanical device, such as a Pyxis machine, by a pharmacy technician. A nurse can then retrieve the medication and deliver it where and when it is needed.

When delivering a drug order or a prescription, the technician is performing an important step in the quality system. Review "The Case of Jimmy's Impatience." The manner in which Jimmy received another person's prescription illustrates the importance of an effective quality system as part of the prescription-delivery process. There are also stories of a nurse giving a patient the wrong medication because the Pyxis was incorrectly filled. Each mechanical system has its own safety system designed to prevent errors. None of these systems, however, are fail-safe. The technician assigned to refill an automated dispensing machine must be familiar with how it works and how to make it almost fail-safe.

Quality Note 2-C   FDA Med-Guides

The Food and Drug Administration (FDA) has the authority to require med-guides to be given to patients with certain drugs. Below is part of an FDA website warning:

"Patient Package Inserts: For some prescription medicines, FDA approves special patient materials to instruct patients about the safe use of the product. These materials may be given to patients by their health care provider or pharmacist, and are considered part of FDA-regulated product labeling.

"Medication Guides: FDA may require distribution of medication guides, FDA-approved patient information, for selected prescription drugs that pose a serious and significant public health concern. Medication guides will be required if the FDA determines that one or more of the following circumstances exist:

- patient labeling could help prevent serious adverse effects;
- the drug product has serious risk(s) (relative to benefits) of which patients should be made aware because information concerning the risk(s) could affect patients' decisions to use, or to continue to use, the product;
- the drug product is important to health and patient adherence to directions for use is crucial to the drug's effectiveness."

A list of the drugs requiring or with available med-guides can be found on the FDA website and can be printed. See: http://www.fda.gov/Drugs/DrugSafety/ucm085729.htm

When Something Goes Wrong

The key to maintaining a successful quality system lies in understanding the problems that occurred in the past and correcting them. If you do not know what went wrong yesterday, you will repeat the same mistake today and tomorrow. A monitoring program is the statistical component of the Deming theory of total quality management and is the key to constant improvement in any pharmacy-quality program. By collecting information on each error and near-miss, the pharmacy can spot vulnerabilities in its workflow and correct errors before they are made. The Achilles heel in most CQI programs is they do not collect enough data to allow them to be continuously analyzed and improved.

Since mistakes can be made anywhere in the workflow, every member of the team must be responsible for collecting and recording information on each near-miss and each error, but most near-misses will be made in the receiving, computer entry, and filling stations of the workflow. These are the parts of the process that are under the control of pharmacy technicians, and hence a large amount of the QRE information should be recorded by them. While many of the QREs will be caught at the pharmacist quality-check station and will be first recorded by the pharmacist there, entering the information into a special database can be a technician function.

Analysis of the information collected will usually be a job assigned to a pharmacist, but gathering the information into a readable format will often be done by technicians. There are times that a technician, under the supervision of a pharmacist, may be the one to perform an initial analysis of the QRE information (review Quality Note 2-A). Technicians collect, gather, and record the information that forms the statistical monitoring program necessary to allow a quality program to succeed and improve.

Using Error and Near-Miss Information

One of the final steps in a quality-assurance plan is recording any mistake that does occur to determine where there are weaknesses within the system. This can lead to steps being taken to improve the workflow and lead to less errors and mistakes. Everyone in the workflow should help collect this information, but the technician is in a position to coordinate gathering the information and entering it into the system.

The CQI program Pharmacy Quality Commitment® (PQC)[9] of the **National Alliance of State Pharmacy Associations (NASPA)** is an example. It consists of two parts. The first part, a quality workflow program called the Sentinel System™, was discussed earlier. The second part, the Quality Manager™, is an error and near-miss recording and analysis system.

Recording QRE in the PQC system is accomplished by documenting selected information on each error and near-miss and noting it on a specially designed chart that uses a simple coding system. Recording a near-miss in the PQC system is designed to take approximately 30 seconds.

At the end of the day, a technician transfers this information into a secured website for this pharmacy that can then be used to prepare charts and graphs each month to allow everyone in the pharmacy to see where mistakes are made and to design procedures to prevent future errors. The key to the system is the pharmacy technician's collecting and recording of information. Unless this is done each day and each month, the system cannot continuously improve.

Quality Information

The **American Society for Health-System Pharmacists (ASHP)** publishes a series of home-study continuing-education modules for pharmacy technicians called "Pharmacy Tech Topics"™. The entire series is highly recommended for all pharmacy technicians, particularly those working in hospital pharmacy. In January 2010, the topic was "Medication Safety and the Role of the Pharmacy Technician." The authors point out that pharmacy technicians should be aware of the types of pharmacy medication errors that may occur. In particular, they draw attention to high-alert medications by drug class or drug name. This information is available from many sources, including ASHP and the **Institute for Safe Medication Practices (ISMP)**. ISMP offers a safety alert newsletter by subscription and many additional items without charge.

One of the registers that ISMP makes available through its website (http://www.ismp.org) is its list of "Error-Prone Abbreviations, Symbols, and Dose Designations."[10] Part of the pharmacy technician's role as quality information organizer may be to collect and disseminate information to all members of the pharmacy staff. This information can be valuable to educate members of the pharmacy team and reduce medication errors.

No individual in a pharmacy, including pharmacists, can hope to be familiar with all information, warnings, and alerts that are published each year in the area of quality assurance or medication errors. However, if all pharmacy technicians work as a team to collect and post such information, the pharmacy can be kept reasonably up to date with this kind of knowledge. Each month, experts in the areas of quality and medication safety publish information that can be put into practice in any pharmacy. There are many sources of the type of material that could be posted in the pharmacy.

For example, the ISMP catalog of "Error-Prone Abbreviations, Symbols, and Dose Designations" lists the abbreviation "hs" as an error-prone abbreviation that should be avoided. ISMP notes that "hs," meaning "at bedtime," could be confused with "HS," which is occasionally used to designate "Half Strength." ISMP suggests that prescribers use "bedtime" and "half strength" instead of the letters "hs." If the pharmacist and the technician are alerted to these possible confusing abbreviations, they can take steps to reduce possible errors.

The pharmacy technician receiving the new prescription that contains "hs" could underline the error-prone abbreviation and write "bedtime" above it on the prescription. This could best be done before the prescription is scanned or moved into the workflow. The technician may feel it is highly unlikely for a member of the team to be confused with the "hs" abbreviation, but if this act prevented only one error some day, the habit developed would be worth the time invested.

ISMP also points out that some prescribers use "BT" for "bedtime" when writing prescriptions or drug orders. This "BT" abbreviation, ISMP notes, has been confused with "BID," which is the common abbreviation for "twice daily." It is better practice, ISMP notes, for physicians to write out the word "bedtime." In the same vein, the abbreviation "QD," used to designate "every day" or "daily," has resulted in errors where a pharmacy technician typed "four times a day" on the label, resulting in a fourfold overdose. These actions may be important for other reasons. The use of "dangerous abbreviations" in hospitals may affect its Joint Commission accreditation status, which in turn would affect Medicare reimbursement.

Another list of helpful tips from ISMP is look-alike drug name sets it compiled with the assistance of the FDA. Most pharmacists and pharmacy technicians are aware that some names of drugs are confusingly similar to other drug names and can result in errors in which the patient is provided with the wrong drug. The results can, of course, be catastrophic, most importantly for the patient but also, to a different degree, for those who filled the prescription. Examples given by ISMP and the FDA are "hydralazine" confused with "hydroxyzine" and "glipazine" mistaken for "glyburide."

ISMP, FDA, APhA, ASHP and other sources make information available that can help the pharmacy reduce the risk of medication errors. Unfortunately, many pharmacists and technicians do not know it exists. Pharmacy technicians can perform a valuable service by making such information available and visible in their pharmacy practice site.

Training Others

Figure 1-6 in Chapter 1 illustrated the risk management process as a series of five steps. The first step in the process is to identify the risk by noting where mistakes in the workflow can be made. The second step is to prepare a plan to reduce the risks discovered in step one. The plan is a designed workflow with a series of best practices that will prevent the mistakes from happening or catch them before they can reach a patient.

The third step is noted in Figure 1-6 as Act. Act is the implementation of the plan. An important part of implementing a plan is the training and testing of pharmacy personnel in the planned quality workflow. A pharmacy technician in each practice site may be designated as a quality workflow trainer. A pharmacist can do this job, but so can a technician. Pharmacy technicians can also make sure the system actually reduces medication errors as they put procedures into everyday practice. Even those steps in the workflow that must be performed by a pharmacist can be tested by a respected and diplomatic technician. Management, in providing the resources to develop and institute a CQI plan, must see, along with staff, that the pharmacy's CQI program is being used.

Participating in Peer Review

Information regarding errors and near-misses can be put together in many ways, but eventually someone has to analyze it and make decisions. The process starts with an analysis of the data. The question that must be answered is: What does the data show? Every member of the pharmacy team should be a part of this process.

When an error reaches a patient, all of those involved in the workflow should participate in a discussion aimed at preventing this error from occurring again. Root-cause analysis is a mechanism whereby everyone involved in filling the prescription in question participates in an attempt to examine possible contributing factors and to find what one factor was the underlying cause of the error. The root cause is the occurrence that, if it had not happened, would not have allowed this error to occur in the first place. Because the pharmacy technicians are the ones on the front line of the receiving, entry, and filling processes, their input is essential.

Because there are more near-misses than errors, this information can be analyzed collectively, looking for vulnerabilities in the workflow and in each process. Again, the pharmacy technician has knowledge of the many parts of the workflow and is well equipped to offer solutions in this process.

Following the Law

Duties legally allowed to be performed by pharmacy technicians are primarily a product of state, rather than federal, law. Pharmacy technicians must be familiar with the laws of every state in which they are licensed or practice. They must also know federal law, particularly in the areas of controlled substances.

Summary

Pharmacy technicians can be instrumental in helping management develop a culture of safety and quality by setting the quality tone. Quality starts with an attitude that the patient occupies the central position in all aspects of professional pharmacy. The only reason for a pharmacy to exist is to serve the patient. If a patient encounters a pharmacy where the pharmacy technicians are rude or the pharmacists are too busy to be bothered with patient questions, that patient should go somewhere else. Each pharmacy has an attitude and, for good or bad, it is contagious.

Setting a quality tone also means making sure that the entire pharmacy is clean and well kept. There is no better indicator of future errors than a messy, cluttered pharmacy counter. Equipment in today's pharmacy is becoming more important in the delivery of quality medications. A good rule for pharmacy equipment is: If you would not use it to cook your family's dinner, do not use it to prepare your patient's medicine.

In 2006, *Drug Store News*[11] asked pharmacists what they would most like to have to improve their working environment. The number one answer was: "more pharmacy technicians." The reasons are clear. Pharmacists want to be able to concentrate on their clinical duties. In order to do that they must have someone they can trust to do the mechanical and support aspects of dispensing medications.

Pharmacy technicians are critical to implementing a quality-assurance system and making it work. Much of the actual workings of any system of continuous quality improvement is in the hands of the pharmacy technicians. Technicians should take ownership of the pharmacy's CQI program to make it work. Programs do not prevent errors; people do. And to a large extent, it is dedicated pharmacy technicians who prevent medication errors. Quality programs save lives. Serious drug errors also affect those making the errors. No one comes to work to hurt a patient. A quality program protects everyone. Pharmacy technicians make quality programs work.

Review Questions

1. The term often used to collectively describe both errors and near-misses is:

    A. Quality-related events

    B. Workflow slips

    C. Process lapses

    D. None of the above

2. The roles in pharmacy used to be considerably different. Typically, in a community pharmacy in the 1970s a prescription was received, labeled, filled, and dispensed to the patient entirely by the pharmacist, often without the aid of any auxiliary personnel. This old method was not very efficient, but in those days it did not matter because

   A. The gross margin per prescription was high
   B. The volume of prescriptions filled was low
   C. There were few third-party payment plans
   D. All of the above

3. The term "mechanical error" was first used in 1990 in a publication of the American Society for Pharmacy Law in connection with the first Pharmacists Mutual Insurance Company claims study. What does the term "mechanical error" refer to?

   A. Wrong drug
   B. Wrong strength
   C. Wrong directions
   D. All of the above

4. Many of the questions that come into a pharmacy may be answered by a pharmacy technician. Some questions, however, are "pharmacist only questions," either because the law restricts who can answer certain types of questions, the questions are pharmacy technical questions, or

   A. Patients want to talk only to pharmacists
   B. They are sufficiently important that the pharmacy must limit the number of persons who can respond
   C. Technicians have not been trained to answer some questions
   D. None of the above; technicians can answer all questions

5. Why is it important for a pharmacy technician to ask a patient with a new prescription what other drugs he or she is taking?

   A. In order for the pharmacist to perform a drug review
   B. To see if the patient is using other pharmacies
   C. In case of litigation involving interactions
   D. For future marketing functions of the pharmacy

6. In order to continuously improve in reducing medication errors, the pharmacy must collect and analyze

   A. Errors
   B. Near-misses
   C. QREs
   D. All of the above

7. Patients are often given information about their medication when they have prescriptions filled. Some written information is required by federal law. What information is that?

   A. Information directed by the physician in the Rx
   B. Med-guides
   C. Manufacturer's package inserts accompanying the stock bottle
   D. None of the above; there is no federally required patient information

8. The ISMP catalog of "Error-Prone Abbreviations, Symbols, and Dose Designations" lists the abbreviation "hs" as one that should be avoided. ISMP notes that "hs," meaning "at bedtime," could be confused with "HS," which is sometimes used to designate

   A. Half Strength
   B. Have sufficient (doses)
   C. Half Split (divide)
   D. None of the above

9. An important role a pharmacy technician can assume in a pharmacy involves making sure each person has all the information necessary to do the job. One way this role can be described is:

   A. Process controller
   B. Organizer-in-chief
   C. Station processor
   D. Workflow manager

10. In 2006 *Drug Store News* asked pharmacists in an online survey what they would most like to have to improve their working environment. The number one answer was

    A. More pharmacy technicians

    B. Fewer prescriptions

    C. More leisure time

    D. More robotics

Endnotes

[1] Pharmacy technicians need to check the law in the states in which they practice for restrictions on the tasks that cannot be performed by a technician. State laws vary greatly in this area.

[2] *Happel v. Wal-Mart Stores, Inc.*, 199 Ill. 2d 179, 186, 766 N.E.2d 1118, 1123 (2002).

[3] This example is from the files of Pharmacists Mutual Insurance Company. The names and locations have been changed to preserve privacy.

[4] See, for example, Monthly Prescribing Reference, Otic Preparations, http://www.empr.com/otic-preparation-medications/article/125864/ accessed July 22, 2010.

[5] This claim is from the archives of Pharmacists Mutual Insurance Company. "Jimmy" is not the real name of the boy who picked up the prescription and "Harold Brown" is not the actual name of the patient whose prescription was taken by the young man. Names have been changed to protect privacy.

[6] All identifying information redacted to protect privacy.

[7] From the files of PMC Quality Commitment, Inc.

[8] See, for example, Flynn, E. A., Barker, K. N., Carnahan, B.J., National observation study of prescription-dispensing accuracy and safety in 50 pharmacies, *JAPhA*, Vol. 43, No. 2, March/April 2003, pp. 191–200.

[9] See http://pqc.net/, accessed 8/10/10. The author of this text was involved in development of the PQC program.

[10] http://ismp.org/communityRx/aroc/files/Appendix_1.pdf Information updated 2009, accessed 8/8/2010.

[11] Drug Store News Retail Pharmacy Customer Service and Patient Satisfaction online survey, October/November 2006.

CHAPTER 3
Role of the Pharmacist

OBJECTIVES

Upon completion of this chapter, the reader should be able to:

1. Explain the role of pharmacists in systems of quality.
2. List the elements of a basic quality workflow in a pharmacy.
3. Describe the role of the pharmacist in overseeing the implementation of a quality assurance system.
4. Discuss the role of the pharmacist in training quality processes.
5. Describe best practices that the pharmacist uses.
6. Explain the importance of the pharmacist in organizing the pharmacy's continuous quality improvement (CQI) system.
7. Discuss duties a pharmacist cannot delegate in a quality system.
8. List ways in which the pharmacist is essential in reducing medication errors.
9. Explain "pharmacist only questions."
10. Explain how pharmacists can analyze error information and direct continuous improvement in the pharmacy's quality system.

KEY TERMS

Accreditation Council for Pharmacy Education (ACPE): A national, independent agency for the accreditation of professional degree programs in pharmacy, providers of continuing pharmacy education and certificate programs in pharmacy.

Common law: Decisions made by courts can have the effect of setting a rule that other lower courts must follow. The court case thus sets a precedent and has the force of law. Court decisions are referred to as the common law.

National Association of Boards of Pharmacy (NABP): A national organization that provides services to state boards of pharmacy. NABP administers testing for pharmacists in most states. It provides many other services including the Verified Internet Pharmacy Practice Sites (VIPPS) program that certifies Internet pharmacies.

OBRA-87 Regulation: The Omnibus Budget Reconciliation Act of 1987 required nursing homes to have all medications for residents who received Medicaid or Medicare reviewed, usually by a pharmacist.

OBRA-90 Regulation: In 1990 the federal government passed the Omnibus Budget Reconciliation Act of 1990 that required, as a small part of the legislation, states to require pharmacists to perform drug reviews, counsel patients, and maintain a patient profile on some patients. By 1993, the states, through their pharmacy practice acts or board of pharmacy regulations had broadened these requirements.

Prescription drug-monitoring program: Online database for tracking controlled-substance prescriptions filled or prescribed by every pharmacy and physician in the state. Pharmacies and physicians are required to report all controlled-substance prescriptions filled or prescribed by them within a specified period of time. Pharmacists are given a code allowing them to log onto the database and check to see if a patient had any controlled substances filled in another pharmacy in the state. The pharmacist can also see how many physicians are prescribing controlled substances for this patient.

OUTLINE

- **The Pharmacist's Evolving Role**
  - Economics
  - Newer, More Powerful Medications
  - Changing Laws and Expectations
- **Judicial Views of Expanded Legal Roles of Pharmacists**
  - The Case of "Don't Use When Climbing a Ladder"
  - The Case of the Alcoholic Patient
  - The Case of the Incomplete Directions
  - The Case of the Asthmatic Boy
  - The Case of "We Did Warn the Doc"
- **Expanded State Statutory Duties**
- **The Importance of the Duty to Warn on Quality**
- **A Quality System from the Pharmacist's End of the Workflow**
- **Overseeing an Increase in Efficiency**
- **Implementing a Quality System**
- **Establishing "Pharmacist Only Questions"**
- **The Pharmacist's Role in Assisting Pharmacy Technicians**
- **The Pharmacist's Quality Check**
- **The Prospective Drug Review**
  - The Case of Allegation of a Deadly Cocktail
  - A Pharmacist Tool—Prescription Drug–Monitoring Program
  - The Case of a Question of Duty to a Non-Patient
- **Education and Counseling: Delivery to the Floor or the Patient**
  - The Case of a Sulfa Allergy and "What If?"
- **Analyzing and Using Error and Near-Miss Information**
- **Training**
- **Following the Law**
- **Summary**

THE PHARMACIST'S EVOLVING ROLE

Due to a number of changes in pharmacy practice including competition among pharmacies, low third-party reimbursement, and increased regulations and new duties for the pharmacist, it is no longer feasible for pharmacists to perform duties that can be accomplished by trained pharmacy technicians. Pharmacists need to concentrate on clinical roles in their practice. Nonclinical jobs and distributive tasks are now delegated to competent, trained pharmacy technicians who, along with other support staff, are supervised by the pharmacists. Five primary challenges have had a dramatic effect on the role of pharmacists in the most visible parts of their jobs. These factors are:

1. Economics
2. Increased prescription volume
3. More powerful medications
4. Changing laws and expectations
5. Judicial recognition of expanded legal roles of pharmacists

Economics

Health care changed dramatically with the almost universal adoption of a health insurance model that altered the way Americans paid for medical care and prescriptions. Health insurance changed the extent and degree to which the public viewed health care. The economics of competition also changed. Patients no longer controlled how much they would pay for a physician's visit or a night in the hospital. The concern became whether procedures were covered by insurance and the amount of co-pay required. Insurance companies, controlling hundreds of thousands of patients, negotiated the prices that would be paid for health care. These health insurance companies were more sophisticated shoppers, driven by profit rather than emotion, when they selected the hospitals and physicians to be included in a health network.

In the past, medications were relatively inexpensive, and few paid attention to pharmacy prices until unions, representing manufacturing workers including the powerful United Auto Workers (UAW), included prescription coverage in their contracts. At first the effect on pharmacy was minimal as the negotiated prices were not much lower than the prices charged for cash-paying customers. Pharmacies, however, began a fierce level of competition among themselves for restrictive and eventually exclusive contracts to service the insured customers. Gross margin was sacrificed for an ever-increasing volume of prescriptions.

New drugs were approved at an increased rate, and more people gained access to health care, resulting in a dramatic, increased demand for prescriptions. This forced some pharmacies out of business and gave increased opportunities to others. Larger chain drugstores bought up independents and smaller chains. Large department stores and grocery stores expanded their presence in the pharmacy business. These large retailers were used to a business model of low margin and high volume. They also appreciated that pharmacy brought shoppers into their stores who would spend money on other items.

While there was a need to cut costs, these pharmacies found they needed an ever-increasing number of pharmacists. Eventually, the limited number of pharmacists in the market led to a pharmacist shortage. Pharmacist wages and costs to the pharmacies increased in accordance with supply and demand.

According to a Kaiser Family Foundation Prescription Drug Trends Report, "from 1997 to 2007, the number of prescriptions purchased increased 72 percent (from 2.2 billion to 3.8 billion), compared to a population growth in the United States of 11 percent. The average number of retail prescriptions per capita increased from 8.9 in 1997 to 12.6 in 2007."[1] Because pharmacies had to fill more prescriptions in order to make a profit, and because prescribers were writing more prescriptions, pharmacies needed to become more efficient. Many of the jobs pharmacists were performing could be done by others. So pharmacies began hiring clerks as helpers. It was eventually recognized that these clerks needed more skills and training; thus, the profession of pharmacy technicians was born.

Newer, More Powerful Medications

Newer, more powerful medications were entering the market in the closing years of the twentieth century. More health conditions could be successfully treated with medications, leading to a reduction in more expensive, inpatient, hospital treatments. This was one more factor leading to increased medication and prescription use. It also meant that the pharmacist's knowledge needed to expand because there would be an increased demand for the pharmacist's clinical skills both in the hospital and in community practice.

Changing Laws and Expectations

In the 1960s, colleges of pharmacy, the **Accreditation Council for Pharmacy Education (ACPE)**, and organized pharmacy saw the need for increased clinical education to meet the newer, professional roles expected of pharmacists. Pharmacists retained their roles in management, oversight, and organization of the distribution of prescription drugs and they expanded into clinical areas. New roles include educating the patient in the use of the drugs, reviewing therapeutic drug use, assisting physicians in product selection, and screening for conflicts among prescribed drugs.

Newer roles have taken on a more defined character and have been recognized as enforceable legal responsibilities. The **Omnibus Budget Reconciliation Act of 1987 (OBRA-87)** is a federal law requiring that nursing home patients in a facility funded by the federal government have their medication use assessed and monitored by an appropriate professional. In most instances this professional is a pharmacist. Pharmacists serve as consultants to the nursing homes, ensuring patients receive proper medication treatment, including[2]:

1. patients must not receive unnecessary medications;

2. patients cannot be prescribed antipsychotic drugs unless they are appropriate for a specific patient condition;

3. patients prescribed antipsychotic drugs will receive gradual dose reductions, or behavioral programming in an effort to discontinue the drugs (unless clinically contraindicated); and

4. the home must have no significant medication-error rates, and patients must also have no significant medication errors.

While pharmacist-consultants do not solve all problems of inappropriate medication use in nursing homes, studies have indicated they improved the situation and saved money.[3] Increasingly, pharmacists are recognized as experts in pharmaceutical care, which is a role far beyond that of dispenser.

In 1990 another federal law, the **Omnibus Budget Reconciliation Act of 1990 (OBRA-90)**, was passed. This legislation had a large impact on community or retail pharmacy practice. OBRA-90, in conjunction with state laws and regulations passed in response, provided a requirement that pharmacists must counsel Medicaid patients concerning their medication. Eventually, by state law, this counseling requirement was expanded to all patients. OBRA-90 also mandates that pharmacies must maintain patient records, and pharmacists must perform a prospective drug review on all prescriptions prior to dispensing.

The Iowa pharmacy regulations passed in response to OBRA-90 are representative of most states. These requirements demonstrate the large resource commitment involved in compliance, and explain the resulting need to find other ways to perform the mechanical functions of the drug-distribution process and why technicians became a necessity. The Iowa regulations[4] provide:

The pharmacist shall be responsible for obtaining, recording, and maintaining the following information:

a. *Full name of the patient for whom the drug is intended;*

b. *Address and telephone number of the patient;*

c. *Patient's age or date of birth;*

d. *Patient's gender;*

e. *Known allergies;*

f. *Significant patient information including a list of all prescription drug orders dispensed by the pharmacy during the two years immediately preceding the most recent entry showing the name of the drug or device, prescription number, name and strength of the drug, the quantity and date received, and the name of the prescriber; and*

g. *Pharmacist comments relevant to the individual's drug therapy, including:*

   (1) Known drug reactions,

   (2) Identified idiosyncrasies,

   (3) Known chronic conditions or disease states of the patient,

   (4) The identity of any other drugs, over-the-counter drugs, herbals, other alternative medications, or devices currently being used by the patient that may relate to prospective drug review.

In addition to the record-keeping mandate, counseling is also required. While many states adopted the federal "offer to counsel" requirement, several states, including Iowa, made counseling mandatory. Counseling or educating patients regarding their medications is not only a legal requirement, but it is also an opportunity for an additional safety check. Consider the Iowa counseling regulations,[5] which have changed a little since 1993:

Upon receipt of a new prescription drug order and following a prospective drug use review pursuant to 657—8.21(155A), a pharmacist shall counsel each patient or patient's caregiver. An offer to counsel shall not fulfill the requirements of this rule. Patient counseling shall be on matters which, in the pharmacist's professional judgment, will enhance or optimize drug therapy. Appropriate elements of patient counseling may include:

a. *The name and description of the drug;*
b. *The dosage form, dose, route of administration, and duration of drug therapy;*
c. *Intended use of the drug, if known, and expected action;*
d. *Special directions and precautions for preparation, administration, and use by the patient;*
e. *Common severe side effects or adverse effects or interactions and therapeutic contraindications that may be encountered, including their avoidance, and the action required if they occur.*

Notice that as part of the Iowa counseling regulations, there is a requirement for a prospective drug use review of the prescription. This is an important part of OBRA-90. Just as OBRA-87 required a review of the medication use of nursing home patients, OBRA-90 provides for a review of medication use in outpatients.

Medicare and Medicaid are insurance programs administered by the United States Department of Health and Human Services (HHS). The HHS Office of the Inspector General (OIG) reported that passage of OBRA-90 "... clearly establishes Congress's desire to involve pharmacists more actively in patient care."[6] With OBRA-87 and OBRA-90, the federal government was interested in saving money. They were also interested in quality of care. The OIG found, "contracted medication reviews revealed potentially serious concerns with residents' drug regimens." In support of its finding, the OIG provided the following statistics:

- 20 percent of the reviewed patient records identified patients receiving at least one drug judged inappropriate for their diagnoses. Additionally, patients' records indicated some residents were taking medications potentially contraindicated by their diet requirements, plans of care, or assessments.

- 16 percent of patients were receiving, without a prescription in their records, drugs for which prescriptions are generally required. Further, 23 percent of the patients were prescribed medications for which the records showed no orders or receipts to indicate the patient actually received the medication.
- Approximately 20 percent of residents received at least one drug considered by experts to be inappropriate for use by the elderly.
- Some patients' records indicate they may be experiencing unnecessary adverse medication reactions as a result of inadequate monitoring.
- 21 percent of patients were receiving drugs that may sometimes negatively interact with other drugs in their regimen.
- Nearly one-third of patients were receiving more than one drug from the same class, sometimes a potential hazard. Drugs from the same class may produce similar side effects that can be additive and need to be carefully managed. Yet 19 percent of all records indicate no monitoring for efficacy.

Pharmacists who perform drug reviews in community pharmacies are likely to find similar prescribing errors. In addition, pharmacists may also find that patients make mistakes, including overdosing and under dosing. Pharmacist drug review of each prescription is part of a quality system. Look again at Iowa regulations as an example. These prospective drug utilization review regulations, unlike the counseling regulations, apply to all aspects of pharmacy, including hospital and nursing home practice. The Iowa regulations provide:

For purposes of promoting therapeutic appropriateness and ensuring rational drug therapy, a pharmacist shall review the patient record, information obtained from the patient, and each prescription drug or medication order to identify:

1. *Overutilization or underutilization;*
2. *Therapeutic duplication;*
3. *Drug-disease contraindications;*
4. *Drug-drug interactions;*
5. *Incorrect drug dosage or duration of drug treatment;*
6. *Drug-allergy interactions;*
7. *Clinical abuse/misuse;*
8. *Drug-prescriber contraindications.*

Upon recognizing any of the above, the pharmacist shall take appropriate steps to avoid or resolve the problem and shall, if necessary, include consultation with the prescriber. The review and assessment of patient records shall not be delegated to staff assistants but may be delegated to registered pharmacist-interns under the direct supervision of the pharmacist.

This regulation does not refer just to new prescriptions, but to all prescriptions. Note also that the pharmacist may not delegate the task to pharmacy technicians. The pharmacist can, however, assign less knowledge-specific tasks to others depending on their skills and training. Drug review can be an important use of the computer software system in that it can be programmed to detect and alert the pharmacist to potential interactions and misuse. However, the computer is not infallible; it may contain false positives and may miss some important drug interactions. In addition to the computer, pharmacist time, training, and experience are required.

Prospective drug utilization review duties are important not only because the laws require them, but also to avoid patient injury where professional liability claims may result if they are not performed and a patient alleges injury because of it. Review the Pharmacists Mutual Claims Study in Chapter 1 (Figure 1-5). Over 8 percent of the claims reported to Pharmacists Mutual Insurance Company during the time of the study involved allegations of inadequate or incorrect drug reviews by a pharmacist that led to harm due to missed contraindications, allergies, interactions, overuse, or underuse of a drug.[7]

OBRA-87 and OBRA-90 were the products of pharmacists themselves. The concepts that became the requirements of OBRA-90 were developed by pharmacists who recognized that they were being underutilized. The actual language used in OBRA-90 was written by a pharmacist who was serving as a staff employee of the Senate Committee on Aging, where the bill originated.

JUDICIAL VIEWS OF EXPANDED LEGAL ROLES OF PHARMACISTS

Since the mid-1980s, state and federal courts across the United States have wrestled with the extent to which pharmacists have a legal duty to patients beyond that of filling the prescription correctly. Even before OBRA-87 and OBRA-90, some state courts began finding that pharmacists had a limited duty to warn patients and physicians of risks associated with drug use. These expanded-duty cases have not been applied universally throughout the states. The concept of "pharmacist duty" is still evolving. The following cases provide a view of the battle within the judicial community.

The Case of "Don't Use When Climbing a Ladder"

In 1985 the Indiana Court of Appeals decided the case of *Ingram v. Hooks*.[8] Ronald Ingram had a prescription for diazepam filled at this local Hooks Drug Store in Ft. Wayne, Indiana. A few days later Mr. Ingram fell from a ladder and was injured. The prescription had been filled correctly in all respects. Mr. Ingram sued Hooks for failing to warn him of possible side effects associated with the drug that he contended caused him to fall. The trial court and later the court of appeals decided that pharmacists in Indiana had no statutory, regulatory, or common law duty to "warn customers of all the hazards associated with a prescription drug." That duty, the court held, was an obligation of the prescribing physician. The holding of the court was: "Accordingly, we hold Hooks Drugs had no duty to warn the Ingrams of the hazards associated with the prescription drug Valium and affirm the trial court's dismissal of the Ingram complaint." (*Ingram v. Hooks* at 887.)

The Case of the Alcoholic Patient

Two years earlier, a New York court had reached a different conclusion. *Hand v. Krakowski*[9] was one of the first court decisions in the country to find a pharmacist could have a duty beyond filling the prescription correctly. In this case the court found the pharmacist could be held liable for failing to warn a customer that he should not take the prescribed medication with alcohol. The court held that because the pharmacist knew the customer was an alcoholic and that the medication was contraindicated for use with alcohol, the pharmacist had special knowledge that he had the duty to share with the patient. While the duty was limited, it was an expansion on the concept that pharmacists would never have a duty beyond that of filling the prescription accurately.

The Case of the Incomplete Directions

Other courts followed suit. In 1986 in the case of *Riff v. Morgan*,[10] a Pennsylvania court found a pharmacist could be sued for failing to warn a patient that the physician's directions on the prescription were incomplete. Mrs. Riff's physician had prescribed Cafergot® suppositories for her migraine headaches. The directions on the prescription and typed by the pharmacy on the label read only "insert one rectally every 4 hours for headache." The patient was not told by either the physician or the pharmacist that the use of these suppositories was to be limited to only two in 1 hour and not more than five in 1 week. Mrs. Riff took much more and was later hospitalized for an overdose of the drug. The court held that the incomplete directions constituted a "clear error on the face of the prescription," and that the pharmacist could be liable for failure to tell the patient or the physician of the potential overdose problem and the limitations on the use of the drug.

The Case of the Asthmatic Boy

In 1990, a Tennessee appellate court[11] also found a pharmacist could be sued for failure to warn either the physician or the patient that two drugs used together could result in one of the drugs building up to harmful levels in the body. The boy had been on an asthmatic drug for 2 years when the physician prescribed an antibiotic to treat an infection. The antibiotic caused the blood levels of the other drug to rise to a dangerous level. There was an allegation that the elevated levels of the asthmatic drug resulted in brain damage.

The court held the pharmacist has a duty to live up to the standards of his profession. It was up to the jury to decide what that standard was and whether the pharmacist met it. The court said: "Therefore, whether the duty to warn of potential drug interaction is included within the pharmacist's duty to his customer is a disputed issue of fact . . . [is for the jury to decide]." (*Dooley v. Everett* at 386.)

Many state courts have been reluctant to find a broad duty for pharmacists to warn, or even, like the *Dooley* case, to send the question to the jury to decide. In the last several years, many courts have applied a legal concept usually used in cases against pharmaceutical manufacturers. Under this theory, the courts have refused to hold pharmacists liable for failure to warn a patient of drug information that the physician did not include in the prescription directions.

The rule called the "learned intermediary doctrine" has been used for several years to insulate drug manufacturers from claims that they had a duty to communicate drug information directly to patients. The drug manufacturer's duty is to tell the prescriber about the drug; it is the prescribers' job to filter that information and decide what they thought a particular patient would need to know. The physicians, courts said, are the learned intermediaries between the patient and the drug manufacturer. Because manufacturers do not have direct contact with patients, they cannot have a duty directly to the patients and thus cannot be sued by the patient directly for failure to provide information about the company's drugs.

Some courts have applied this learned intermediary doctrine to pharmacist-patient cases. The court in *Ingram v. Hooks*, cited above, explained its reasoning for applying the doctrine by saying pharmacists do not have detailed medical knowledge about each patient and therefore:

> *The injection of a third party in the form of a pharmacist into the physician-patient relationship could undercut the effectiveness of the ongoing medical treatment. We perceive the better rule to be one which places the duty to warn of the hazards of the drug on the prescribing physician and requires of the pharmacist only that he include those warnings found in the prescription.* (Ingram v. Hooks *at 886.*)

The courts that have applied the learned intermediary doctrine to the pharmacist-patient relationship have started to find exceptions. Illinois courts have adopted this doctrine and applied it in pharmacy cases. In the *Happel v. Wal-Mart Stores*[12] case discussed earlier (see Chapter 2), the court found that the doctrine did not apply where the pharmacist had special knowledge. The pharmacy in *Happel* had knowledge in its computer system that the patient was allergic to aspirin. The pharmacist testified that she knew there was the potential for an allergic reaction if someone who was allergic to aspirin also took Toradol, the drug prescribed for Mrs. Happel.

The Case of "We Did Warn the Doc"

In 2010, the Illinois court applied the learned intermediary doctrine in *DiGiovanni v. Albertson's, Inc.*[13] In that case, the court noted that the pharmacist had warned the prescriber.

> [The physician] prescribed Tenoretic[14] to treat high blood pressure while she was already taking lithium for manic depression. The two drugs were apparently known to have a negative interaction, and the computer indicated so when the Tenoretic prescription was being filled. <u>The record indicates that the pharmacist called the physician prior to filling the prescription regarding the potential interaction, and the physician indicated that he would monitor Laverne.</u> Making a notation in the file, the pharmacist filled the prescription for the Tenoretic. When the lithium prescription was refilled, the pharmacist saw the note regarding notification to the physician about the interaction and that the physician would monitor the patient. <u>We find that the pharmacist properly filled the prescriptions that the physician wrote, took notice of the warning in the system regarding a possible interaction between the two drugs, and notified the physician of the potential interaction prior to filling the prescription. The physician then indicated that he would monitor the usage, so the pharmacist filled the prescription and made a notation.</u> Under these circumstances, as in Eldridge, Leesley, and Fakhouri, *we find that the pharmacist was under no duty to warn the customer of the possible interaction between the two drugs under the learned intermediary doctrine. To hold otherwise would impose a greater duty on the pharmacist than on the drug's manufacturer, as the duty of extending warnings to patients concerning prescription drugs belongs with physicians.* (DiGiovanni v. Albertson's, Inc., 940 N. E.2d 73 {2010}) (footnotes omitted; underlining emphasis added).

> **RxErcise 3-A   What if?**
>
> Discuss what you think would have been the result in the *DiGiovanni v. Albertson* case if the pharmacist had not called the physician? What if the pharmacist had called but had not documented the phone call?

EXPANDED STATE STATUTORY DUTIES

The National Association of Boards of Pharmacy (NABP) publishes proposed rules and regulations that are used by many of the states as templates. Many states follow these suggestions. If the courts have had reluctance mandating that pharmacists increase their intellectual, nondispensary duties, state boards of pharmacy have not. The Iowa Board of Pharmacy OBRA-90 regulations are an example of these requirements. Like Iowa, almost every state expanded the federal OBRA-90 duties to all patients, not just Medicaid patients. The boards have also been willing to enforce the stricter rules in disciplinary actions against pharmacists.

The Importance of the Duty to Warn on Quality

In Chapter 1 we looked at a world-wide recognition of the need for quality systems throughout all industries. The lessons of the need for a quality system have not been lost on the profession of pharmacy. Medication errors are increasingly seen as a preventable problem, and pharmacies are adopting CQI as a way to reduce them. Many states have passed laws requiring pharmacies to institute quality methods.

As the role of the pharmacist continues to evolve and as new roles for pharmacy technicians are developed, the role of the pharmacist in the pharmacy workflow is becoming one of oversight, organization, management, and monitoring the quality program. Pharmacists still have a role in dispensing, but it has moved to the end of the workflow.

A Quality System from the Pharmacist's End of the Workflow

With increasing pressure on the pharmacist to provide counseling for each patient and perform a prospective drug utilization review, pharmacists have been forced to move their activities to the end of the workflow. The pharmacist's role begins primarily after the prescription has been completely filled, labeled and coupled with a receipt. In addition to counseling and drug review, it remains the pharmacist's responsibility to be certain that the prescription is correctly filled. In the prescription workflow, this is referred to as the "pharmacist quality-check station."

While it is not always possible to maintain a strict separation of duties, placing pharmacists in a quality-check role may increase overall accuracy and reduce the risk of medication errors. A check by a different person than the one who performs the task (a "second set of eyes") may provide a better way of catching mistakes.

The OBRA-90 prospective drug utilization review may be performed at the pharmacist quality-check station. Here the pharmacist reviews the patient's list of current and past medications for potential problems, and considers any warnings given by the computer such as allergies, incompatibilities, overuse of the drug according to the prescribed directions, and any patient-compliance problems.

At this point in the workflow, the pharmacist may consider the need for patient counseling. Counseling requires preparation. If the patient is on other medications, the pharmacist must consider the effects of taking the two drugs together. The technician can assist the pharmacist by providing any alerts noted by the computer when the prescription was filled. Some pharmacies print a copy of alerts and the patient's recent profile that then are placed with the prescription to be used by the pharmacist during the prospective drug review. When technicians assist, pharmacists can efficiently do their job at the end of the workflow.

Overseeing an Increase in Efficiency

The combination of high prescription volumes and economic pressures requires that the pharmacy team operates as efficiently as possible. Efficiency is more than working quickly. Efficiency is much more likely to result if the workflow is managed intelligently by avoiding rework. This means avoiding mistakes and near-misses that result in time lost by filling prescriptions more than once.

The pharmacist in charge may appoint someone to coordinate the pharmacy's CQI program so that everyone in the workflow understands the tasks that they are to perform. The person who acts as coordinator may be a pharmacist or a highly respected pharmacy technician with the duty to understand the CQI system and to assist all members of the staff to perform within it. The coordinator may also be in charge of training new staff members in the CQI system and testing staff to ensure the program is operated efficiently.

Implementing a Quality System

Edwards W. Deming in his Total Quality Management program taught that it was management's role to provide the correct tools to the workers. Once management has provided the CQI program, staff must implement it. In most pharmacies this initially is the job of the pharmacist in charge. All pharmacists have a role in overseeing the system during their shift.

Establishing "Pharmacist Only Questions"

A part of the CQI workflow involves establishing rules, policies, and procedures that everyone must follow as part of overall quality. One important rule is that there are certain tasks that only a pharmacist should perform. The law in each of the states contains board of pharmacy regulations regarding tasks that are reserved for a pharmacist, pharmacy intern, or pharmacy students. All members of the staff should understand these important laws and regulations and abide by them at all times.

There are some pharmacist-only tasks that are not promulgated as law but are implemented as quality procedures. One of these involves a set of "pharmacist only questions," which are best practices that become integral parts of the CQI workflow. Several questions may fit this category such as:

- Will this drug interact with anything else I am taking?
- I am allergic to ____. Is that a problem with this drug?
- This medication is a different color than the one I got last month.

> **RxErcise 3-B   Pharmacist Only Questions**
>
> List other "pharmacist only questions" and discuss how they should be handled if the situation arises.

THE PHARMACIST'S ROLE IN ASSISTING PHARMACY TECHNICIANS

As pharmacists' duties evolve into more clinical applications, there is less time available for pharmacists to fill prescriptions. Increasingly, pharmacy technicians have the task of filling prescriptions correctly with pharmacists assisting in these first stations in the workflow, seeing that the technicians have adequate space and a clean, neat environment in which to work. Pharmacists provide the final quality check for each prescription and may sometimes find a mistake. This can provide an opportunity for training, teaching, and helping technicians.

THE PHARMACIST'S QUALITY CHECK

A final quality check is among the pharmacist's most important tasks. This embodies the first duty of every health care professional: First, do no harm.

There should be a separate area set aside for the pharmacist quality check. The technician can assist the pharmacist in seeing that this area is kept clear and reserved only for those prescriptions that have not yet been checked or are in the process of being checked. It is also important that all prescriptions for one patient be separated so that they are not confused or coming led with another patient's medication order. This often involves using a basket for each patient.

When a patient's order is first received in the pharmacy, it is placed in a basket. As a prescription moves through the assembly part of the workflow, the label, receipt, prescription container, and the stock bottles are placed in the basket. The technician has the task of being certain that all the items the pharmacist needs, including any special instructions, are delivered to the final quality-check area.

THE PROSPECTIVE DRUG REVIEW

Following the pharmacist's quality check, the pharmacist performs a prospective drug utilization review. This is a part of the OBRA-90 regulations in each state. As discussed earlier, the pharmacist's purpose is to review the prescription order looking for, among other things:

1. Overutilization or underutilization of the prescribed drug;
2. Therapeutic duplication between any of the drugs ordered and dispensed this day and any other drugs the patient may be taking;
3. Drug-disease contraindications, including any drugs that should not be taken or require special precautions when taken by a patient who has a particular condition;
4. Drug-drug interactions for any combination of drugs the patient may be taking that when used with other drugs, including over-the-counter drugs, could result in harm;
5. Incorrect drug dosage or duration of drug treatment, which may indicate a prescriber error;
6. Drug-allergy interactions, checking the patient's known allergies against any drugs that may cause a particular problem;
7. Clinical abuse/misuse, which may be indicative of a patient error, either accidentally or because the patient is abusing the medication.

The Case of Allegation of a Deadly Cocktail

The technician should be aware of what the pharmacist is doing in the final-check area and why it is important. Action by pharmacists during drug review may save lives. Consider the case of *Powers v. Thobhani*[15] in Florida. According to the appellate court:

> Gail Powers, age 46, collapsed, unconscious, in her home on October 21, 2002, and died the next day at the hospital, having never regained consciousness. An autopsy indicated that the cause of death was "Combined drug overdose (oxycodone and diazepam)." Lab results were positive for atropine, diazepam, nordiazepam, oxycodone, benzodiazepines and opiates, all prescribed by Thobhani and all allegedly filled by Your Druggist and The Medicine Shoppe.

Gail Powers's husband brought suit against the physician, Dr. Thobhani, and the pharmacy. He alleged that the pharmacy should have warned Mrs. Powers that she was taking too many drugs. He also alleged that some drugs should not have been prescribed together nor as often. The judge recited the facts from Mr. Powers's complaint:

On April 5, 2002, Gail Powers began receiving treatment from her primary neurologist, Dr. Thobhani, for ongoing neck and back pain. Thobhani treated Gail on at least 25 occasions during the 6-month treatment period. Over the 6 months, Thobhani prescribed a minimum of six varieties of drugs and narcotics, including oxycontin/oxycodone, Percocet, soma, Xanax, and diazepam. During the 6-month period, Thobhani allegedly repeatedly prescribed these narcotics and other medications days before Gail should have depleted the preceding prescription. Thobhani also allegedly prescribed two or more narcotics at a time along with other contraindicated drugs.

Powers alleged that Your Druggist and The Medicine Shoppe filled every prescription written by Thobhani, without question. The pharmacies also allegedly filled numerous prescriptions for these narcotics too closely in time, within days of having filled previous prescriptions. Powers alleges that this prescription-filling pattern continued until the day of Gail's death. (Powers v. Thobhani, 903 So.2d 275 at 276–277 {2005}) (footnotes omitted).

For our purposes here, the important thing is not the legal issue decided in this case, but the example of the value of a pharmacist's prospective drug review. The allegations in this case had not been proven at the time of this preliminary court ruling. What the court here was citing was what the patient's husband alleged in the complaint. For our purposes, however, let us assume that the allegations in the case are true. Physicians do occasionally overprescribe, particularly when it comes to drugs for pain relief, as in this case. If physicians never made mistakes, pharmacists' job of drug review would be much simpler. One of the items pharmacists may catch in a drug review is a potential harmful overdose. When a possible overdose is noted, or when a patient is refilling the prescription too early, the pharmacist may decide to call the physician and/or have a discussion with the patient. The pharmacist should document his actions. These interventions can save lives.

A Pharmacist Tool—Prescription Drug-Monitoring Program

Sometimes patients get prescriptions for controlled substances, such as the drugs being taken by Gail Powers, at more than one pharmacy. A few years ago a pharmacist would not have known if a patient was going to more than one physician and more than one pharmacy. Now, in most states, the pharmacist has a tool that can provide such information. All but a few states have a **prescription drug–monitoring program**. When these programs are instituted in a state, pharmacies and physicians are required to report controlled-substance prescriptions filled or prescribed. During prospective drug utilization review, the pharmacist can log onto the program and check to see if this patient has had any controlled substances filled in another pharmacy in the state. The pharmacist can also see how many physicians are prescribing controlled substances for this patient.

The Case of a Question of Duty to a Non-Patient

One of the first states with a prescription drug–monitoring program was Nevada. The Nevada Board of Pharmacy, which monitors the program in that state, notified a group of pharmacies that one of their patients ". . . had obtained approximately 4,500 hydrocodone pills at 13 different pharmacies."[16] A year after the letter to these pharmacies was sent, the patient was allegedly still using large quantities of controlled substances obtained from most of the same pharmacies.

While driving under the influence of these drugs, it is alleged this patient struck and killed a delivery man and injured a second person who was helping unload the truck. Because of the way the law in Nevada was written, the pharmacists in this case were found to have no duty to the non-patient delivery person. The case illustrates, however, the importance of a pharmacist's review.

> Quality is more than preventing pharmacy mechanical-dispensing errors. Quality is the totality of the function of providing medication to patients and includes preventing, with the assistance of pharmacy technicians, prescriber and patient errors.

EDUCATION AND COUNSELING: DELIVERY TO THE FLOOR OR THE PATIENT

> Counseling is an important part of the CQI process. A hospital pharmacy's drug order or a community pharmacy's prescription is not complete until it is delivered to the patient. In hospitals this means that the pharmacy technician ensures that the medication is available for nurses to administer. Special instructions often appear on the medication administration record (MAR) and patient information is often available from the computer system or the automated dispensing machine. Some hospitals employ floor pharmacists who educate both nursing staff and patients with medication information. In a community pharmacy this means presenting the final prescription to the patient or caregiver with sufficient information for proper use.

The Case of a Sulfa Allergy and "What If?"

Counseling is the job of the pharmacist and it is best accomplished when a pharmacy technician has prepared all the material needed. A case out of the superior court of Connecticut provides a good example. The allegations in the case are relatively straightforward. The case is *Levesque v. Cluett*, 44 Conn. L. Rptr. 633 (2007).[17] The patient, Mary Ellen Levesque, was having symptoms of a urinary tract infection and called her physician. The physician prescribed Bactrim®, a sulfa containing an anti-infective commonly used to treat such symptoms. The prescription was called into Mrs. Levesque's pharmacy where it was filled as ordered. After she took the medication, she "experienced severe muscle discomfort."

The problem as alleged by Mrs. Levesque in her lawsuit was that she was allergic to sulfa. As a result, she claimed ". . . she suffered injuries and damages, some or all of which are permanent: peripheral neuropathy; sensory polyneuritis; chronic severe pain; chronic numbness, tingling and burning; diminished sensation in fingertips and the soles of her feet; hypersensitivity to touch and temperature; loss of sleep; and continual fear and discomfort."

Mrs. Levesque filed a lawsuit against both her physician and her pharmacy. Against the pharmacy, she alleged failure to perform a proper drug review, saying her allergy had been disclosed to the pharmacy and should have been in its records. She also complained that the pharmacy should have asked if she had an allergy before filling the prescription, and should have warned her of possible harm from taking sulfa when she picked the prescription up. Based upon these allegations, the court decided she had shown enough to proceed to discovery and perhaps eventually to a trial.

RxErcise 3-C What If?

Levesque v. Cluett, 44 Conn. L. Rptr. 633 (2007)

Let us use this case as the basis of an illustration of the importance of counseling and preparing for counseling. Although we do not know all of the facts, from what we have, consider a hypothetical "What if?"

- What could a pharmacy have done for a similar patient when the prescription was phoned in?
- What steps could a pharmacy technician have taken before the filled prescription was given to the pharmacist for quality check, drug review, and counseling?
- What information might a pharmacy technician have given to a pharmacist allowing him/her to effectively counsel the patient?

Pharmacies are required to keep a record of all patients' medication use as well as disease states and allergies. In this case, the physician called in the prescription, which the pharmacist would have taken and written the information on a prescription blank before handing it to a technician to enter into the computer system. The technician would complete the computer entry and review it to make sure this is the correct patient. (Today, the prescription might have been entered directly into the computer database through electronic prescribing and transmission.)

From the information in the computer, a label with proper directions would be ready to print. If Mrs. Levesque's allergy was already noted in the pharmacy computer, an alert should show up on the screen when the information is entered. Since this is a high-level alert, most pharmacy computer software would require a pharmacist to clear the system before a technician could go further with the prescription. A printout or a note would be placed in the basket with the new prescription for further review by the pharmacist during final check.

Many alerts given by computer software can be overly cautious and may be overridden when proper questions have been asked and fears alleviated. The prescription may, depending on the pharmacy's quality protocols, be moved to a special area so questions can be resolved. The pharmacist may call the physician's office to inquire about the allergy information in the computer. Or the pharmacist may discuss the information with the patient prior to calling the physician.

If the physician has said it is permissible to give the medication to the patient in spite of the allergy warning, the pharmacist may speak to the patient regarding the conversation with the physician. Counseling is important in this case as questions need to be answered and the patient needs to be given specific information.

Quality Note 3-A   If We Filled Mrs. Levesque's Rx

Let us go further with our example and review what might happen in a hypothetical pharmacy filling Mrs. Levesque's prescription.

- The pharmacy technician places the filled prescription with the label attached into the patient's quality workflow basket. Also in the basket is the original telephoned prescription transcribed by the pharmacist. The basket may contain a printout with the allergy alert from the computer.

- There may be a special sticker placed on the prescription bag informing the pharmacist that "Counseling is required." Everyone on the pharmacy staff knows when this sticker is placed on the bag, a patient may not receive the medication until a pharmacist has counseled the patient.

- The technician has highlighted the "allergic to sulfa" note on the printed alert and has printed the patient's profile from the database for the pharmacist to review. The physician's telephone number is also available for the pharmacist in case a call is necessary.

- In this case, the pharmacist has decided to question the patient about the allergy before calling the physician, knowing the information could be old or that the physician and the patient may have already discussed the situation. (Sometimes allergies may be suspected at first but later discovered to be incorrect.)

(Continues)

> **Quality Note 3-A   If We Filled Mrs. Levesque's Rx (Continued)**
>
> - Remember in this case Mrs. Levesque said the pharmacy already had the allergy information in the computer before she came into pick it up. What if it was not? The computer would not have given an alert.
> - When the patient arrives at the pharmacy the technician, or sometimes the pharmacist, would ask and record the new prescription questions:
>   1. "Date of birth?"
>   2. "Do you have any allergies?"
>   3. "Are you taking other medications?"
> - The pharmacy technician's role in gathering needed information and supplies for the pharmacist can increase efficiency and save patients from undue harm or risk of harm.
> - Document information necessary to show what was asked and answered.

ANALYZING AND USING ERROR AND NEAR-MISS INFORMATION

Anytime errors reach the patient, everyone on the staff has an obligation to learn from the experience. The pharmacist's role is to coordinate a root-cause analysis of the error to make sure lessons are learned that could avoid a repeat of the same mistake in the future. A root-cause analysis begins with a determination of what was the initial mistake or mistakes, which, if eliminated, would prevent the error from being made.

Once the causes have been determined, the questions are:

1. What procedures can be put in place to *stop it* from happening again? (Careful! This is for teaching, not punishment—a good quality system must be nonpunitive.)

2. What other procedures can be put in place to *catch such a mistake* before it reaches the patient, if step 1 is not completely successful?

We will study this type of analysis later. For now, we need to understand that the pharmacist bears primary responsibility for seeing that an analysis occurs. He or she may delegate that job to another member of the staff, but the pharmacist will usually be responsible for the process.

Training

Another role of the pharmacist involving quality is to oversee the training for the quality-assurance system. Regular and continuous training for all members of the staff should include sharing results of any analysis, working together to use those results, and, prior to the institution of a new procedure, discussing it to ensure a buy-in from all. Deming Principle number seven reads: "Focus supervision on helping people do a better job; ensure that immediate action is taken on reports of defects, maintenance requirements, poor tools, inadequate operating definitions, or other conditions detrimental to quality."

Part of a pharmacist's job is to see that every member of the staff receives the best training available from the company. This includes feedback on every QRE in order to learn from each mistake. The pharmacist on each shift should make sure that all near-misses and errors (QREs) are reported so the information can be used.

Following the Law

An important part of every workflow is to see that the law is observed. This is true for all statutes and regulations pertaining to the practice of pharmacy, including federal law, controlled-substance law, state law, as well as state regulations passed by the board of pharmacy. While everyone involved in pharmacy has an obligation to follow the law, it is particularly important for the pharmacist on duty.

CHAPTER 3 • Role of the Pharmacist

Summary

The role of the pharmacist is critical in maintaining quality in any pharmacy-practice setting. At some points the pharmacist is part of supervision, and at some points the pharmacist is part of staff. Perhaps the best way to think of the pharmacist's role in the day-to-day operations of the pharmacy is as "team leader." In the final analysis, it is the team made up of the pharmacist, technicians, clerks, managers, and support staff who determine whether medication errors will be reduced to the minimum in a particular pharmacy. As leader of the team, the pharmacist must accept the overall responsibility for how well the system works.

Review Questions

1. What is meant by the term "common law?"
   A. Laws that are the same in all states are referred to as the common law.
   B. Appellate court decisions are referred to as the common law.
   C. FDA and other federal laws are referred to as the common law.
   D. State board of pharmacy regulations or rules are referred to as the common law.

2. What is the particular importance of how the common law is applied?
   A. An appellate court ruling sets a precedent that the lower courts must follow and thus the decision has the force of law.
   B. It is a way of making sure that all states apply pharmacy laws uniformly throughout the United States.
   C. It ensures that in a state the board of pharmacy rules are applied the same for all pharmacies.
   D. Federal laws are the same for all pharmacists in the United States.

3. What is the Omnibus Budget Reconciliation Act of 1987?
   A. A federal law that restricts compounded prescriptions for Medicaid or Medicare patients.
   B. A state law that directed how Medicaid or Medicare prescriptions were to be paid.

C. It was an earlier version of OBRA-90.

D. A federal law that requires that nursing homes have a person (usually a pharmacist) review all medications for residents who receive Medicaid or Medicare benefits.

4. According to a Kaiser Family Foundation Prescription Drug Trends report, from 1997 to 2007, the number of prescriptions purchased increased

   A. From 3.7 billion to 3.8 billion.
   B. From 3.5 billion to 3.8 billion.
   C. From 3.0 billion to 3.8 billion.
   D. From 2.2 billion to 3.8 billion.

5. Which of the following is *not* a reason why the role of the pharmacist has changed, causing pharmacy technicians to perform more of the mechanical dispensing functions in pharmacy today?

   A. Increased prescription volume
   B. More powerful medications
   C. An increase in the number of pharmacy schools in the United States
   D. Judicial recognition of expanded legal roles of pharmacists

6. As an example of a state board of pharmacy OBRA-90 regulation, Iowa rules say that as part of a prospective drug review, a pharmacist is required to review the patient record and other information available to identify, among other things, which of the following:

   A. Overutilization or underutilization
   B. Therapeutic duplication
   C. Drug-disease contraindications
   D. All of the above

7. According to the Pharmacists Mutual Insurance Company Claims Study, what is the fastest growing claim against pharmacists and pharmacies?

   A. Mechanical dispensing errors
   B. Wrong drug errors

C. Drug review claims

D. Unauthorized release of confidential information

8. What is the learned intermediary doctrine as it applies to pharmacy law cases?

   A. A legal theory holding that, because physicians are learned intermediaries between the patient and the pharmacist, pharmacists do not usually have a legal duty to warn about potentially harmful effects of a drug.

   B. A legal theory holding that pharmacists are learned intermediaries between the patient and the manufacturer of a prescription drug.

   C. A legal theory holding that pharmacists have a duty to warn their patients of the most common side effects of the prescribed drug dispensed to the patient.

   D. It has no bearing on pharmacy law.

9. As the pharmacist moves away from the mechanical dispensing functions involved in filling a drug order or prescription, which of the following duties are the most important for the pharmacist?

   A. Final quality check

   B. Prospective drug review

   C. Counseling the patient (or educating medical and nursing staff) on new prescriptions

   D. All of the above

10. What does it mean to say the pharmacist is his or her "brother's keeper"?

    A. A pharmacist has the obligation of safeguarding patients against all adverse medication events.

    B. It is the name of a popular pharmacy CQI program.

    C. A part of the pharmacist's role, as part of a health care safety net, is to discover and correct mistakes of prescribers or nurses.

    D. This is a religious term that does not have a place in the discussion of professional roles.

Endnotes

[1] http://www.kff.org/rxdrugs/upload/3057_07.pdf September, 2008, accessed January 2, 2011.

[2] Department of HHS, Office of the Inspector General (OIG), Prescription Drug Use in Nursing Homes, Report 3: A Pharmaceutical Review and Inspection Recommendations, June 1997.

[3] Trygstad, T. K., Christensen, D., Garmise, J., Sullivan, R., and Wegner, S. E., Pharmacist Response to Alerts Generated from Medicaid Pharmacy Claims in a Long-term Care Setting: Results from the North Carolina Polypharmacy Initiative, *Journal of Managed Care Pharmacy (JMCP)*, Vol. 11, pp. 575–583, No. 7, September 2005.

[4] IAC 657–6.13(155A).

[5] IAC 657–6.14(155A).

[6] Department of HHS, Office of the Inspector General (OIG), Prescription Drug Use in Nursing Homes, Report 3: A Pharmaceutical Review and Inspection Recommendations, June 1997, Executive Summary, i.

[7] See Drug Review Claims on Pharmacists Mutual website: http://www.phmic.com/phmc/services/RM/profliab/claimsstudy/Pages/DrugReviewClaimsbyYear.aspx accessed December 8, 2010.

[8] *Ingram v. Hooks*, 476 NE2d 881 (Ind. App. 1985).

[9] *Hand v. Krakowski*, 89 A.D.2d 650, 453 N.Y.S.2d 121 (1982).

[10] *Riff v. Morgan*, 353 Pa. Super. 21, 508 A.2d 1247 (1986).

[11] *Dooley v. Everett*, 805 Sw2d 380 (Tenn. App 1990).

[12] *Happel v. Wal-Mart Stores, Inc.*, 199 Ill.2d 179, 262 Ill.Dec. 815, 766 N.E.2d 1118 (2002).

[13] *DiGiovanni v. Albertson's, Inc.*, 940 N.E.2d 73 (2010).

[14] Tenoretic is the brand name for a combination of atenolol (a beta-blocker) and chlorthalidone (a diutetic). It is usually used to treat hypertension (high blood pressure).

[15] *Powers v. Thobhani*, 903 So.2d 275 (2005).

[16] *Sanchez ex rel. Sanchez v. Wal-Mart Stores, Inc.*, 221 P.3d 1276 (2009).

[17] *Levesque v. Cluett*, 44 Conn. L. Rptr. 633, 2007 WL 4305676 (Only the Westlaw citation is currently available.) Not reported in A.2d (2007).

CHAPTER 4

Prescription Workflow
The Basics

OBJECTIVES

Upon completion of this chapter, the reader should be able to:

1. Study the basics of a pharmacy prescription workflow.
2. Describe the importance of best practices in reducing medication errors
3. List the typical stations that make up a pharmacy workflow.
4. Describe how e-prescriptions may impact medication errors.
5. Discuss the importance of stations in a risk-management workflow.
6. Explain how the Shewhart cycle is used in risk management.
7. Describe the use of the term "preventable adverse medical event."
8. Explain the risk-management process and its steps.
9. Describe the use and importance of national drug code (NDC) numbers in reducing medication errors.
10. Discuss the pharmacist's stations in the pharmacy workflow and how technicians can assist.

KEY TERMS

Best practice: A technique or procedure used and developed over time that has been proven to either stop an error before it begins or to catch a mistake before it can reach the patient and become an error.

CQI station: A CQI station is a stage within a series of steps designed as part of a planned workflow. A pharmacy workflow is made up of a series of processes. At each station a person performs tasks leading to the dispensing of medication. Typical stations within a pharmacy workflow are: receiving the prescription, entering information into the computer, filling the prescription, pharmacist final check, DUR, counseling, and delivery.

Electronic prescribing (e-prescribing): A method of writing and transmitting a prescription through the use of a computer or handheld personal digital assistant (PDA). The prescriber enters the information into a device and sends it in electronic form directly to the pharmacy. E-prescriptions replace writing, telephoning, or faxing the prescription.

Preventable adverse medical event: An adverse medical event is an injury resulting from a medical intervention, not due to the patient's underlying condition. An adverse medical event is preventable if it is attributable to an error.[1] Not all adverse medical events are preventable.

Preventable adverse medication event: Any incident in which the use of a medication (drug or biologic) at any dose, a medical device, or a special nutritional product (e.g., dietary supplement, infant formula, medical food) may have resulted in an adverse outcome in a patient.

Risk-management process: A continuous cycle of identification, planning, acting, monitoring, changing and then beginning again with identification of the risks that remain. It may be represented in four or five steps.

Shewhart cycle: A planning process developed by Dr. Walter Shewhart. It is a way of looking at quality improvement as plan, do check. The Shewhart cycle is sometimes called the "Deming Cycle" or simply PDCA.

Workflow: A series of stations designed as a plan for efficiently and correctly filling a prescription order. The workflow begins when a drug order arrives at the pharmacy and ends when the patient receives the correct medication with information for use.

OUTLINE

Risk Management and the CQI Workflow
The Shewhart Cycle
   Plan
   Do
   Check
   Act
Workflow
Stations—Laying Out the Processes
Introducing Best Practices into the Workflow
   NDC Check
   The Basket System
   The 2-Second Rule
   The Case of "His and Hers"
   Final Bag Check
   Verify the Patient
   Triple Check
   Original Only When New
   "Take 5"
   Other Meds
   Allergies
   Unusual Dose
Building Quality Habits into the Workflow
Putting Best Practices to Work
Receiving the Prescription
   The Case of the Two Kay Wilsons
   Saving Young Lives
   The Case of Grandma's Digoxin
Data-Entry Station
Filling the Prescription
The Pharmacist's Final Quality Check and Drug Review
Delivery
Counseling
Special Problems Station
Summary

Risk Management and the CQI Workflow

The risk-management process is a continuous cycle of identification, planning, acting, monitoring, changing, and then beginning again with identification of the risks that remain. In pharmacy the system resulting from employing the risk-management process is called continuous quality improvement (CQI). Following the adage, First, do no harm, the initial focus in pharmacy is in reducing the risk of a medication error reaching a patient. Not only because mechanical errors are most likely to result in claims, but, more importantly, a patient could be injured. In addition, the pharmacy could be sued; the pharmacist and pharmacy technicians could have action taken against their licenses.

Owners of businesses must concern themselves with many more risks including floods, fires, costs, competition, and more. Each of these involves the study of risk management. The risks we explore in this text are limited to how medication errors occur and how they can be avoided. The first step in risk management is to identify those risks associated with potential medication errors.

Once we have identified the risks that may result in a QRE, we must decide what steps may be taken to reduce those risks. A CQI program will incorporate a series of **best practices** as part of a prescription-dispensing and clinical pharmacy workflow. Best practices are proven techniques that can prevent a mistake from occurring or can catch a QRE before it reaches a patient. For simplicity, practicing pharmacists and pharmacy technicians call a mistake that does not reach a patient a "near-miss." They call a mistake that does reach a patient an "error."[2]

Selected best practices are combined into a **workflow** that begins when a prescription or drug order enters the pharmacy and ends when the completed product is delivered to the correct place in the health care facility or to the patient. The workflow is laid out, approved, and taught to all members of the staff.

No workflow plan is perfect. The pharmacy must monitor the workflow and use the information received to determine changes needed to further improve the CQI system. A CQI plan is never complete. It constantly evolves and improves.

As an example, consider a program available through the National Alliance of State Pharmacy Associations (NASPA). This association of 50 state pharmacy organizations provides a quality assurance program called Pharmacy Quality Commitment® Sentinel System ^{TM}.[3] The Sentinel System^{TM} sets up a method of process controls throughout the workflow. NASPA's Sentinel System^{TM} incorporates more than 20 best practices, some used multiple times, to prevent or capture mistakes before they reach a patient. Each best practice is designed to make it increasingly difficult for a mistake to reach a patient.

The most challenging problem involves training and implementation of the workflow to ensure that each best practice is used each time. Training and implementing the CQI program are roles that the pharmacy technician can perform.

THE SHEWHART CYCLE

There are many tools that can be used to implement a quality program. One of the tools Dr. Deming used is the Shewhart Cycle, a planning process developed by Dr. Walter Shewhart.[4] The Shewhart Cycle can be used to organize and develop a workflow to reduce errors.[5] The steps in this tool are illustrated in Figure 4-1 and simply stated as:

Plan

Do

Check

Act

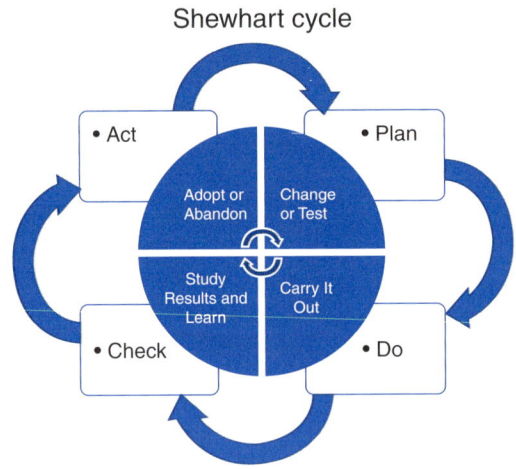

Figure 4-1 Shewhart cycle
© Cengage Learning 2013

Plan:

- Plan a change or test aimed at improving the workflow or a single station in the workflow.
- The planning phase involves identifying the problem or risks in the system.
- Next, the causes of the problems are identified.
- Each process is then mapped with best practices and steps designed to reduce the risks identified either from occurring or from reaching the patient if one does occur.

Do:

- The plan is first implemented in a limited manner to allow it to be tested before being expanded completely.
- Train those who will be testing the plan to carry out the steps and best practices in the order designed.
- At this stage the pharmacy may use check lists to learn each step.
- Quality habits will be acquired when the plan has been proved and put into full practice.

Check:

- Study the results of the trial plan.
- What was learned from the small scale test?

- Did it work?
- Check for reduction in variability, which is the measure of improvement.
- If the test is successful, proceed to step 4 (Act) and implement the workflow on a full-scale basis.
- If the test is not successful, return to step 1 (Plan) and use new solutions.

Act:

- Adopt changes.
- Standardize the policy and the proven workflow.
- Continuously monitor the system.

Workflow

When a drug order or prescription arrives at the pharmacy, a series of processes begin that ends with delivery of the medication. What happens between is referred to as the "pharmacy workflow." A workflow is more efficient if it proceeds in a linear fashion. This chapter examines a basic, simplified workflow and how it is designed to reduce medication errors.

> **RxErcise 4-A   Observe a Pharmacy Workflow**
>
> Visit a hospital or retail (community) pharmacy and observe the workflow.
> Make notes as to whether the workflow proceeded in a straight line, or whether it flowed in some other manner. Was the workflow efficient? What best practices did you observe?

Typically, in a community pharmacy, the prescription will be delivered to the pharmacy staff through a window in the "drop off" area. A prescription may also be called in by a physician or, if the prescription is a refill, by a patient. Increasingly, prescriptions arrive in a pharmacy through e-prescribing, that is, from the physician's computer or PDA. It is interesting to note that while e-prescriptions may reduce the risk of incorrectly reading a physician's written prescription, the practice may increase other risks such as a physician selecting a wrong line on the PDA.

Let us observe a workflow in a hypothetical pharmacy. For simplicity, presume the prescription enters from one end of a long counter. At entry, a pharmacy technician receives the prescription and then delivers it to the next step, which is usually the computer-entry station. Each prescription will then stop at a number of stations, at each of which several steps will be performed according to the workflow plan.

STATIONS—LAYING OUT THE PROCESSES

The most convenient way to examine a pharmacy workflow is to divide it into a series of stations, looking at what happens at each station. A typical workflow is illustrated in Figure 4-2.

At each step in the process a mistake could result in a **preventable adverse medical event**.

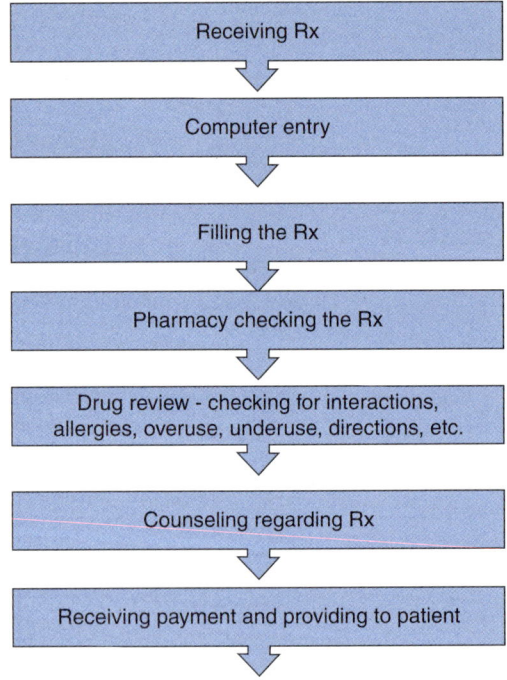

Figure 4-2 Illustration of stations as part of pharmacy workflow
© Cengage Learning 2013

INTRODUCING BEST PRACTICES INTO THE WORKFLOW

The purpose of the workflow is to provide an efficient and uniform method of moving the prescription through the system. Each step should be performed by the technicians and pharmacists in the same manner each time. Designing a workflow with scripted steps allows the staff to learn the process in a manner that makes it more unlikely that steps will be omitted.

It is important that all steps be performed as designed. The workflow will have a number of **best practices** that make up the individual steps. A scripted workflow will also facilitate training and testing of technicians. By having a set procedure, the pharmacy can certify that all members of its staff use each best practice. This can provide an element of proof that any errors reaching a patient were in spite of its training and workflow, not because either was deficient.

A basic pharmacy workflow incorporates the theories that underlie the risk-management process in order to reduce the risk of a medication error reaching the patient. Best practices are key to building an effective system that can accomplish this goal. This text will not try to provide a comprehensive list of best practices because pharmacists and technicians will continue to discover new best practices and to drop some as newer systems or technologies replace older ones.

What is important is that students understand the role of best practices and why they must be used in an organized fashion. The most effective are ones that become habits, making them difficult to ignore or skip. This is itself a best practice referred to as "building quality habits."

NDC Check

One of the best-known and most widely used best practices is the NDC check. Every drug manufactured in the United States is assigned a unique national drug code (NDC) number, a ten- to eleven-digit[6] number divided into three sets.

- The first set of numbers identifies the manufacturer, repackager, or distributor of the drug.

- The second set of numbers identifies the specific strength, dosage form, and formulation of the particular drug for that company.

- The third set of numbers identifies the package size and type.

An NDC number is printed numerically and by bar code on drug packages and stored in the pharmacy's computer system. By design, all computer pharmacy software causes the NDC number to be printed on the receipt or printout. The NDC number may be used as a double check that the drug pulled from the pharmacy shelf is the same drug that was entered into the computer.

Consider a simple example. A technician in a community pharmacy types "cilostazol tablets 100 mg" into the computer when preparing a new prescription and, from a list on the computer screen, selects the brand manufactured by Sandoz, Inc. The name of the drug and its strength will be printed on the label. The name of the drug along with the lot number will be printed on the receipt. The receipt will then accompany the label and the prescription to the place where the prescription is to be filled.

The NDC bar code and number printed on the receipt would be 0185–0223–60. The first set of numbers, 0185, indicates the drug is manufactured or distributed by Sandoz, Inc., a drug manufacturer located in Princeton, New Jersey.[7] The second set of numbers, 0223, tells the technician that the drug is cilostazol tablets 100 mg. The final set of numbers, 60, indicates the bottle size; in this case the bottle contains 60 tablets.

Continuing with this example, a technician places the receipt, the original prescription (since this is a new prescription), and the label into a basket (another best practice) and places the basket in the area where the prescription is to be filled. The bottle is pulled from the shelf and is placed into the basket. Before the technician opens the stock bottle, he or she will check the NDC number on the receipt against the NDC number on the stock bottle. By using a number of best practices, the technician continues to reduce the risk that an error will be made. The more times a prescription is checked, the more difficult it is to make an error that reaches the patient.

Note that in this example the technician is assured only that the product entered into the computer is the same as the product pulled from the shelf. The technician who entered the information into the computer could have made a mistake. If the product is taken from the shelf using the incorrect information printed on the label, the QRE may not be caught. This is the reason a workflow will contain a number of best practices each designed to catch all mistakes before they reach a patient.

Return to the example of the cilostazol 100 mg prescription. Presume the technician pulled a bottle of Sandoz's cilostazol 50 mg tablets from the shelf instead of the correct 100 mg strength. When the technician checks the NDC number on the receipt, 0185-0223-60, the number on the stock bottle will not match. The NDC number for Sandoz cilostazol 50 mg is 0185-0123-60. The first four numbers are the same because both products are manufactured by Sandoz. The last two numbers are the same because both products come in the same size container, in this case 60 tablets. The middle numbers that indicate the product, dosage form, and strength are different.

An NDC check has proven to be an effective way of avoiding a mistake. Today many pharmacies use a scanner that will read the NDC barcode on the receipt and the NDC barcode on the stock bottle. The NDC barcode check is essentially the same check as the visual NDC check. Many pharmacy workflows will repeat an NDC check at least once more prior to delivery of the medication to a patient or nursing station.

> **RxErcise 4-B   Researching Drug Knowledge: What Is Cilostazol?**
>
> Look up a brand of cilostazol 100 mg. Who is the manufacturer and what is its NDC number? What is cilostazol used for? Name the two common side effects of cilostazol.

The Basket System

When a pharmacy is busy, there may be several prescriptions on the counter waiting to be filled. A common QRE may result when a prescription bottle, or its corresponding paperwork setting on the counter, is inadvertently moved from one place to another. This could result in a label from one person's prescription, or a stock bottle from one person's prescription, being moved. If that happened, a technician filling a prescription could affix the wrong label to a bottle or place the wrong drug in a bottle. A technician could also pick up a finished prescription and place it into a sack with another patient-receipt attached. The patient could then be given a bag containing another patient's prescription.

In order to avoid this type of migration of items from one portion of the counter to another, many pharmacies use small plastic baskets in which are placed all of the items belonging to one patient. Some pharmacies will use color-coded baskets to differentiate one type of patient from others. A white basket may signify the patient is waiting. A green basket may mean these prescriptions require some additional work, such as calling the physician, before they can be filled. Many pharmacists and technicians find the basket system to be a successful best practice that can avoid errors. Others, however, do not like it, believing it causes confusion. This latter group is a minority; the basket system is widely used.

The 2-Second Rule

A modern pharmacy tends to be hectic from time to time. It is easy to become distracted in the middle of a task. Several errors in pharmacies have occurred when tablets are placed into an unlabeled prescription bottle and the pharmacy technician is called away or distracted. The problem is a filled prescription bottle sitting on the counter without a label. When the technician returns to complete the prescription, a wrong label is affixed to the bottle.

To overcome this potential error, technicians and pharmacists may adopt a "2-second rule" that states no bottle is to be left with medication in it for longer than 2 seconds before a label is attached. This rule trains technicians and pharmacists to affix the label to the bottle prior to moving to another job. Most phone calls and other distractions can wait until the label is placed on the bottle.

The Case of "His and Hers"

Mr. and Mrs. Jackson[8] are elderly patients suffering from several ailments that require medication. Both use the same pharmacy and often come to the pharmacy together to pick up their medication. They have absolute trust in everyone at the pharmacy. It never crossed their minds that their pharmacy could make a mistake. On this day, Mrs. Jackson ordered two prescriptions to be refilled and Mr. Jackson ordered one refill.

When the prescriptions were filled, all three were filled accurately and all three were checked. The three prescriptions were sitting together along with the three receipts. Mrs. Jackson's two receipts were placed in a bag that contained Mr. Jackson's one prescription. Mr. Jackson's one receipt was attached to a bag which contained Mrs. Jackson's two prescriptions. Both bags were then placed in "will call" to be picked up by the Jacksons when they came into the pharmacy later that day.

The Jacksons picked up their prescription refills and went home. Later Mrs. Jackson opened her bag, retrieved the one prescription in it, and for the next 30 days took Mr. Jackson's prescription. Likewise, Mr. Jackson took Mrs. Jackson's two prescriptions for the next 30 days. It was only when Mr. Jackson became ill that the mistake was discovered. After an investigation, it was determined that indeed the prescriptions had been placed in the wrong bags by the pharmacy.

Many claims against pharmacies have come from a correctly filled prescription being placed in the wrong prescription bag. There are several ways this mistake can happen, but usually the mistake takes place when the finished prescription bottles are placed in the bag to be given to the patient. In many cases the prescriptions have already been checked and approved.

Final Bag Check

Like most best practices, "final bag check" is simple and yet effective. Before any bag is sealed or stapled, one final check is made of the contents. Final bag check is performed by the pharmacist during the final quality check, or by a technician following the pharmacist's final quality check. The bag is then marked to indicate that the final bag check has been made, either by applying a sticker to the bag, writing the initials of the person who checked, or in other ways.

Verify the Patient

Occasionally a correctly filled prescription is given to the wrong patient. A pharmacy quality plan should include a method of verifying that the patient receiving the prescription is the correct patient.

Verification may be made by using the patient's telephone number or address. One physicians' clinic in the Midwest asks patients to pronounce their name and date of birth as a method of verifying this is the correct patient.

The date of birth is a more unique identifier than a telephone number or an address, since several people may live at the same residence. However, the date of birth is not always readily available in the pharmacy when delivering a prescription to a patient. Some pharmacies have the technician state the patient's name, telephone number or address, and ask the patient to verify that information. The problem with this method is that the patient may not have understood what was said and simply respond with a "yes." A better technique is for the technician to say to the patient: "Please say your name and your address."

Triple Check

The NDC check is used to verify that the drug entered into the computer is the same drug used to fill the prescription. In addition, the best practice "triple check" checks the name three times in three different places.

1. When the technician filling the prescription retrieves the stock bottle from the shelf, he or she checks the name on the receipt or label against the name on the stock bottle. *Note:* if the prescription is new, the check is made against the original prescription rather than the receipt or label, providing a double check against the computer technician's entry (see "Original Only When New" below).

2. When the technician takes the stock bottle from the shelf to the counter, he or she performs a second name versus name check immediately before the product is counted or poured.

3. Finally, the third check of the drug name on the receipt, label, or original prescription is made after the filling is completed and the label has been placed on the bottle.

In a planned workflow all steps are performed at the same place each time. Occasionally, however, a technician will be busy and skip one or more of these checks. By developing a standard protocol for when each check takes place, the technician should develop a habit that becomes more difficult to skip.

Note that with the NDC check and the triple check the technician has verified four times that the product being used to fill the prescription is exactly the one that was entered into the computer. Redundancy and multiple best practices in the workflow design make making a mistake increasingly difficult.

Original Only When New

Trying to discover where most of their mistakes come from, one pharmacy recorded all errors and near-misses for a 30-day period, noting where in the workflow each mistake was made. They found that 42 percent of all the mistakes were made during computer entry. The results are shown in Figure 4-3.[9]

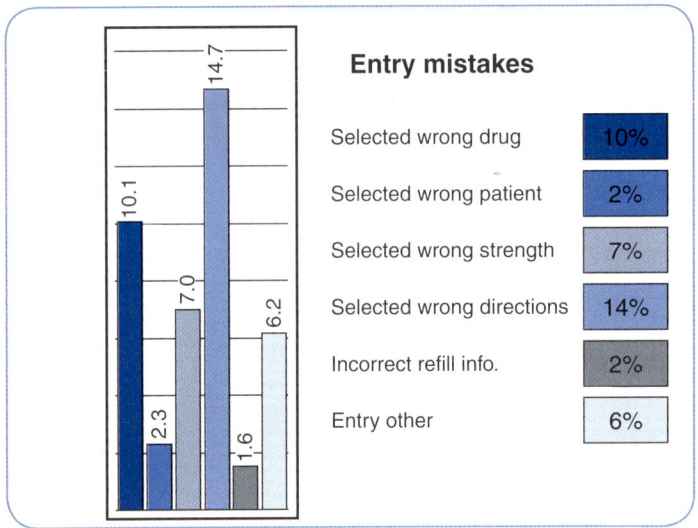

Figure 4-3 Entry mistakes
© Cengage Learning 2013

Other data from pharmacies using a similar system to capture near-misses and errors suggest this pharmacy's findings were not unusual. If the wrong drug is entered into the computer, the best practices of NDC check and triple check may not prevent the mistakes from reaching the patient.

Judging from the results in Figure 4-3, an additional best practice is necessary to ensure that correct information is entered into the computer. When a technician types in the original information from a new prescription, the original prescription is placed in the basket for the filling technician.[10]

The filling technician uses for the first time the original prescription to perform the name versus name check. The new prescription is not filled from the receipt or the label, forcing a second reading and interpretation of the prescription. This best practice is to ensure the correct drug is pulled from the shelf and used to fill the prescription.

If incorrect information is entered into the computer, the NDC check will fail, indicating the drug selected using the original prescription is different from the drug indicated on the label/receipt.

This will cause the filling technician to question the information on the label. A mistake caught at this point is sent back to the computer-entry technician for correction. The information regarding the near-miss is recorded. Next month's statistics will reflect this event.

"Take 5"

"Take 5" is a simple concept. At each station in the workflow, the first step is to take a small amount of time (5 seconds) to check what was done at the preceding station. For example, the first step in filling a prescription is to check the printed label for four prescription-dispensing "rights."

- right patient
- right drug
- right strength
- right directions

Note in Figure 4-3 that 14 percent of all QREs in this pharmacy were caused when incorrect directions were placed into the computer. In addition, 10 percent of the QREs in the pharmacy workflow were caused when the wrong drug was typed into the computer. If this pharmacy is typical, "Take 5" at the beginning of the filling process would be a valuable addition to the workflow.

"Take 5" is also used at the beginning of the pharmacist quality check. After the prescription is filled, the pharmacist performs a comprehensive check prior to approving the finished prescription. The more times a prescription is checked the less likely it is that an error will reach a patient.

Quality Note 4-A   *Learning from Nurses*

The 5 Rs of Medication Administration

When working in a hospital, you will notice nurses speak of the 5 Rs of administration:

- Right patient
- Right route
- Right dose
- Right time
- Right medication

While these are slightly different than the four prescription-dispensing rights mentioned above, they are similar. Pharmacists and pharmacy technicians should be familiar with what the nurses mean when they speak of the "5 Rs of medication administration."

Other Meds

To perform a prospective drug review as required by OBRA-90, the pharmacist must know all other medications the patient is currently taking. This is particularly important for new prescriptions.

Patients will often use more than one pharmacy. Pharmacists and pharmacy technicians cannot presume that all prescriptions a patient is taking are in this pharmacy's database. Therefore, it is important to include a procedure asking a patient for a list of all medications the patient is taking. As indicated in Chapter 2, a good place to do this is during the intake process with the pharmacy technician saying: "Please tell me what other medications you are currently taking." The information must then be documented.

If the patient's response to the pharmacy technician's question is, "I'm not taking any other medication," the technician will mark in large capital letters NOM in red, which means "no other meds." If the patient is taking other medications, the technician will mark a large capital M on the front of the prescription and write the list of medications on the back of the prescription. When the prescription is delivered to the computer-entry technician, he or she will check to make sure the list of medications in the computer matches what is written on the back of the new prescription. If this is done with each new prescription, the patient profile should be current.

Not all other medications are prescription items. Many over-the-counter (OTC) drugs such as aspirin can also react with prescription drugs and should be checked by the pharmacist during prospective drug utilization review. For example, if aspirin is taken by a patient who also takes warfarin, the time that it takes for the blood to clot will be affected. Many patients incorrectly do not consider herbal products and vitamins as drugs. For example, a patient who is taking a vitamin-mineral product that contains calcium may inadvertently reduce the effectiveness of some antibiotics. Herbals, which many people consider safe because they are "natural" products, can affect high blood pressure medications, antidiabetic medications, anti-infective medications, and others.

The pharmacist will not rely solely upon the list on the other side of the prescription, but may also want to review the patient's computer profile and any computer-generated warnings. Asking about other medications and making a visible notation on the front of the prescription can assist the pharmacist in the very important job of prospective drug review.

Allergies

If a patient has allergies, it is important for the pharmacist to know that when performing a drug review.[11] The pharmacy's computer needs to contain allergy information for each patient, and the workflow should provide for collecting and documenting information concerning allergies. A notation of NKA on the front of a new prescription means "no known allergy." If the patient indicates he or she has allergies, it should be noted on the face of the prescription with a note on the back detailing what the patient said. This practice allows the pharmacy's computer to remain up-to-date.[12] Patients may not know or be aware of all allergies at the time they become new patients, so they are asked again when every new prescription is presented.

Unusual Dose

As part of the workflow, pharmacy technicians are trained to recognize a simple definition of "unusual dose." By documenting this on the face of new prescriptions, the pharmacy staff is alerted to a prescription that may be out of the ordinary, even if only slightly so.

Most prescriptions are for oral medications. For the purposes of a quality workflow, an unusual dose may be defined as a prescription other than one to be taken orally. A prescription for a rectal suppository, an otic drop, an ophthalmic drop, or an injection would be "unusual." A simple way to note this on the new prescription so it is easily recognized is to circle the dose with a red pen. The second type of unusual dose would be any medication taken more than two tablets, capsules, or units at any one time. When more than two doses are given at any time, an error involving the medication will be more likely to cause harm. Therefore it is prudent to alert everyone in the filling process that this prescription is for an unusual dose and should be checked at least once more.

The workflow is designed to call special attention to any part of the prescription that may be unusual or that needs special attention. Note the prescription in Figure 4-4. The red letters stand out. The technician who enters the information into the computer, the technician who assembles and fills the prescription, the pharmacist who checks the prescription, and the pharmacist who counsels the patient will all be aware of certain things about the prescription when they handle it.

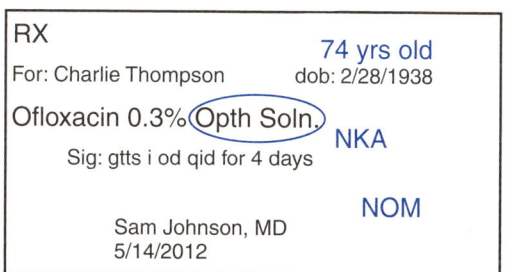

Figure 4-4 Charlie Thompson's prescription
© Cengage Learning 2013

Each member of the pharmacy staff will note that Charlie is 74 years old and considered a vulnerable patient according to the pharmacy's "under 6 / over 60" rule. Each member will also note that Charlie has no known allergies and is not on any other medications at the present time. They will see that the prescription is considered an "unusual dose" because it is not taken orally; in this case it is used in the eye. If Charlie had allergies a large, red "A" would have been written on the prescription. If he was taking other medications, a large "M" would have been written on its face. In either or both of those cases, staff would have known to turn the prescription over to see what information was provided regarding allergies and/or other drugs that Charlie was taking.

> **Quality Note 4-B   Documentation on Charlie's Prescription**
>
> There may be other advantages and uses for the documentation on the front of Charlie's prescription. Pharmacists may be sued if they fail to alert a patient to a warning of an interaction. Ofloxacin has a warning regarding a condition called tendinitis. The warning says, "Tell your physician and pharmacist if you are taking oral or injectable steroids such as dexamethasone (Decadron, Dexpak), methylprednisolone (Medrol), or prednisone (Sterapred)."
>
> What if Charlie sued the pharmacy a year later saying he was taking dexamethasone at the time he had this prescription filled and the pharmacist should have warned him of the danger of taking the two drugs together?
>
> The pharmacy could use the documentation on the prescription to prove the technician asked Charlie if he was taking other drugs and he said, "No." This prescription could be introduced into court and shown to the jury.

BUILDING QUALITY HABITS INTO THE WORKFLOW

The best practices reviewed above work because they decrease the risk of a QRE being made. If a QRE is made, best practices increase the likelihood that the mistake will be caught before it reaches the patient and becomes an error. Best practices work unless the pharmacist or technician forgets to use them. A problem with workflows is designing a system where each step is used each time.

When a claim was reported to a pharmacy's insurance company, the investigator asked the pharmacist, who filled the prescription with the wrong drug, if he had used the NDC check that was a part of the pharmacy's CQI system. The pharmacist answered, "Yes, I always do." Regardless of the pharmacist's belief, it was obvious that an NDC check had not occurred. If it had, the mistake would have been revealed immediately and the error would not have reached the patient.

Most pharmacists and pharmacy technicians believe they "always" use an NDC check. It is not always true. A pharmacy can assist the staff to develop habits in the use of each best practice. Habits make it less likely that a best practice will be skipped or forgotten. This will be discussed as part of training.

PUTTING BEST PRACTICES TO WORK

When a pharmacist or a technician first enters a new pharmacy, he or she needs to study the workflow and understand each of the steps and best practices built into each station.

The easiest way to understand the workflow is to study it in smaller parts. Each of these parts is a station along a road from where the prescription enters the pharmacy to where it exits. Figure 4-2 examines a very simple outline of a series of stations. At each station there is a set of steps that can be thought of as a mini workflow, as well as best practices that have been developed and implemented as part of the system.

RECEIVING THE PRESCRIPTION

In a community pharmacy, the first station in the workflow is usually the drop-off window. While a prescription may enter the pharmacy in several ways, often it is by a patient walking up to the drop-off window and handing a new prescription to the pharmacy technician.

In this first station, there are several places in which a mistake could be made, so a CQI system must take steps to avoid possible mistakes. Under Deming's theory, all QREs can be viewed as coming from or as caused by one of five factors: people, method, material, machine, or environment. So we must note what we believe to be the cause of the mistake. This is important because we will use the information identified at this point to later design the workflow to reduce the risk of these mistakes occurring.

There are a lot of steps in what at first instance appears to be a simple process.

The Case of the Two Kay Wilsons

Kay A. Wilson's husband entered the pharmacy and handed a new prescription to the pharmacy technician. Approximately 15 minutes later, her husband was called to the pickup window and told the prescription was ready. As he was paying for it, he noticed that the middle initial printed on the receipt was "J." Earlier the pharmacist had counseled on the new prescription, but at that time neither Kay's husband nor the pharmacist noticed the incorrect middle initial.

It was later discovered that the pharmacy had two patients named Kay Wilson. The prescription for Kay A. Wilson had been entered into the record belonging to Kay J. Wilson. The medication and the directions were correct, but according to the record, Kay A. Wilson had never received this medication. The pharmacist's prospective drug utilization review was incorrect. The pharmacist had reviewed the list of drugs in the records of Kay J. Wilson. Future drug reviews for both Kay Wilsons would also be incorrect.

The mistake in Wilson's prescription was traced back to the computer-entry technician. Learning this allowed the technician and the pharmacy to institute steps that could prevent future errors of this type. As with most best practices, the solutions instituted were simple. In the future, additional identifying information will be entered on the prescription.

The pharmacy in this case used a solution similar to that used in Charlie's prescription shown in Figure 4-4. Review the red notations the technician made on that prescription. In the Wilson case, the pharmacy added steps that called on the receiving technician to double check the patient's address, phone number, and date of birth to make sure the correct patient was selected. The steps taken in receiving the prescription went beyond the problem illustrated by the Wilson case.

In Chapter 2 under Pharmacy Technicians–First in the Workflow we identified steps that can be taken at the first station to reduce the risk of an error reaching the patient. In thoses steps we prepared the prescription with information which the pharmacy staff could use to reduce the risk of medication errors. The information and notations made by the pharmacy technician at this station will be used throughout the workflow.

It is tempting to think of this receiving station as less important because it is merely where we take the prescription. The work performed here, however, can ensure that the patient receives the medication exactly as ordered by the prescriber. It also allows the pharmacist to perform an effective DUR and counsel the patient.

Review the steps taken by the pharmacy technician in Chapter 2 when receiving a prescription. In each of the following cases ask how the error might have been avoided by taking extra time at the receiving station. The list in Chapter 2 is not a complete workflow and more details can be added. It is important that the steps outlined in receiving the prescription be implemented into the overall workflow. Prescriptions may also be received other than through the "drop off" window. The workflow needs to accommodate each of these alternatives. There will be times that other members of the pharmacy staff received the prescription, including the pharmacists. For that reason every member of the pharmacy staff should be instructed in these steps and trained to be certain that each new prescription contains all information needed to reduce medication errors throughout the process.

Saving Young Lives

In 1970 the federal government passed the Poison Prevention Packaging Act.[13] The federal Poison Prevention Packaging Act requires that all prescriptions be placed in a child-resistant safety container unless the patient or the prescriber requests otherwise. The stated purpose of the law was "to protect children from serious personal injury or serious illness . . . ." The act was broader than prescription drugs and covers many products sold in a typical pharmacy.

It required, with a few exceptions that all "household substances" be packaged in "special packaging" designed to protect young children. Household substances was defined in the statute:

(2) The term "household substance" means any substance which is customarily produced or distributed for sale for consumption or use, or customarily stored, by individuals in or about the household and which is—

(A) a hazardous substance as that term is defined in section 2(f) of the Federal Hazardous Substances Act (15 U.S.C. §1261(f));

(B) a food, drug, or cosmetic as those terms are defined in section 201 of the Federal Food, Drug, and Cosmetic Act (21 U.S.C. §321); or

(C) a substance intended for use as fuel when stored in a portable container and used in the heating, cooking, or refrigeration system of a house.

To meet the Act, the product, including prescriptions, had to be in a container "designed or constructed to be significantly difficult for children under five years of age to open or obtain a toxic or harmful amount of the substance contained therein within a reasonable time and not difficult for normal adults to use properly, but does not mean packaging which all such children cannot open or obtain a toxic or harmful amount within a reasonable time."

Exceptions are provided in the law for prescriptions for "elderly or handicapped persons unable to use such substance when packaged" as required. In order to dispense a prescription in a non-child safe special container either the patient or the physician must request it.

Failure to abide by this law can result in discipline for the pharmacy, the pharmacist, and the pharmacy technician. The workflow should have procedures that can provide proof that a non-safety cap was requested by the patient or physician anytime one is not used.

How can a pharmacy prove 2–4 years after a prescription has been filled that it was the patient who requested a non-safety cap? No person on the pharmacy staff is likely to remember exactly what happened that long ago. The answer is to build a best practice that can document that the patient or caregiver requested the non-safety cap by signing a statement with the request. Many pharmacies use a rubber stamp with words: "I requested this prescription (or all of my prescriptions) be filled without a safety cap." If at some point in the future there is a question, the pharmacy can present the patient's signature as proof. In addition to the legal implications of a patient's request for no safety cap, consider "The Case of Grandma's Digoxin."

The Case of Grandma's Digoxin

Pharmacies should encourage all patients to use child-resistant safety containers for all prescriptions. A pharmacy's first duty is to safeguard its patients, and that includes small children who live with or visit the patient. Pharmacist Jim Johnson learned this lesson in a most difficult manner.[14] Jim received a phone call from one of his elderly patients who asked why her digoxin prescription did not have a safety cap on it. Jim pulled the prescription from the file and on the back was a rubber stamp that Jim had designed with the words, "I requested my prescription not be dispensed in a child-resistant special container." The patient's signature was below the stamped statement. When Jim told his patient that she had signed the request, she began to cry. She told Jim that her grandson had just died after getting into her bottle of digoxin. It was a difficult lesson for all concerned, including Jim and his entire staff. Jim said later, "In the future, if a patient doesn't want a safety cap, I will honor their request, but, I will *always* recommend that they think about it one more time."

DATA-ENTRY STATION

In our hypothetical community pharmacy we are building a basic workflow moving from one station to the next. At each station we are building a set of steps into a process incorporating best practices designed to reduce the risk of an error reaching a patient. A hospital pharmacy could also be used as a hypothetical, where the steps would be slightly different, but the ideas would be similar. In most community pharmacies, the second step in a workflow would be entry of the information into the pharmacy's computer system. This station is often referred to as Data Entry.

The exact steps at this station will be dictated to a large extent by the software used in the computer. As at each station, the first step in building this mini workflow is to step back and observe, in order to identify any potential risks that could lead to a mistake and perhaps eventually an error.

This is an important part of filling any prescription or drug order. It is here that information is entered and patient records updated by a technician who then enters the name of the drugs prescribed and the directions into the patient's records. As shown in Figure 4–3, it is also an area in which mistakes can be made that can result in errors.

When a pharmacy builds its workflow, it will identify risks at this data-entry station. To counter them, the pharmacy will add best practices to this station's workflow. Other best practices will be added at later stations in the workflow as additional checks on QREs that may occur during data entry.

The computer software will determine how the pharmacy technician enters the prescription information into the correct patient's record. Typically it will be to type in the first few letters of the patient's name and then select from a list displayed. The name and strength of the drug is entered in a similar manner. The prescription directions are typed in along with the refill and any special information. The software usually provides shortcuts for entering the directions, which are often referred to as "SIG codes."

The data-entry technician prints the label and the receipt, which are placed in the basket and sent to the assembly or filling area. The prescription label and the receipt will have a unique prescription number assigned by the computer. A tag from the receipt with this unique prescription number will be placed on the original prescription.

If the prescription is a refill, information is entered into the computer using the prescription number that was assigned when the prescription was new. The old prescription bottle will either be thrown away at this point or will go in the basket with the new label and receipt to be sent to the filling area. An old prescription bottle should not be reused.

If the pharmacy's computer software allows, the pharmacy technician at the receiving station will scan the original prescription into the computer system whereby it can be viewed from anywhere in the workflow where a terminal is located. If the pharmacy does not use scanning technology, the new prescription is placed in a basket along with other necessary information and the basket is delivered to the computer entry station.

When a pharmacy builds its CQI system, it will add more detail and several more steps than discussed here. The order of the steps is less important than that each member of the staff follow the steps each time as outlined.

FILLING THE PRESCRIPTION

If the original prescription was scanned into the computer system, it will be available for viewing by the pharmacy technician who fills the prescription. If not, the original prescription will be placed in the basket along with the label and receipt. The basket is delivered to the area for filling. The technician who fills a new prescription uses the original prescription when selecting the correct drug and strength from the shelves. In some pharmacies, the plan will call for the original prescription to be retrieved from the prescription drawer and used for the first refill. After the first refill, the label and receipt can be used to fill the prescription.

The pharmacy technician pulls the correct stock bottle from the shelf and, depending on the form of the drug, will either count out the number of tablets or capsules required, or will pour the amount of liquid prescribed into a prescription bottle. The label is placed on the bottle and the completed prescription along with the stock bottle and the receipt are placed back in the basket and sent to the pharmacist for the final check. The prescription has now been filled and the receipt prepared. Once the pharmacist has made sure everything is correct, the prescription will be placed in a bag for delivery to the patient. Also at this point the stock bottle can be returned to the shelf. Checking the NDC number on the stock bottle, or scanning the number, is important, but if the stock bottle must be returned earlier, the pharmacy can design an alternative method to be used. Other methods may be less efficient and could lead to omitting this important check.

The Pharmacist's Final Quality Check and Drug Review

The pharmacist is ultimately responsible for ensuring each prescription is filled correctly. Edwards Deming taught in Total Quality Management that quality does not rely upon a system of 100 percent inspection.[15] This part of his teaching must be modified in the practice of pharmacy. Each prescription must be checked for final accuracy by a pharmacist. In some instances, state law allows a "tech check tech" system, but only selectively. This is currently allowed in only a few hospitals and in only a few states. Unless policies and procedures and state law specifically allow this procedure, it may not be used.

The pharmacist reviews all elements of each prescription:

- correct patient
- correct drug
- correct strength
- correct directions

At the same station, the pharmacist performs a prospective drug utilization review on new prescriptions, looking at other drugs the patient is taking, available information regarding medical conditions, allergy information, and other relevant data.

The pharmacy technician can be an important assistant for the pharmacist at this stage of the workflow. For example, a technician may be directed to print out and place in the basket warnings given during the computer-entry process, or, if the pharmacist does not have a terminal at the final check area, provide a list of current drugs the patient is taking. The pharmacist may also need access to the original prescription in the case of a new prescription.

Delivery

After the prescription has been filled and checked, it can be prepared for delivery to the patient or a nursing floor. In the hospital, this may mean placing the completed order into an automatic dispensing machine such as a Pyxis®, where it will be available when needed. If the completed orders are to be delivered to a nursing home, the drugs may be placed in special dosing units depending on the nursing unit's equipment. The technician needs to learn and study the policies and procedures for each of these delivery processes.

In the community pharmacy, the prescription is usually delivered directly to the patient. If the patient is to pick up the medication later, it is sent to a "will call" holding area. Occasionally, prescriptions will be delivered directly to the patient's home. In each of these cases there should be a written process established.

Counseling

The technician's assistance can be valuable in preparing information necessary for pharmacist counseling. The computer will print patient-information sheets to be provided to the patient along with the medication. These need to be available for the pharmacist at the time of counseling. Some drugs, by federal law, are required to have special patient-information leaflets and some require federally mandated med-guides. It may be the technician's job to see that printed materials are available for the pharmacist at the time the prescription is delivered for checking, review, and counseling.

Special Problems Station

Occasionally a prescription or drug order cannot be filled immediately. The prescribing physician may have to be called because of a question regarding an allergy, an interaction with another medication, or for any number of other reasons. In these cases, it is usually a good idea to remove this prescription drug order from the regular workflow so that it does not cause confusion. The area to which waiting prescriptions are delivered may be referred to as a "problems station" or a "special attention area." The procedures in this special station will be different in various pharmacies. The pharmacy technician needs to be familiar with these rules and directions.

SUMMARY

At times it will be convenient to think of the pharmacy workflow as a single procedure beginning when the prescription is delivered to the pharmacy and ending when it is delivered to the patient or other professional. In most cases, however, it is better to consider the workflow as a series of work stations. At each one of these stations there will be a mini workflow defined by steps and best practices. The pharmacy technician should examine each of these processes and be able to perform each of the steps and best practices exactly as they are designed. It is through the use of a structured plan that the risk of medication errors can best be reduced to the minimum.

REVIEW QUESTIONS

1. The best practice known as "Take 5" is used in which risk-management workflow?
   A. Computer data-entry station
   B. Filling/assembly station
   C. Pharmacist final check station
   D. All of the above

2. The risk-management planning tool often known by the initials PDCA is also known as the
   A. Shewhart cycle.
   B. Planning cycle.
   C. Risk-management process.
   D. Planners' working tools.

3. What does the first set of numbers in the NDC list identify?
   A. Manufacturer
   B. Repackager
   C. Distributor
   D. All of the above

4. What is the significance of all the numbers of an NDC code match except the third set?
   A. The drug is different.
   B. It is a generic.

C. The manufacturer, drug, and strength are correct, but the bottle size is different.

D. The drug is distributed by a repackager.

5. What is the best practice called that teaches that no bottle may be left with medication in it for more than a short period of time before a label is attached?

   A. "Take 5"
   B. "The 2-second rule"
   C. "The ½-minute label"
   D. None of the above

6. A way to verify that the prescription is being delivered to the correct patient is by asking the patient for what?

   A. Telephone number
   B. Address
   C. Name
   D. All of the above

7. The best practice called "Original Only When New" refers to what practice?

   A. Any new prescription is filled using the original new prescription, not from the information on the receipt or label.
   B. The original prescription is pulled from the records when refilled.
   C. Certain prescriptions may not be refilled.
   D. All of the above

8. What information should pharmacy technicians receiving a new prescription from a patient in a community pharmacy be trained to ask for?

   A. Are you taking any other prescription medications?
   B. Are you taking any other OTC medication?
   C. Do you have any allergies?
   D. All of the above

9. What is the main requirement of the Poison Prevention Packaging Act?

   A. Amber prescription bottles are required for all prescription drugs.

   B. All prescriptions must be placed in a child-resistant safety container unless the patient or the prescriber requests otherwise.

   C. All prescriptions must be placed in a child-resistant safety container.

   D. All prescription drugs on a special FDA list (poisons) must be placed in a safety container.

10. What concept in Deming's original Total Quality Management system must be modified when incorporated in pharmacy practice?

    A. The concept that the business should not perform 100% inspection of all output

    B. The concept that statistical control may be used to monitor the CQI system

    C. The concept that some risks may be avoided completely

    D. The concept that some errors are acceptable

Endnotes

[1] Kohn, L. T., Corrigan, J. M., and Donaldson, M. S., Eds., 2000, *To Err Is Human: Building a Safer Health System*, p. 4. Washington, DC: National Academy Press, 2000.

[2] See Chapter 1, Key Words: **Medication error** for a more complete definition of medication error.

[3] The author of this textbook was one of the primary authors and designers of the original Pharmacy Quality Commitment® program before it was purchased by NASPA. Originally designed for use by Kmart pharmacies and Eckert Drug Stores, it was later part of PMC Quality Commitment, Inc., a subsidiary of Pharmacists Mutual Insurance Company. See http://www.pqc.net

[4] Dr. Walter Shewart was a statistician who developed a way of looking at quality improvement while he was employed at Western Electric, a division of AT&T. Dr. Shewhart presented what became known as the Shewhart Cycle in the early part of the twentieth

century. The Shewhart cycle, sometimes called the "Deming Cycle" or simply "PDCA," is still used and can be seen in ISO 9000 and Sigma Six training as well as other programs used today.

[5] See http://asq.org/learn-about-quality/project-planning-tools/overview/pdca-cycle.html accessed 2/13/2011; also see http://www.sixsigmaspc.com/dictionary/PDCA-plan-do-check-act.html accessed 2/13/2011

[6] The FDA standard for NDC numbers is 10 to 11 digits. For further explanation see http://www.fda.gov/Drugs/InformationOnDrugs/ucm142438.htm. (accessed January 20, 2011).

[7] Previously this NDC number was used by Eon Labs, Inc., which merged into Sandoz, a division of the Novartis Group.

[8] The names have been changed. The facts are taken from an insurance claim.

[9] Identifiable information has been removed. From the files of PMC Quality Commitment, Inc. with permission.

[10] If the prescription is scanned into the computer, the scanned image is used instead of the paper prescription, which will be filed.

[11] See Chapter 2, The Pharmacy Technician and the Prescription Workflow: Receiving the Prescription/Drug Order.

[12] Review the case of Heidi Happel, Chapter 2.

[13] Poison Prevention Packaging Act of 1970, 15 USC §§ 1471–1477.

[14] From a Pharmacists Mutual Insurance Company claim. Names have been changed, and all identifying information omitted.

[15] Deming E. W., 1986. *Out of the Crisis*. Cambridge, MA: MIT Press, pp 266, 410, et seq,; also see Fourteen Points, Point 3, "Cease dependence on inspections to achieve quality," p. 14.

CHAPTER 5

Identify the Risks
Determining Where Mistakes Could Be Made in the System

OBJECTIVES

Upon completion of this chapter, the reader should be able to:

1. Study the role of pharmacy technicians in identifying risks in pharmacy.
2. Understand how potential risks of error can be identified.
3. Explain the five causes of medication errors.
4. Discuss the Health Insurance Portability and Accountability Act (HIPAA) as a risk-management concern in pharmacy.
5. Discuss the importance of observation of workflows in designing a CQI system.
6. Explain how a pharmacy can test its system for vulnerabilities to medication errors.
7. Determine which drugs should be included in special risk-management prevention techniques.
8. Explain the concept of using a claims study to determine which risks are more likely to result in injury to a patient.
9. Discuss how look-alike, sound-alike product risks can be reduced through best practices.
10. Discuss the concept of patient responsibility as it impacts a pharmacy CQI system.

KEY WORDS

Causes of errors: W. Edwards Deming taught that causes of quality-related events can be categorized into five factors. Using these five factors provides a convenient method of identifying the sources of QREs. Once the source is known, it can be eliminated, thereby reducing potential future errors. Deming referred to these five causes as "P, 3 Ms, and E", for:

People: Usually not a specific person, but the position, such as entry technician.

Method: The manner in which a job is being preformed such as the workflow, a process, the "will call" procedure, or the delivery service; it could include software.

Material: All materials used in dispensing a prescription, including shelves, packaging, bottles, caps, and stock bottles.

Machine: Anything electronic or mechanical, including the computer, scanner, cash register, or even the telephone system. It would also include robotics; it could include software.

Environment: Anything that affects what is happening around the pharmacy, including lighting, loud radios, people talking, staff moving through the pharmacy, or any element that could be considered attractive.

Covered entity: A covered entity is an organization or individual that uses electronic means to transmit health care information about its patients. A covered entity and everyone working for it is subject to HIPAA privacy rules.

Health Insurance Portability and Accountability Act of 1996 (HIPAA): HIPAA is a federal law protecting patient privacy of health care records. Violations can result in fines and even imprisonment. Broadly speaking, release of confidential information is a medical error that should be addressed as part of a pharmacy's CQI program.

Intellectual error: A name given to claims that are not mechanical in nature, such as placing the wrong drug in the prescription bottle or typing the wrong directions. Intellectual errors may involve an error in judgment or omission of an act requiring judgment. Intellectual errors include release of confidential information, drug review errors, and lack of counseling.

Prothrombin time (Pro Time) and international normalized ratio (INR) tests: Two tests used to determine the time it takes blood to clot. One of these tests is used for patients on warfarin therapy as a way of determining the amount of this drug in their system and adjusting their dosage from that information. The more common of these two tests used today is the INR. Good INR values are considered as being between 2 and 3.

CHAPTER 5 • Identify the Risks

OUTLINE

Identifying Risks
    Locating Vulnerabilities
    The Case of the Bleeding That Would Not Stop
    ID: A Powerful Drug—Special Attention

Step Back and Observe
    The Five Causes of All Mistakes

Observing Station by Station

Receiving the Prescription
    Look Alike—Sound Alike
    The Case of "I don't have a cough!"

Computer Data Entry
    Caution: For Each Problem Solved—A New One Created

Filling the Prescriptions
    Manual Filling
    Robotic Filling
    The Cases of One Mistake, 17 Wrong Prescriptions

Pharmacist Final Check Station
    Two Cases of Bypassing the System
    Studying the Outlier
    Identify by Tracking Success

Delivering the Rx to the Patient
    Can the Patient Be at Fault?

Identifying a Special Risk: HIPAA and Privacy
    The Case of the High School Student

Counseling

Summary

IDENTIFYING RISKS

Continuous quality improvement (CQI) systems are designed using a series of best practices to stop or at least reduce the risk of medication errors. The concept is to prevent mistakes that may lead to the errors or by catching quality-related events before they reach a patient. Best practices and other steps in a pharmacy workflow are selected depending on the risk identified. In this chapter we will look at the simple workflow example discussed in Chapter 4 and identify with more precision what and where the risks of a mistake occurring may be in the system.

When pharmacists or pharmacy technicians begin working at a pharmacy, they will usually find a CQI system in place that they will need to learn and use. However, that preexisting system will require changes over time, for no matter how good a CQI system is, it will never be perfect. Their previous study of how to design a system will enable them to later make changes or improve a system. In this chapter we will not identify all problems or all mistakes that could be made in a pharmacy workflow since there are many variations to be found in the world of pharmacy practice. Changes in workflow occur rapidly as more efficient systems are introduced. This chapter intends for the student to consider and analyze how mistakes can be made and to identify potential areas for change when analyzing a pharmacy workflow.

Locating Vulnerabilities

In order to reduce the risk of a medication error reaching and potentially injuring a patient, we need to determine where a mistake is likely to happen. Every system has vulnerabilities, that is, places where the system can break down. By locating and fixing these places, we can reduce the risk of a mistake occurring. We know that the best way to prevent a medication error is by preventing the mistake or QRE that can lead to it. There are many places where a mistake can be made, some at greater risk than others. The first step in establishing a quality improvement program is to identify where in the workflow a mistake is most likely to occur.

The Case of the Bleeding That Would Not Stop

Mrs. Franks was a 70-year-old patient who had been diagnosed with atrial fibrillation. In order to avoid a possible stroke, Dr. Johnson, Mrs. Franks's physician, prescribed warfarin 1 milligram, a low dose of an anticoagulant.[1] The prescription was called into Mrs. Franks's regular pharmacy by a nurse in Dr. Johnson's office. Mrs. Franks's son picked up the prescription that same day and she took her first dose that evening. For the next 2 weeks, she continued taking her medicine at the same time every evening, just as Dr. Johnson had prescribed. It was at the end of the second week that, while preparing a meal, Mrs. Franks accidently cut her finger with a knife. Applying pressure did not stop the blood flow. Nothing she did stopped the bleeding. She became concerned and called her son, who picked her up at her home and took her to the emergency room. She took her warfarin prescription with her to the hospital along with her other prescribed medications and showed them to a nurse at the hospital when she checked in. The warfarin prescription was correctly labeled as 1 milligram dosage, but the nurse quickly identified the tablets in the bottle as 5 milligram warfarin.

Mrs. Franks was treated and returned home with the correct medication, filled free of charge by the pharmacy and delivered along with sincere apologies. A claim was made on behalf of Mrs. Franks against the pharmacy asking for compensation for the hospital charges, other expenses she incurred, and an additional amount for her pain and suffering. The pharmacy's insurance company settled quickly. After 15 years as a loyal customer, Mrs. Franks changed pharmacies.

While Mrs. Franks's injuries were relatively small, the error had the potential of being catastrophic. A fivefold overdose of warfarin could have resulted in internal bleeding. If the bleeding went into the brain, it could have caused a stroke, leaving her a bed-ridden invalid dependant on continuous care by nursing staff for several years. While the cost in dollars might have been high, human cost, including the quality of Mrs. Franks's life in her remaining years, would have been even higher.

> **RxErcise 5-A** *Identifying the Risk*
>
> **Where Did the Error in Mrs. Franks's Prescription Occur?**
>
> Before we can fix the problem and avoid another prescription error such as the one that occurred to Mrs. Franks, we must identify where the mistake or mistakes might have occurred. The problem is not unlike that in the television program CSI, where the scientists must first decide what happened.
>
> Follow the workflow. In each station, make a note where the mistake in filling Mrs. Franks's prescription *could have* occurred.
>
> Assume for the purpose of this exercise that the physician's office called in the prescription correctly. For each possiblity, note how we might determine if the mistake did or did not occur at that place. For example:
>
> **Data Entry Station:**
>
> The technician could have entered the wrong strength of drug into the computer. But in Mrs. Franks's case, we know that did not happen because the label was correct, indicating the computer entry was correct.
>
> The technician could have entered information into the patient profile for the wrong Mrs. Franks. Solution: We can discover this by checking the computer records under the correct Mrs. Franks's record.
>
> **Filling Station:**
>
> Mistake could have happened when _____ (fill in the blank). Compare your answers with what actually happened in Mrs. Franks's case below. What actually happened will be only one of the possible problems.

ID: A Powerful Drug—Special Attention

Warfarin is a powerful drug that does exactly what it is supposed to do: retard the coagulation of the patient's blood. When used correctly, it can save lives and reduce the risk of potentially dangerous blood clots. When used in the wrong dose, it can be deadly. Warfarin is one example of a powerful drug that warrants special attention. There are many others.

The best known brand of warfarin is Coumadin, currently manufactured by the pharmaceutical company Bristol-Myers Squibb. Coumadin (warfarin sodium) is available in several strengths.[2] (See Figure 5-1).

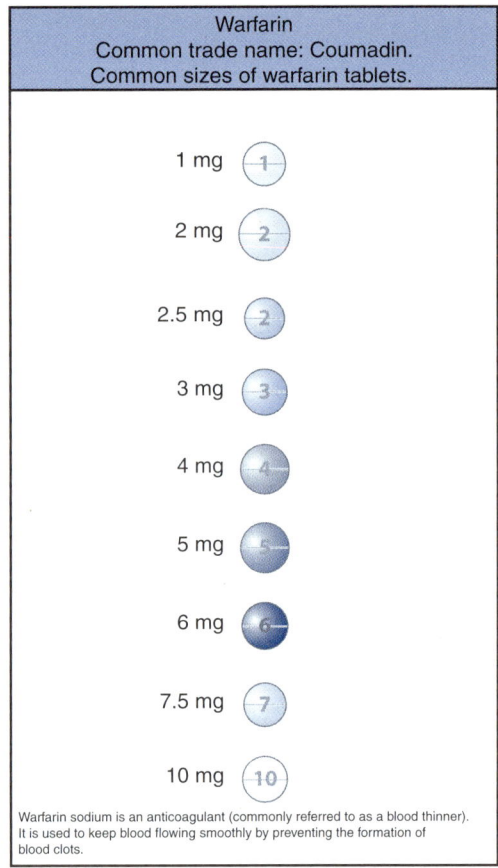

Figure 5-1 Strengths of Coumadin
© Cengage Learning 2013

According to one insurance company study, warfarin is involved in more claims than any other drug. At the request of a division of the DuPont Company, a former manufacturer of Coumadin brand of warfarin, Pharmacists Mutual Insurance Company reviewed its mechanical-error claims to determine how often Coumadin (warfarin sodium) was involved in pharmacy medication-error claims as compared to other drugs.

Pharmacists Mutual found that for a 3-year period of time, warfarin (although not necessarily the brand name Coumadin) accounted for 7 percent of all mechanical-error claims against pharmacists and pharmacies[3] reported to the insurance company (see Figure 5-2).

This does not mean that more mistakes are made with warfarin than with other drugs. According to a report of near-misses compiled by pharmacies, mistakes involving warfarin were not among

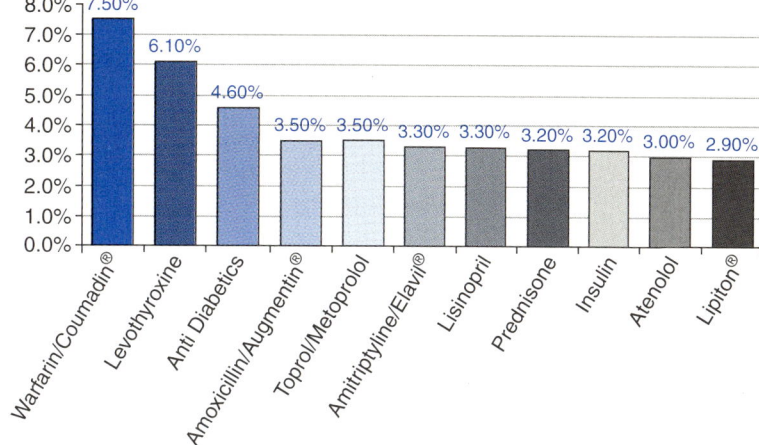

Figure 5-2 Pharmacists mutual claims study drugs most often involved in mechanical error claims
© 2011, Pharmacists Mutual Insurance Company, used with permission
http://www.phmic.com/phmc/services/RM/profliab/claimsstudy/Pages/
DrugsMostInvolvedinMechanicalErrorClaims.aspx (accessed November 8, 2010)

the top 10 of mistakes recorded. This would suggest that warfarin may be involved in fewer mistakes but more claims when compared to other drugs. The difference in these findings may be explained by the increased relative potential for injury; thus, an increased number of claims will result when warfarin is given in error. Warfarin is a powerful and dangerous drug when administered incorrectly. This type information is important in identifying risks in a pharmacy.

It is important for the pharmacy involved in Mrs. Franks's medication error to discover what happened in order to avoid a repeat

> **Quality Note 5-A**   *Each Pharmacy Should Make Its Own List of "Problem Drugs"*
>
> Pharmacists Mutual's list of Drugs Most Involved in Mechanical Error Claims is compiled from claims filed with the insurance company. As mentioned these are not the drugs most often involved in mistakes or even errors. Rather than relying completely on the Pharmacists Mutual list, each pharmacy may wish to make its own "Top 10" list of drugs that cause problems or lead to mistakes. A list of more than 10 may dilute the sense of "special" drugs reserved for special treatment. Remember, however, the Pharmacists Mutual list is valuable because it shows the drugs that may lead to most significant injury if involved in an error, such as warfarin.

of the same error in the future. The pharmacy needs to identify where this error occurred, investigate where the risk of similar future errors is the greatest, and then use that information to prevent them.

The first step in instituting a quality-improvement program is to identify where a mistake could be made. There are two primary times while working with a CQI program when a pharmacy will systematically take this step. One is after an error or a near-miss has occurred, such as in the Franks case. The other is when the program is first designed and implemented. Future chapters will examine identifying risks by studying errors. This chapter will discuss the identification of potential risks when a system is designed or implemented into a pharmacy workflow.

Step Back and Observe

An important way to identify risks is to observe what happens during the pharmacy's normal workflow. It is difficult to develop a complete understanding of the workflow when the observer is actively involved in the process.

Use Mrs. Franks's case as an example of an observational RxErcise. Step back and observe Mrs. Franks's prescription from the time it leaves the physician's office until Mrs. Franks arrives in the hospital following the error. The question we are asking throughout this process is: Where could a mistake occur? The suggestion in RxErcise 4-A in Chapter 4 was to visit a hospital or community pharmacy and make notes while observing each step from the time a prescription or drug order arrived in the pharmacy until it left the pharmacy. In this RxErcise, we will go beyond the pharmacy and expand our observations to a time before the order reaches the pharmacy and continue to observe what happens after Mrs. Franks's prescription leaves the pharmacy. This expanded observation can be used later when the question becomes: How can I prevent an error from reaching and injuring a patient? Occasionally, there may be more than one mistake that can be identified. If there are multiple QREs, the question may be: Which mistake(s) could the pharmacy have prevented?

When Mrs. Franks's physician first decided to use warfarin to prevent future possibilities of a blood clot or stroke, the physician was required to engage in some educated guesses. With warfarin there are no exact formulas for the initial dose. There are many factors to take into consideration including the individuality of the patient, the patient's diet, and how the patient may react to the warfarin. An initial dose could be as low as a half milligram every other day to something much higher. The physician will, shortly after beginning therapy, order tests to determine how the patient's body is reacting to the drug.[4]

The physician will order a **prothrombin time (Pro Time) test** or an **international normalized ratio (INR) test** to determine whether the dosage of the anticoagulant (blood thinner) needs to be increased or decreased. Eventually, by using diet and by adjusting the dose, a patient will become stabilized on a dosage regimen. Because there is often an initial adjustment period and because the dosage of warfarin is sometimes sensitive, Mrs. Franks's physician should have carefully gone over with her the initial dosage and what she should expect. We have now identified at least one potential source of error: it is possible that either the physician did not make certain that Mrs. Franks knew her initial dose, or that Mrs. Franks did not understand what the physician told her. Although neither of these would be pharmacy errors, the pharmacy is in a position to influence a positive outcome to reduce the risk of injury. The pharmacy's CQI system should take such possibilities into consideration when it is designed.

The physician wrote Mrs. Franks's new prescription and it was sent to the pharmacy. Another potential source of error is that the physician or the nurse who called in the prescription could have made a mistake by communicating a 5 mg dose to the pharmacy rather than the 1 mg dose it should have been. From the facts that were given, however, this does not appear to be the case. We know the prescription was correctly entered into the computer because the label correctly stated the dosage as 1 mg.

Consideration of these possibilities shows where a potential error could have been made and provides information we can use in designing a workflow. Knowing that an error could have been made during computer entry, we can design the computer-entry station workflow to safeguard against such a mistake. Other mistakes could also have been made during the computer entry part of the workflow.

When observing the workflow and looking for vulnerabilities or risks, we note the cause of each risk we identify. We may identify several possible causes. Each possible cause that is identified may eventually be determined to be significant or not. Such determination will be made during a later analysis. In the identification phase, we are concerned only with finding possible risks and possible causes.

The Five Causes of All Mistakes

Professor Deming said the causes of all problems in the workflow can be categorized into one of the following factors:

People[5]

Material

Machine

Method

Environment

Most mistakes made in the pharmacy workflow are the result of either a flaw in the system or a human error. The system is designed to prevent or catch both of these.

When we use the term **people** as a cause, primarily we are identifying the position in which the person is working, such as the technician pulling the stock bottle from the shelf. All human beings can be distracted, confused by similar names, or misidentify boxes that look alike. Assume in Mrs. Franks's case that our later analysis shows that the 5 mg stock bottle was pulled mistakenly because all of the warfarin bottles of different strengths looked alike. So our later fix may involve one or both of the two following best practices designed to overcome this problem.

Certain drugs cause more problems than others. Figure 5-2 shows a study of claims against pharmacies in which the drug warfarin accounted for 7 percent of all mechanical-error claims. When the cause in these cases is found to be human error, it is identified as "Person." In the majority of cases, it does not matter whether John or Emily made the mistake. For purposes of designing a CQI system, the significant factor is that it was a technician or pharmacist retrieving the wrong bottle from the shelf.

Stock bottles and the shelving are part of the **materials** category. This may also include prescription bottles and safety caps. When we look at materials as one of the potential causes, we should consider all materials used in dispensing a prescription.

The **machine** category is anything electronic or mechanical including the computer, scanner, cash register, and even the telephone system. In a hospital pharmacy, this can include the Pyxis machine or any other mechanical device that could affect pharmacy operations. Robots and any type of automatic filling devices are important parts of the machine category. Software systems used by the computer are also in this category of cause factors.

The **method** refers to the manner in which a job is being preformed. In the case of the pharmacy, it includes the CQI workflow and the flow within each individual station. The prescription "will call" procedure and the pharmacy's delivery service are methods. A mistake in these areas can be a cause or contributing factor leading to an error.

The **environment** includes any part of the pharmacy's background that affects workflow or people in the pharmacy. Environment includes lighting; sounds, such as loud radios; people talking; staff moving through the pharmacy; and any element that could be considered distracting. The environment also includes physical aspects of the pharmacy such as clutter on the shelves or in the workflow area.

When determining what factors may have caused or contributed to a particular problem, it is not necessary to place something in each category of the factors. The importance of looking at these five elements is to allow us to concentrate on and consider all possible causes and solutions. When investigating the causes of an error, it is possible we could find that the computer software is the sole cause, or that there were deficiencies in the whole workflow, or that a mistake was made by the entry technician. It is important only that we consider everything that contributed, or could have contributed, to the problem we need to solve.

Observing Station by Station

When pharmacists or pharmacy technicians begin working in a pharmacy, they will probably discover the pharmacy already has a CQI system in place. So they will not be called upon to design a system from scratch. Instead, they will look at a functioning pharmacy workflow and study how it was constructed in order to understand why individual steps are in place and how they were designed to reduce the risk of QREs.

Let us study a workflow in a community pharmacy to identify where mistakes or QREs could be made. The same exercise would work if we used a hospital workflow.

The prescription process begins when the order or prescription enters the pharmacy department. From there we will follow the prescription through the workflow until it is delivered to the patient. In each step we ask what mistake could happen at this stage of the process. Once we have identified potential mistakes (QREs), we can further refine the workflow and build a system to prevent future mistakes from happening. Even the best systems will not prevent all mistakes, so we will also build systems to intercept mistakes that do occur. In this way we can prevent a prescription error from being delivered to the patient.

On a more limited scale we will perform the same identification process whenever an error is made so we can prevent future errors. This practice will be discussed in later chapters. The lessons associated with identifying risks learned here can also be applied in investigating and performing a root-cause analysis on individual errors.

Receiving the Prescription

There are several ways for a prescription to enter the pharmacy. We will not examine all, but will look at some of the most common.

The prescriber may call a prescription into the pharmacy and it may be received on a recording that is then transcribed by the pharmacist onto a prescription pad. As an alternative, the pharmacist may speak directly to the physician or nurse, writing the information directly on the prescription blank. If the prescription is a refill, it may enter the pharmacy by electronic order directly into the computer or on a voice-mail system. A voice recording may be taken off the system by the technician and either written or typed directly into the computer. A patient may also call the pharmacy directly for a refill order during business hours, either leaving it on a recording or speaking directly to a member of the pharmacy staff. As an exercise, let us identify where a mistake could be made in each of these situations.

Look Alike—Sound Alike

When the pharmacist listens to a recording or talks to the prescriber, he or she could hear the instructions incorrectly or write them down wrong. The Institute for Safe Medication Practices (ISMP) has a list of drug names that often cause confusion, either because they sound confusingly similar to another drug or because two drugs look alike.[6] Two of the drugs listed by the ISMP as ones that can be confused because they sound alike are Adderal® and Inderal®. These two drugs could not be more unlike each other in actions.

Adderal® is a combination of dextroamphetamine and amphetamine.[7] This is a powerful central nervous system stimulant drug and is classified as a schedule II controlled substance. Adderal® can be habit forming. It is prescribed as a treatment for the symptoms of attention deficit hyperactivity disorder (ADHD) in both adults and children. It is also used to treat a condition called narcolepsy, a disorder that causes one to fall asleep during the day.

Inderal® contains the drug propranolol, which is a beta blocker. According to *PubMed Health*, a National Institutes of Health publication, it can be prescribed for "high blood pressure, abnormal heart rhythms, heart disease, pheochromocytoma (tumor on a small gland near the kidneys), and certain types of tremor. It is also used to prevent angina (chest pain) and migraine headaches."[8]

Since Adderal® is a central nervous system (CNS) stimulant, it could cause a rise in blood pressure. If either drug were given by mistake and taken for an extended period of time, the problems could be more serious than just the effects of the drug. Adderal® can be habit forming, so sudden discontinuation of the drug when the error is discovered could result in symptoms of withdrawal. Inderal® contains a warning in the official FDA-approved literature that reads, "Do not stop taking propranolol without talking to your physician first. If propranolol is stopped suddenly, it may cause chest pain or heart attack in some people."

The Case of "I don't have a cough!"

Occasionally, a mistake is made by the prescriber. A physician in Iowa called in a prescription for promethazine with codeine syrup, used to treat a cold with a cough. When the patient came to pick up her prescription, a pharmacy student waited on her and, as trained in her classes at the pharmacy school, asked, "What did the physician tell you this was for?" She expected the answer to be "for my cough." Instead the patient said, "It is for my female problems." The student and the pharmacist-on-duty called the physician who, after checking his charts, explained that this patient was to have gotten a female hormone product. When he called in the prescription, he had the wrong chart in his hand. While the error in this case was the physician's, it was a preventable error. Because of the workflow in this pharmacy, the staff was in a position to prevent this potential error.[9]

COMPUTER DATA ENTRY

In a standard workflow, after a prescription is received in the pharmacy it is usually then delivered to the data-entry or computer-entry area where a pharmacy technician enters the information. The data-entry station is a place in the workflow where a large percentage of QREs occur (refer to Figure 4–3 in Chapter 4). By listing the potential risks that may happen here, we can later use this information to design a system that will reduce the risk of error at this station.

Potential risks that may occur in the computer-entry station include the following:

- entering the name of the wrong patient
- entering the wrong drug
- entering the wrong strength of the drug
- typing in the directions incorrectly

- entering the wrong physician's name
- entering the wrong refill information, depending on the method used
    - mistyping the prescription number
    - entering the name incorrectly
    - entering the name correctly, but selecting the wrong individual from the list of names on the computer screen

There are several ways that data entry may be performed, many of which will be dictated by the software the pharmacy uses to fill prescriptions. Potential QREs will be affected by the particular manner in which the software functions and allows entry of the information. Most commercial pharmacy software will allow the drug name to be entered either by typing in the name or by entering the NDC number. Either method could result in an error.

Refer again to Figure 4–3 in Chapter 4, which shows one pharmacy's 30-day results when it tracked all errors and near-misses. At the end of 30 days, the pharmacy used its online software to prepare a graph showing where in the process each mistake was made. The pharmacy found that 42 percent of its QREs in the entire workflow that month were made during data entry. Seventeen percent of all QREs were a combination of selecting the wrong drug and selecting the wrong strength.

Caution: For Each Problem Solved—A New One Created

New technology allows e-prescribing. A physician using e-prescribing enters the prescription directly into the computer. When e-prescribing is fully implemented, the two functions of receiving the prescription and entering the data are combined into one step. The physician can type directly into her or his computer or PDA. The information is then sent directly to the pharmacy's computer, thereby avoiding the necessity for a pharmacy technician to enter the information into the pharmacy's computer. With this new technology, it is less likely an entry error will occur.

One risk of error is reduced by introducing e-prescribing. It, however, introduces other potential problems. The prescriber may click on the wrong line in the handheld PDA and send the wrong drug information to the pharmacy's computer. From the patient's point of view, either error is equally injurious. If the pharmacy technician makes the mistake, it is easier for the pharmacy to design a workflow to catch and rectify it before it reaches the patient. If it is discovered that the cause is in the prescriber's workflow, he or she must be alerted. When any new technology is introduced, the pharmacy staff should discuss and prepare for any foreseeable problems.

FILLING THE PRESCRIPTIONS

After information is put into the computer, a new label is generated along with a receipt. This information and each of these items are then delivered to the assembly or filling station. In many pharmacies this is still done by hand, but increasingly, robotics perform much of the mechanical aspects of selecting and placing the drugs into the container and affixing the label to the bottle. With any system, mistakes are possible.

Manual Filling

Along with a label and receipt, other printed materials are prepared, for example, a patient-information leaflet. With some prescriptions there may also be FDA-mandated patient material and warnings. Accompanying the other material for a new prescription will be the original prescription. In an increasing number of pharmacies, however, the new prescription is scanned into the computer and the paper prescription is filed since it is not needed; an image of the original prescription is now on the computer screen.

If the pharmacy is using a best practice basket[10] procedure, the printed material will be placed in the basket and delivered to the technician in the filling or assembly area. If there is only one technician working at the time, this could be the same technician who received the prescription from the patient and who entered the information into the computer. Even if one technician is performing all tasks, the workflow should still move laterally to separate stations located in each area.

The filling technician will check the label[11] and, if the order is for a new prescription, will use the new prescription to identify the drug called for and pull the stock bottle from the shelf. This may be the original prescription or the scanned image, depending on the system the pharmacy is using. If the order is a refill, the technician will use the label or receipt to identify the correct drug and strength.

When the stock bottle is placed into the workflow, the technician will use best practices that are a part of the pharmacy's CQI system to fill the prescription. The finished prescription bottle or product is now ready to advance to the next station in the workflow, which is usually the pharmacist's final check area.

Experienced pharmacists and technicians often voice the opinion that most mistakes are made in the filling procedure. It is likely that there are an equal number of QREs made at the filling station and the data-entry station.[12] Whichever station produces the higher source of mistakes, studying the processes of the filling station is important in identifying risks of potential errors.

During the manual filling of prescriptions, many mistakes are possible. Listed below are just a few.

- The technician could misread the order, causing him or her to pull the wrong drug from the shelf.
- The technician could inadvertently select the wrong drug or the wrong strength of drug from the shelf.
- The technician could place the wrong label on the bottle, resulting in medication either provided to the wrong patient or incorrect directions provided for the same patient.
- A finished prescription bottle could be placed in the wrong basket or with the incorrect receipt, causing the wrong prescription to be delivered to the patient.
- A technician, having correctly decided which drug is needed to fill the prescription, inadvertently picks up the bottle beside it, which may be the wrong strength of the correct drug.

All of these quality-related events are possible. During one 3-year period in which pharmacy mechanical-dispensing claims were studied by Pharmacists Mutual Insurance Company, 2 percent of all claims involved amitriptyline 100 mg tablets dispensed in place of the 10 mg tablets that had been prescribed.[13] A similar percentage of those mechanical-error claims were for an otic (for the ear) preparation dispensed instead of an ophthalmic. While these QREs could have been made at either the computer-entry station or the filling station, most of the claims studied found the mistake was made during filling.

Warfarin, which accounted for the largest number of claims in this and later studies at 7 percent, often involved either the wrong strength or the entirely wrong drug. Many of these errors were made during filling. Some robotic systems do not include warfarin in the list of products that should be dispensed by robot.

Robotic Filling

Even with the most advanced robotic-filling systems, only about 60 to 70 percent of the prescriptions are usually dispensed by the robots. The rest are still dispensed manually. The risk of errors can be reduced through the use of robotics, but that does not mean a system using robotics will be error-free or that all risks are eliminated. There are special risks of error associated with robotic systems. For example, most robotic systems are filled from stock bottles that are poured into a large bin from which the prescription drug is counted by the robot. The filling is customarily performed by a technician and checked by a pharmacist, and each system has safety features to prevent inaccuracies when filling the robot's bins. But consider the following case. Pharmacies need to realize that with any system, mistakes are possible.

The Case of One Mistake, 17 Wrong Prescriptions

In the mid-1990s, a pharmacy was using an early mechanical system that counted the number of tablets of the drug to be placed into a prescription bottle from a large bin. During computer entry, a pharmacy technician or pharmacist entered the name and quantity of the drug. If the prescribed drug was one that was in the mechanical system, the computer sent a message to the system directing it to count the correct number of tablets. After the tablets were counted, they were dropped into a lower portion of the bin where, once delivered, the technician could open a door allowing the counted tablets to be poured into the bottle the technician held below the door on the bin. While many of these older systems have been replaced by modern robots, many remain in use. This pharmacy reported 17 misfilled prescriptions within a 2-day period of time. The QREs resulted from filling the system's large bin with the wrong drug during a recent replenishing process. Digoxin (heart medication) tablets were accidentally placed in the bin that should have contained high blood pressure tablets.[14]

One problem with robotics may stem from the fact that they are presumed by everyone to be incapable of making an error. That leads to a confidence that may cause technicians and pharmacists to skip much of the checking process. Even if "the robot is always right," it is able to perform only the task assigned to it by the operator or the computer. Should the wrong drug be entered by a technician during data entry, the wrong drug will be dispensed by the robot. Because "the robot is always right," many of the checks performed by the filling technician during a mechanical fill may be omitted for these prescriptions.

PHARMACIST FINAL CHECK STATION

Just as "the robot is always right" syndrome could lead to errors that may have otherwise been caught, a similar problem may exist for a pharmacist who comes to believe "the technician is always right." The problem is that technicians and robots are *almost* always right. A pharmacist checks 200 prescriptions and they are all correct. The pharmacist may become more lax when checking the two hundred first and two hundred second prescriptions.

The pharmacist final check area is a critical part of a pharmacy's continuous quality system. There are some machines that can now be employed to assist the pharmacist with the final check. Such machines do what they are programmed to do. They act mechanically, performing the same task over and over and never becoming acclimated to the belief that anything is "always right." They do not learn or adapt.

Pharmacists are human beings whose minds can be compared to a much more sophisticated computer. The human mind can learn, grow, adapt, and change. One lesson the human mind may learn is that since there were no mistakes in the last 200 prescriptions, it is unlikely there are any in the next two prescriptions. That marvelous ability of the human mind may occasionally become its "Achilles' heel."

To most laypeople observing a pharmacy operation, it appears easy for a pharmacist to check each prescription and ensure that it contains the right drug, in the right strength, with the right directions, for the right person, and exactly as the prescriber ordered. Most times, even if a mistake has been made earlier in the system, the pharmacist does catch it. In a study of near-misses caught before they reach a patient, consistently 75 to 80 percent were caught by a pharmacist in a final quality check. Some near-misses are caught in other parts of the workflow and occasionally, some avoid all detection and are delivered to the patient.[15]

If the pharmacy can identify how pharmacists at the final quality check station miss some mistakes that should have been caught, it can modify its CQI workflow system to reduce the risk of other mistakes in the future. Before the pharmacy can redesign its system, it must identify what could go wrong.

Two Cases of Bypassing the System

I. One problem discussed earlier can be described as "the technician is always right" syndrome. There is a flip side of that interesting phenomenon. In a case before a state board of pharmacy, when the technician was questioned regarding an error, the technician involved said, "I thought if I did make a mistake the pharmacist would catch it. They always do."[16] If both of these "I thought the other guy would be right" conditions can be accepted as correct, a cause has been identified. This information can be used to improve the pharmacy's CQI system.

II. One large pharmacy chain implemented a new, efficient, technologically sophisticated CQI workflow. When errors continued to occur, the pharmacy sought the causes in order to improve the system. One problem identified was that the chain's pharmacists were not checking the label against the new prescription. In some cases pharmacists were missing technician-entry mistakes. Checking should not have been difficult because each new prescription was scanned and easily available on the computer screen at the pharmacist's final check station.

The analysis disclosed that when the pharmacists were busy, they tended to skip the required procedure of pulling up the scanned prescriptions on the pharmacists' computer terminal. The system did not work because it could be bypassed. One cause for bypassing this step in the workflow may be explained by the pharmacists' expectation that prescriptions, entered and filled by the technicians, were almost always correct.

Studying the Outlier

One way to identify a problem is to study outliers. Outliers are items in a set that are different; they do not fit the observed pattern. The solution in the second case above, the pharmacy chain, came from one of its pharmacies that was an outlier. This pharmacy was not having the same problem, nor did it have as many errors as its sister pharmacies in the same chain. In this outlier pharmacy, when the technician delivered a prescription to the pharmacists' station for checking, something different happened. In this pharmacy the technician was trained to automatically pull up the image of the scanned prescription on the pharmacists' terminal.[17] This step was not part of the chain's workflow; it had been added by the technicians. The technicians in this pharmacy decided this was a way to assist the pharmacist.

The chain identified the problem in the other pharmacies by looking at the outlier. The key to finding the answer was in identifying the problem. It took a group of executives and specialists hours to identify the problem that technicians had solved before it became a problem.

Identify by Tracking Success

Some pharmacies have the capability to track near-misses and use the information to identify vulnerabilities in the pharmacy's CQI workflow. Almost all pharmacies tracked their errors, that is, mistakes that reached the patient. Fewer can tell

1. How many of their near-misses are caught before they reach the patient;
2. When near-misses occur and are caught;
3. Where near-misses occur and where they are caught; and
4. Who catches near-misses.

Since most pharmacies do not track near-misses in addition to errors, they cannot know statistically how often their quality system was successful in preventing QREs from becoming errors. One pharmacy found that they caught two thirds of their QREs before they reach the patient. One pharmacy in Iowa consistently caught 98 percent of all QREs.[18] Most pharmacies can be expected to fall somewhere in the middle of these two examples. Unless a pharmacy tracks its successes (near-misses caught), it cannot identify its success rate. Such pharmacies miss a useful tool that can identify potential risks and vulnerabilities.

Delivering the Rx to the Patient

One pharmacy that did track near-misses as well as errors, and then used the information to graphically display the causes, found that, during 1 month, 4 percent of all QREs involved a patient receiving someone else's prescription. These prescriptions had been filled correctly, but were either given to the wrong patient or almost given to the wrong patient.

RxErcise 5-B   Awarding Damage in the Case of "His and Hers"

In Chapter 4 we examined the case of "His and Hers," involving Mr. and Mrs. Jackson. Review what happened in that case and add a couple of additional facts.

Mildred and James Jackson[19] were both in their seventies and had been married for almost 50 years. On the day in question, Mildred had one prescription refilled and James had two.

When the prescriptions were placed in the prescription bags for delivery to the patients, Mildred's was placed in James's bag with its two receipts, and both of James's prescription bottles were placed in Mildred's bag with one receipt.

For almost a month, until the mistake was caught, Mildred took both of James's prescriptions and James took Mildred's prescribed drug. During that time, neither was taking their own medication.

You are on the jury and you must render a verdict. Using the limited facts available to you, decide the percentage of negligence that should be assigned to each person in the lawsuit, including the patient. Before making your decision, read and consider the information in "Can the Patient Be at Fault?" that follows this RxErcise.

Complete the jury verdict form in Figure 5-3. Assume, in your deliberations, the following hypothetical facts to be true:

- You must apportion fault among
    - the *pharmacist* who checked the prescriptions;
    - the *pharmacy technician* who put the prescriptions in the bags;
    - the *patient Mildred* who picked up the prescriptions and incorrectly placed them into two boxes at home that were marked "Mildred's Meds" and "James's Meds" (in doing so Mildred used the receipts on the bags rather than the labels on the bottles);

> ○ the *patient James* who took the wrong medication from the box marked "James's Meds." (The prescription bottle in the box had Mildred's name on it. The drug looked entirely different from anything James had taken before. Mildred did the same when she took her medication.)
>
> - You and your fellow jury members unanimously determined the damages suffered by Mildred and James to total $100,000.00.

Can the Patient Be at Fault?

Often in a medication-error malpractice trial, more than one person may be found to be negligent and each of their negligences may be determined to have contributed to the plaintiff's injuries. This may be the pharmacy technician who entered the information, the pharmacy technician who filled the prescription, and/or the pharmacist who was responsible for checking. Each person will be judged by the legal standard of negligence. In order to be sued and found liable, the individual must be shown to be negligent. All four of the following elements must be proven in order to find any person negligent.

1. The person must owe a duty to the other party (e.g., a pharmacy technician and a pharmacist have a duty to each patient to fill the prescription correctly).

2. The person must have failed in that duty owed to the other (e.g., the pharmacy technician and/or the pharmacist failed to perform a required task that led to the prescription being filled incorrectly).

3. The other party must have been injured.

4. The other's injury must have been a result (even if only partly) of the person's failure to properly execute his or her duty. (This is often called the "but for" test—"But for" the pharmacist's negligence, the plaintiff would not have been injured.)

A plaintiff (patient) may also be negligent and the plaintiff's negligence may have contributed to his or her own injury. Since the jury cannot award more than 100 percent of what monetary damages it assesses, the jury must divide the amount of the total damages awarded among all those it finds to have negligently contributed to the injuries (damages).

In a case like the one in RxErcise 5-B, the jury will be given a verdict form such as the one in Figure 5-3. Using such a form, the jury will divide the percentage of fault among all of the defendants and, if the facts of the case warrant, the plaintiffs. If the jury finds the plaintiffs' negligence contributed to their own injuries, the amount paid by the defendants to the plaintiffs will be reduced by that percentage.

This doctrine is called "Comparative Fault." In most states, if the plaintiffs' negligence is over 50 percent, they will not collect any money from the defendants. In other states, there is no 50 percent rule and the percent by which the plaintiffs are at fault is just subtracted from the total awarded.[20]

Jury Verdict Form

State of Columbus
County of Amerigo Vespucci
IN THE SUPERIOR COURT

Mildred Johnson   Case # 12-1003
and
James Johnson

                                                       Plaintiffs

Vs

Hometown Pharmacy
Angela Brown, pharmacist
and
William Martin, pharmacy technician

                                                       Defendants

                        Verdict

We the jury, having found that all defendants were negligent and all contributed to the injuries suffered by the plaintiffs, and having further found that the plaintiffs' negligence contributed to their own injuries, now render the following verdict in the total amount of $100,000.00, proportioned in the following manner:

Hometown Pharmacy	_____ %
Angela Brown, pharmacist	_____ %
William Martin, pharmacy technician	_____ %
Mildred Johnson, plaintiff	_____ %
James Johnson, plaintiff	_____ %
Total	100%

NOTE: Should the jury find that the plaintiffs' negligence in total contributed to more than 50% of the total, by the laws of this state, plaintiffs shall not recover any amount from the defendants.

Figure 5-3 Jury verdict form
© Cengage Learning 2013

The case in RxErcise 5-B, although based on a real claim, is an extreme example of what can happen. A patient's prescription may be placed in the wrong bag and thus given to the wrong patient. A pharmacy technician could misunderstand a patient's name or there could be two patients with similar names. In one case, a delivery person left the prescription at the wrong house. The occupants of the house were not home at the time, so the delivery person put it into a mail slot. The family's dog chewed through the packaging and the plastic bottle and consumed all of the drug. The dog died.

Consider the pharmacy that found that 4 percent of its QREs occurred during delivery. While the percentage is small, it is a mistake that should not happen. When a prescription has been filled correctly, the pharmacy should have a system that can ensure it reaches the right patient.

When we think of identifying the risks in a prescription workflow, we usually think of mechanical medication errors—wrong tablet in the bottle, wrong directions, wrong strength, wrong delivery to the wrong patient. There are, however, other risks that should be considered at the end of the workflow after the pharmacist has checked the prescription and it has been placed in the prescription bag for counseling and delivery to the patient.

Identifying a Special Risk: HIPAA and Privacy

One risk that is not often considered as a quality concern is a violation of the patient's privacy rights, including violation of the HIPAA federal regulations. Every state board of pharmacy has a regulation protecting the privacy of patients. A violation of these regulations can result in a complaint to the state board of pharmacy in addition to a lawsuit, if the patient can show injury resulting from the release of his or her confidential records.

In addition to concern over state regulations, a CQI plan needs to consider federal laws and regulations. In 1996, concerned about the amount of patient health information that private insurance companies and others had in their files and how this information could be misused or inadvertently released, the United States Congress passed HIPAA. This legislation was designed to protect not just the information collected by insurance companies, but all health care records of any health care provider that used electronic transmission for any health care documents. Up to the implementation of HIPAA, there had been no uniform laws among the states or any federal regulations that controlled how such information would be protected and under what circumstances it could be used or released.

The main concern that prompted HIPAA was electronic records. With electronic records the problem of privacy became more acute. The legislation became effective upon the passage of regulations by the United States Department of Health and Human Services (HHS). The federal law, entitled Health Insurance Portability and Accountability Act of 1996, or HIPAA, took effect in 2002. Some parts of HIPAA, however, did not become effective until 2005.

HIPAA was about more than privacy. A primary reason for the underlying legislation was to ensure that insurance benefits would be portable from one group insurance plan to another. The law placed limits on the manner and extent to which group health insurance plans could exclude people or pre-existing medical conditions from its policies.

In pharmacy we primarily consider HIPAA a privacy protection rule. HIPAA did not replace all state privacy regulations. It only replaced those state rules that were less strict than the federal regulations. In pharmacy, therefore, we need to consider both sets of laws and comply with both. If we cannot comply with one because it would not allow us to follow the other, then the federal law takes precedence.

Under federal law a pharmacy, if it uses electronic means to transmit health care information, is a **covered entity**, meaning it is covered by the HIPAA rules along with everyone working for the pharmacy. A full study of HIPAA regulations is beyond the scope of this text, but we should review some of the basic rules and exceptions that relate to preventing medication errors.

The failure to protect a patient's medical information is, in its broadest sense, a medical error. In pharmacy terms, an error is preventable if the pharmacist, pharmacy technician, or the pharmacy can influence its effect on the patient. A malpractice claim involving the unauthorized release of medical information is, like counseling and drug utilization review claims, considered to be an **intellectual error**.[21]

HIPAA sets a national standard designed to protect patients' health care information. The material protected by HIPAA is information that could be used to identify the patient, including the patient's name, address, telephone number, and even the patient's prescription number.

Pharmacy technicians should also be aware that HHS, the federal department charged with implementing HIPAA, has said that the regulations are not intended to prevent necessary use of medical information or to make the use of medical information unduly burdensome. HHS has published frequently asked questions (FAQs) and answers to provide the agency's interpretations of the HIPAA regulations. These FAQs can be found on the HHS website: http://www.hhs.gov/ocr/privacy/hipaa/faq/index.html Below are just two of the hundreds of questions answered on this website.

FAQ: *My state requires consent to use or disclose health information. Does the HIPAA Privacy Rule take away this protection?*

Answer: *No. The Privacy Rule does not prohibit a covered entity from obtaining an individual's consent to use or disclose his or her health information and, therefore, presents no barrier to the entity's ability to comply with state law requirements.*

FAQ: *Can a patient have a friend or family member pick up a prescription for her?*

Answer: *Yes. A pharmacist may use professional judgment and experience with common practice to make reasonable inferences of the patient's best interest in allowing a person, other than the patient, to pick up a prescription. See 45 CFR 164.510(b). For example, the fact that a relative or friend arrives at a pharmacy and asks to pick up a specific prescription for an individual effectively verifies that he or she is involved in the individual's care and the HIPAA Privacy Rule allows the pharmacist to give the filled prescription to the relative or friend. The individual does not need to provide the pharmacist with the names of such persons in advance.*

HIPAA regulations do not require prior patient authorization before some disclosures can be released. It depends on the use and the purpose of its use by the pharmacy.

Under HIPAA, all patient-identifiable information is private except information that is provided to the patient himself or herself or information that is disclosed pursuant to HIPAA regulations. A patient may allow the use or release of his or her information by signing an authorization that must be voluntary and written in plain language. All other disclosures under HIPAA are considered permitted rather than required.

Pharmacists and pharmacy technicians will generally be concerned with three permitted disclosures under HIPAA, commonly referred to as TPA:

1. Treatment—information used to properly care for the patient (e.g., a physician calls in a prescription and the pharmacist shares with the physician information about other medication the patient is taking that was prescribed by a different physician)

2. Payment—information necessary for the pharmacy to secure payment for its services (e.g., sending patient information to the third-party payer organization that will authorize payment from the patient's insurance company to the pharmacy)

3. Health care operations—information the pharmacy is required to use as part of the pharmacy's regular operations (e.g., prescription records in the pharmacy are audited)

If the state has a prescription monitoring program, the pharmacy is required by law to provide some patient information to the database maintained to provide a record of all controlled-substance prescriptions prescribed and filled in the state. Use of this information is restricted. One use is to provide pharmacies and physicians with a record of all controlled-substance prescriptions being taken by their patients. This use is permitted under HIPAA.

HIPAA also allows other release of information when it is required by law. Depending on state law, examples may include releasing records pursuant to court orders or when a statute or regulation requires it. For example, if a couple is involved in a divorce, one party may ask the court to compel the pharmacy to release records to the other spouse. The release may be allowed under state law pursuant to a court order. In most states a subpoena is not a court order. A subpoena is usually an order to bring the records to the court. State laws vary. A subpoena may not itself authorize the pharmacy to send the records unless a signed authorization from the patient is attached. Pharmacies should consult an attorney when a subpoena is received. Otherwise, there may be a risk of a lawsuit for unauthorized release of records.[22]

HHS lists six circumstances under which otherwise-protected information may be released without the patient's direct authorization:

1. as required by law (including court orders, court-ordered warrants, subpoenas) and administrative requests;
2. to identify or locate a suspect, fugitive, material witness, or missing person;
3. in response to a law enforcement official's request for information about a victim or suspected victim of a crime;
4. to alert law enforcement of a person's death, if the covered entity suspects that criminal activity caused the death;
5. when a covered entity believes that protected health information is evidence of a crime that occurred on its premises; and
6. by a covered health care provider in a medical emergency not occurring on its premises, when necessary to inform law enforcement about the commission and nature of a crime, the location of the crime or crime victims, and the perpetrator of the crime.

HIPAA also recognizes that there are times when protected health information may need to be used in order to prevent a "serious and imminent threat" to a person or the public.[23] Patients may authorize another individual to act for them, usually called a "personal representative." Not every caregiver has been given the legal authority to receive all information that the patient could receive. A personal representative is one who has been legally authorized to act on behalf of the patient, or sometimes the patient's estate. There should be a signed document from the patient appointing a personal representative.

Pharmacies have policies and procedures regarding how to deal with confidentiality issues. These may be part of the pharmacy's CQI plan or part of a general policy and procedure manual. If a situation is not specifically covered by a pharmacy rule, the question should be referred to the pharmacist-in-charge or management to make the decision.

Compliance with privacy rules is a part of a pharmacy's risk management plan. Every pharmacy technician and pharmacist must be trained in the principles of HIPAA and state privacy laws. And training in privacy rules should expand beyond the prescription department.

The Case of the High School Student

In one pharmacy, when the pharmacy was busy, prescriptions could be rung up on one of the registers in the front of the pharmacy. Usually these registers were manned by clerks who were not pharmacy technicians. On one busy day, a mother took her daughter's prescription to the front cash register where she was waited on by a young high school student. This student clerk knew the mother's daughter and recognized the name on the receipt. The prescription was for birth control pills, as the young clerk knew from the receipt and the feel of the bag when she was ringing it up. The prescription was not prescribed for contraception, but was for an acne problem. The next day, the high school clerk spread the "news" throughout the school that this high school patient was on birth control pills. According to later testimony and records presented, the embarrassment caused great mental stress to the high-school-age patient and the pharmacy was sued. Following the incident, the pharmacy instituted new training techniques. The pharmacy probably hired a new clerk.[24]

COUNSELING

One of the final steps in the delivery of a prescription to the patient involves pharmacist counseling. Counseling and prospective drug utilization review can result in intellectual claims. Increasingly, pharmacists and pharmacies are being held to their responsibility to warn regarding the use of prescribed medications, potential side effects, allergies, and interactions. Lack of or inadequate counseling is a medication-error risk that can be identified and protected against. Counseling should be a part of a CQI program.

Only a pharmacist may counsel a patient, but there are things that a pharmacy technician can do to make the pharmacist's job of counseling the patient more efficient, for example, assembling all necessary information and materials. A pharmacy needs to identify risks associated with counseling.

Counseling is more than telling a patient something about the prescription he or she is receiving; it is an educational process. It can take several forms:

- words spoken by the pharmacist
- printed material provided with the prescription
- videos provided for patients to be viewed in the pharmacy or for loan to the patient
- websites designed to educate the patient about a drug or disease

The risk is in failing to provide a patient with information needed to avoid some problem associated with the medication. Rarely have there been claims alleging that the pharmacist counseled a patient after a physician or caregiver (usually a spouse) "ordered" the pharmacist not to do so. Most of these have been dismissed without payment. The other risk is lack of documentation providing proof as to what material the patient was provided with when the prescription was dispensed.

One particular risk regarding education of the patient should be discussed as part of a medication-error risk-management plan. The federal government and the Food and Drug Administration (FDA) require certain information and documents to accompany specific medications. This information is usually provided by manufacturers, and pharmacies are required to dispense it along with the prescription. These documents are called Medication Guides or "med-guides." If not given, the pharmacy could face penalties. Pharmacy technicians and pharmacists should know which drugs require federally mandated med-guides. Technicians should make sure all required material is available for the pharmacist during the final check, counseling, and delivery to the patient.

On its website, the FDA provides the following information about med-guides:

Medication Guides are paper handouts that come with many prescription medicines. The guides address issues that are specific to particular drugs and drug classes, and they contain FDA-approved information that can help patients avoid serious adverse events.

> *FDA requires that Medication Guides be issued with certain prescribed drugs and biological products when the Agency determines that:*
>
> - *certain information is necessary to prevent serious adverse effects;*
> - *patient decision making should be informed by information about a known, serious side effect with a product; or*
> - *patient adherence to directions for the use of a product is essential to its effectiveness.*

Currently, the FDA lists over 280 products, plus their generics, that require med-guides.[25] An example is Ritalin®. This med-guide is four pages long, which is much longer than the standard patient-information leaflet printed by most prescription computer software. It includes a description of the tablets and storage information such as the temperatures within which the tablets should be stored. One section of the Ritalin med-guide is entitled: "What is the most important information I should know about Ritalin?" Other sections discuss "What is Ritalin?" and "Who should not take Ritalin?" There are questions about other medications that can be taken with this drug, how it should be taken, and what are common side effects associated with Ritalin. It has been reported in the pharmacy press that in 2005, in one small undercover shopping study of 20 pharmacies, only 5 percent provided the required med-guide for the product being shopped.[26]

Summary

The workflow in a typical pharmacy, hospital or community, is relatively simple as compared to most manufacturing processes. It is surprising, however, how many risks of medication QREs are present in the pharmacy workflow. All errors can be prevented, but no system is perfect and there will always be errors. We can reduce the risk of errors if we can identify where the risks are in the workflow. Once identified, we can then select best practices to reduce the likelihood of errors—or even better, underlying mistakes—happening or reaching the patient. This is the first step in reducing medication errors.

Review Questions

1. According to the Pharmacists Mutual Study, what drug or class of drugs is involved in most mechanical-error claims?
    A. Coumadin®
    B. Otic preparations
    C. Insulin
    D. Lipitor®

2. There are two primary times when, working with a continuous quality improvement (CQI) program, a pharmacy should systematically try to identify where mistakes can be made in the pharmacy workflow. One is when the program is designed and implemented. When is the other?
    A. Before a board of pharmacy inspection
    B. After an error or a near-miss has occurred
    C. Before each prescription is filled
    D. None of the above; the only time this step is used is when the CQI program is first designed

3. What is considered the first step in instituting a quality improvement program?
    A. Identifying the risk of where a mistake could be made
    B. Reviewing all prior claims over the past year
    C. Monitoring the current workflow
    D. Training

4. A patient on warfarin will usually be given tests to determine clotting time as a way of adjusting his or her dosage. The most common today is the INR. Which of the following would be considered a good INR value?

   A. 1.5
   B. 2.3
   C. 6.8
   D. 12.1

5. Which of the following is *not* one of the factors Deming said we should look at when analyzing the cause of an error?

   A. People
   B. Method
   C. Machine
   D. Extrinsic factors

6. What does HIPAA stand for?

   A. Health of Individual Privacy Accounts
   B. Health Insurance Portability and Accountability Act
   C. Healthcare Individual Privacy Assurance Act
   D. None of the above

7. What organization is covered under HIPAA?

   A. A covered entity
   B. A pharmacy that does not use any electronic means to store or transmit health care data
   C. A veterinarian
   D. All of the above

8. What disclosures under HIPAA are specifically permitted by the regulations?

   A. Payment
   B. Treatment
   C. The pharmacy's health care operations
   D. All of the above

9. How many products require med-guides to be given when they are dispensed?

   A. None
   B. 120
   C. 280
   D. 540

10. One problem that can be identified regarding robots in a pharmacy is:

    A. They occasionally make mistakes.
    B. The pharmacy staff may consider them as "fool proof" and not carry out some required steps in checking prescriptions.
    C. Patients may consider them as replacements for humans.
    D. Completed prescriptions lack sufficient documentation.

Endnotes

[1] An anticoagulant drug is often referred to as a blood thinner. While technically not accurate, it is a convenient term and one that is used by lay patients.

[2] Because of the significance of warfarin in claims and pharmacy errors, technicians should be familiar with the drug, including why its use is problematic with several other drugs, such as aspirin. To learn more about Coumadin and warfarin, visit the manufacturer's website http://www.coumadin.com/ or do an internet search for warfarin.

[3] See Pharmacists Mutual Insurance Company study on its website: http://www.phmic.com/phmc/services/RM/profliab/claimsstudy/Pages/DrugsMostInvolvedinMechanicalErrorClaims.aspx accessed April 6, 2011.

[4] For a good general description of warfarin use and testing, see HealthPoint website: http://www.heartpoint.com/coumadin.html and Drug Information Online website: http://www.drugs.com/warfarin.html accessed January 2, 2011.

[5] Deming originally used the term "man" in the generic sense of "mankind." Today the term "people" is substituted.

[6] For ISMP's List of Confused Drug Names, visit the ISMP website: http://www.ismp.org/tools/confuseddrugnames.pdf accessed March 9, 2011. Every pharmacy should keep a copy of this list where the staff can easily refer to it.

[7] See http://www.ncbi.nlm.nih.gov/pubmedhealth/PMH0000166/ accessed March 9, 2011.

[8] See http://www.ncbi.nlm.nih.gov/pubmedhealth/PMH0000727/ accessed March 9, 2011.

[9] This incident was reported to the author by the pharmacy student involved in the counseling and later by a call to the physician.

[10] The basket procedure is described in Chapter 6. It is a best practice that many pharmacies use to ensure that all material (label, receipt, stock bottle, prescription bottle, patient information leaflets, etc.) remain together. The purpose is to prevent material from one person's prescription being comingled with another patient's material.

[11] See the best practice "Take 5" described in Chapter 6.

[12] From the files of PMC Quality Commitment, Inc. The study referred to here was not scientific but was a collection of data from several pharmacies using the company's Pharmacy Quality Commitment® system and its Quality Manager™ component. This system is now owned by the National Alliance of State Pharmacy Associations (NASPA). See http://www.pqc.net

[13] See Pharmacists Mutual Claims Study at http://www.phmic.com The 3-year study referred to was done at the request of DuPont Pharma, the company that at the time was the manufacturer of Coumadin® brand of warfarin. Pharmacists Mutual looked at the 10 drugs most often involved in its claims during that 3-year period. The fact that the 10 drugs, or drug classifications, were cited in the study does not mean they were the drugs most often involved in mistakes or errors, but in reported claims. A later study of near-misses showed that neither amitriptyline nor warfarin were in the top 15 drugs involved in near-misses.

[14] From the files of Pharmacists Mutual Insurance Company.

[15] Data from the files of PMC Quality Commitment, Inc., a subsidiary of Pharmacist Mutual.

[16] Heard by the author during an investigation before a state (unrevealed) board inquiring into a wrong drug complaint. The testimony was unsworn and was during an informal portion of the investigation. The quote presents the essence of the technician's statement and is not meant to be portrayed as an accurate, verbatim quotation.

[17] This discussion and informal analysis were heard by the author during a board of pharmacy meeting. The discussion involved company pharmacists and managers and members of the state board. It was prompted by reports of several errors within a relatively short period of time, all from the same chain, and within 3 months of the company explaining its new system to reduce errors.

[18] Both figures are from PMC Quality Commitment, Inc. files. Both pharmacies tracked their near-misses and errors through a system called The Quality Manager™. In the first month, pharmacy one caught only 67% of the near-misses. Pharmacy two consistently, for several months, caught over 98%.

[19] From the files of Pharmacists Mutual Insurance Company. These are not the real names. As with all examples from these files, no information is given identifying the pharmacy, pharmacists, or patients.

[20] If any of the pharmacy's employees are negligent, the pharmacy is also negligent because the acts of an employee who is working in the course of his or her employment are attributed to the employer. In the case in RxErcise 5–2, we added a percentage for the pharmacy in order to consider the question of any independent negligence on the part of the pharmacy for having, among other things, a CQI system that allowed this error to occur.

[21] See Pharmacists Mutual Claims Study: http://www.phmic.com/phmc/services/RM/profliab/claimsstudy/Pages/CounselingClaims,PersonalInjuryClaims,Other.aspx

[22] See *Washburn v. Rite Aid Corp*, 695 A.2d 495 (R.I. 1997). In this case, the Washburns were in a contested divorce. Mr. Washburn's attorney subpoenaed Mrs. Washburn's prescription records from Rite Aid. Rather than bring the requested records to the deposition as stated in the subpoena, the pharmacy mailed copies of the records directly to Mr. Washburn's attorney. The court concluded that this action by the pharmacy was an unauthorized release of confidential records and the court said that Mrs. Washburn could sue the pharmacy for damages.

[23] See HHS summary of HIPAA, http://www.hhs.gov/ocr/privacy/hipaa/understanding/summary/index.html accessed February 28, 2011.

[24] From the files of Pharmacist Mutual Insurance Company. All pharmacy and patient information has been excluded or changed to protect those involved. It is unknown whether the high school clerk was fired.

[25] The list and the med-guides are subject to change. The pharmacy should check the FDA website regularly to update its list of required medication guides. See http://www.fda.gov/Drugs/DrugSafety/UCM085729 accessed March 15, 2011.

[26] Sasich, L. D., and Sukkari, S. R., Viewpoint: Don't forget to give out med-guides, *Drug Topics*, April 3, 2006.

CHAPTER 6

Best Practices and Other Tools
Practices to Reduce the Risk of Errors

OBJECTIVES

Upon completion of this chapter, the reader should be able to:

1. Study the use of best practices to reduce medication errors.
2. Understand how best practices are used as part of a pharmacy workflow.
3. Describe the application of best practices to errors.
4. Discuss the use of scanners in a pharmacy workflow.
5. Describe how robots are becoming a part of pharmacy practice.
6. Discuss the rise of e-prescribing in pharmacy.
7. Understand the drawbacks to e-prescribing and problems that can arise.
8. Describe how pharmacy technicians can assist pharmacists to prepare for counseling.
9. Study the pharmacist prospective drug review and the role technicians can play in assisting the pharmacist.
10. Discuss electronic forms of prescription verification to reduce medication errors.

KEY TERMS

Best practices: Techniques that have been proven to be effective. When best practices are used in the dispensing of medications, they help in stopping or catching dispensing mistakes before they reach patients.

Centers for Medicare and Medicaid Services (CMS): An agency of the federal government that oversees the rules and regulations associated with federal health care programs, including Medicare and Medicaid.

E-prescribing: A method by which a prescriber can electronically send a prescription directly to a pharmacy from the physician's computer or handheld personal digital assistant (PDA) device.

Indian Health Service counseling: An agency of the federal government charged with health care services for Native Americans and Alaska natives. Its mission statement says: "Our mission . . . to raise the physical, mental, social, and spiritual health of American Indians and Alaska Natives to the highest level." In the 1960s, its officers developed a pharmacy-counseling model using open-ended questions. That model is now taught in all pharmacy colleges in the United States.

Verifiers: An electronic scanner that uses overlapping systems to verify that the drug in the finished prescription bottle is what was entered into the computer. The primary system is spectrographic analysis of the medication in the prescription bottle and comparison of it with a database of most commonly used drugs.

OUTLINE

Risk Management Tools
Best Practices
    The Case of Mrs. Franks—The Rest of the Story
    The Analysis
        Applying Tools: Mark It

The Case of Molly's Bedtime Overdose
    Applying Tools: Unusual Dose
    Applying Tools: Two Sets of Eyes
    Applying Tools: "Show and Tell" Counseling
    Preparing for Counseling
    Applying Tools: Prospective Drug Review

Collecting Knowledge to Assist in the Prospective Drug Review
Documentation—Protecting the Pharmacy
Applying Tools: "Take 5"
Everyone Corrects Their Own QRE
Triple Check
Placing Best Practices in the Workflow
Cool Tools
   Scanners
   Robot
      ScriptPro, LLC
      Parata Systems, LLC
   Verifying Systems—Pass Rx
E-Prescribing
Summary

Risk Management Tools

Earlier chapters introduced selected **best practices** that could be made a part of a pharmacy's workflow to stop or catch mistakes. This chapter expands the discussion and studies their development and use in a CQI workflow as well as other tools that can be used. Included are samples of electronic and robotic tools, which can themselves be considered best practices. These tools and best practices are an important part of most CQI workflows.

We study these tools in order to learn how best practices work and why they can reduce the risk of an error. While it may be beneficial for pharmacy technicians to study several best practices, it is much more important for them to understand the purpose and mechanism of risk-management tools. Most pharmacy technicians in their careers will need to adopt new practices that will improve the quality systems in the pharmacy environment in which they work.

Tools are adopted because they have proven their value in the past in preventing mistakes. However, the exact tool is less important than understanding why a particular tool or practice works and how it can be improved. Some of the tools discussed are simple forms that can help organize a particular task; others are sophisticated mechanisms such as robots and scanners. For example, one machine uses a spectrometry authentication sensor system to scan and test filled prescriptions before the medication is delivered to the patient. This machine can alert the pharmacist about any discrepancy or questions of accuracy.

Best Practices

Over the years, pharmacists and pharmacy technicians have learned different techniques to help them avoid mistakes. When one worked, they told their colleagues who would try them as well.

The most successful of these tricks and techniques, called "best practices" because they work, have been widely accepted by more and more members of the pharmacy community.

Best practices are usually simple techniques; they are not complicated. When you hear of one, you usually do not have to write it down. Instead, you might say, "Of course, why didn't I think of that!" This is why they work—they are simple and easy. In this chapter we will explore several best practices. Many you will put to use; many you already know; some will not fit your practice environment. The best practices discussed here do not form an exhaustive list, but are representative of those used in pharmacy today. For most there are no scientific test results proving they work. Best practices are proven by common sense and repeated use.

The Case of Mrs. Franks—The Rest of the Story

Most best practices begin with a mistake that usually becomes an error. Earlier we studied the case of Mrs. Franks, a 70-year-old patient who was prescribed warfarin 1 mg daily because of her atrial fibrillation. She took her medicine for 2 weeks, exactly as prescribed. When she accidently cut her finger with a knife, she could not stop the bleeding. In the emergency room it was discovered that her warfarin prescription, while correctly labeled as 1 mg, actually contained 5 mg warfarin tablets. The pharmacy's insurance company settled Mrs. Franks' claim against the pharmacy for her time, pain, suffering, and medical costs. After 15 years as a loyal customer, Mrs. Franks changed pharmacies.

That, however, should not have been the end of the story. Mrs. Franks' misadventures provide a valuable lesson that can be used by the pharmacy staff to improve the pharmacy's CQI workflow to prevent a repeat of similar incidents.

From this point on the story is hypothetical. We do not know what the real pharmacy did, or what their investigation found, or if they made any changes. Using the few facts we know, however, we can study steps to reduce the risk of errors occurring in the future. We begin with an analysis of what happened, and then end with the addition of best practices to the workflow.

The Analysis

We know the label was correct on Mrs. Franks' prescription, so the mistake was not made when the information for this new prescription was entered into the computer. It appears the wrong strength of warfarin was taken from the shelf at the time the prescription was filled. The mistake was not caught during the pharmacist's final check or during counseling. With these few facts, let us look at some best practices generally and apply them to Mrs. Franks' case. When studying these, ask how they work and what is the purpose of each.

Applying Tools: Mark It

In every pharmacy, certain drugs repeatedly cause problems. Pharmacists and technicians can often list certain drugs they consider particularly bothersome because they feel they are the ones most often involved in mistakes. Some drugs are a special concern because an error can cause particularly dangerous results. These drugs may not be the same for every pharmacy, but there are some that would appear in most pharmacies' lists. Such lists can be found in several places including the ISMP website and the Pharmacists Mutual Claims Study of Drugs Most Involved in Claims.

Pharmacists Mutual looked at several years (1996–2009) of mechanical-error claims for the drugs or classification of drugs involved most often in claims. The results are shown in Figure 6-1. The significance of the claims study is that it shows, not which drugs are most often involved in misfills, but which drugs are more likely to be involved in a claim. These are errors that cause significant injuries.

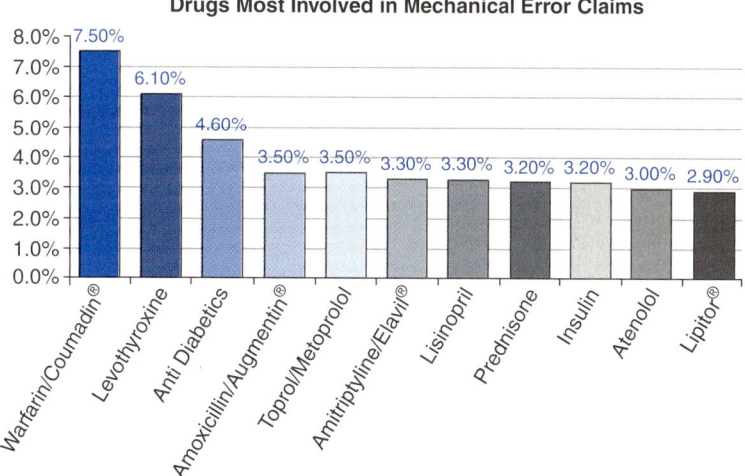

Figure 6-1 Pharmacists Mutual Claims Study: Drugs Most Involved in Mechanical-Error Claims
© 2011, Pharmacists Mutual Insurance Company, used with permission
http://www.phmic.com/phmc/services/RM/profliab/claimsstudy/Pages/DrugsMostInvolvedinMechanicalErrorClaims.aspx (accessed November 8, 2010)

To alert its staff that a selective list of drugs deserves special caution, a pharmacy can mark that part of the shelf containing these drugs in a manner that differentiates it from the hundreds of other drugs in the inventory. That is the simple idea behind "Mark It."

The pharmacy selects a limited number of drugs or categories that it decides should be double-checked before they are pulled from the shelf. All drugs will be subjected to a number of best practices and double and triple checks, but these drugs are given an additional check at the time they are taken from the shelf.

> **Quality Note 6-A   Be Selective Marking Shelves**
>
> When deciding which drugs should be highlighted, be careful not to mark too many. If too many drugs are selected for this special treatment, the marking may fail over time to fulfill its purpose because the selected drugs are no longer special.

The shelf can be marked by using brightly colored paint or tape applied along the shelf edge. This makes this shelf stand out. When reaching for a stock bottle on this marked shelf, the technician should be trained to stop, think—"This is a drug I need to be especially careful of when filling"—and check one more time. While this takes only a few seconds, it can reduce the risk of pulling the wrong drug or wrong strength.

Warfarin and Coumadin® serve as good examples of drugs that might be selected by pharmacies for the best practice "Mark It." The shelves with these drugs would be marked with a colored tape. Since warfarin accounts for over 7 percent of all mechanical-error claims, its selection for special attention appears likely. It is not just that warfarin is involved in claims against pharmacies, but, more importantly, the risk of injury is high if it is dispensed incorrectly. It is unlikely that there are more mistakes with warfarin than with other drugs; there may be fewer. But if a mistake is made with this drug, it is more likely to be significant.

In Mrs. Franks' case, the most likely scenario is that a technician or pharmacist took the 5 mg stock bottle of warfarin from the shelf rather than the 1 mg bottle. The same person probably opened the bottle and counted out the required number of tablets. Again, the technician did not notice the mistake. There were other places where this mistake should have been caught. Each of these missed opportunities was a quality related event (QRE) and a mistake.

> **RxErcise 6-A   How Many Mistakes Make an Error?**
>
> Review what you know about Mrs. Franks' case. List how many mistakes it took to get the prescription from computer-entry through to the time Mrs. Franks took the medicine.

If the shelf in front of the warfarin stock bottle had been conspicuously marked with red colored tape, there was a chance the person filling it would have stopped and checked one more time. Marking the shelf may not have helped in avoiding the error, but the risk of the error occurring would have been reduced. No best practice will avoid all errors, and for that reason several are used in a well-designed CQI workflow. The National Alliance of State Pharmacy Associations' (NASPA) Sentinel System™, which is the workflow part of its Pharmacy Quality Commitment® quality system, uses over 20 best practices. Many of them are used more than once. It is the combination of best practices that makes a system successful.

> **Quality Note 6-B   Using Multiple Best Practices to Stop One Error**
>
> Study Figure 6-1, the case of Molly's bedtime overdose, and Quality Note 6-A. Consider the drug amitriptyline. Note the second-best practice used for the same purpose. This case illustrates the use of multiple best practices.
>
> Most amitriptyline claims involve a prescription for amitriptyline 10 mg incorrectly filled with amitriptyline 100 mg.[1] In this case, the pharmacy may decide to mark only the 100 mg strength stock bottle in a manner designed to draw attention to it. The pharmacy may decide not to mark the entire shelf containing the other strengths. In this case it added a second-best practice. Why would the pharmacy use both?

The Case of Molly's Bedtime Overdose

Molly had been depressed, so her physician wrote a prescription for amitriptyline 10 mg with the directions to take three tablets at bedtime.[2] The information was entered into the computer correctly, but when the technician pulled the product from the shelf, he pulled a bottle of 100 mg amitriptyline instead of 10 mg. Both the technician and the pharmacist who checked the prescription missed the error.

That night Molly took three tablets as indicated on the label. Instead of the intended 30 mg dosage at bedtime, she took 300 mg. The next morning Molly's husband was unable to wake her and called "911." Molly woke up in the ambulance on the way to the hospital.

Below we will use Molly's case as an example of "Applying Tools: Unusual Dose." Complete RxErcise 6-B.

Applying Tools: Unusual Dose

The incident with Molly illustrates how several best practices may overlap and serve the same purpose. When we discussed the duties of pharmacy technicians in Chapter 2, we described information the technician could note when receiving a new prescription. The list included:

- allergy information
- other drugs being taken by the patient
- patient's address and phone number

- date of birth, with a note if the patient is under 6 or over 60 years old
- any unusual dose (any medication taken other than orally or taken more than two at a time)

In the case of Molly's bedtime overdose, the claim gave rise to the best practice of instructing the intake technician to note any "unusual dose" on the prescription. Three doses of any drug at one time would fit this definition. Pharmacy technicians can be trained to identify potential problems such as an "unusual dose." The dose could be wrong and the pharmacist may wish to discuss it with the prescriber and the patient.

RxErcise 6-B Molly's Prescription

Study Molly's prescription in Figure 6-2.
- Discuss the items the technician has written on the new prescription.
- What purpose is served by each of the technician's notations?

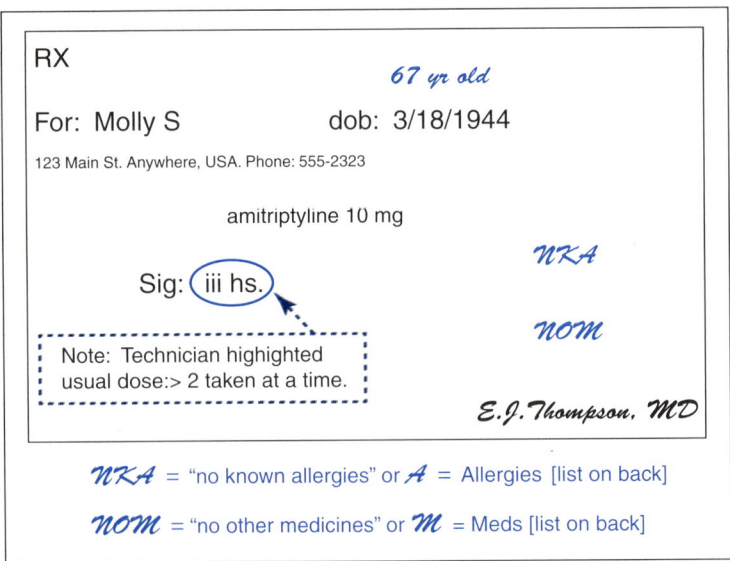

Figure 6-2 Molly's Prescription
© Cengage Learning 2013

The "unusual dose" best practice alerts the intake technician to highlight the dose, by drawing a circle around it, so that everyone in the workflow will know to give this prescription an even higher level of scrutiny than normal prescriptions. Each of the best practice notations added by the technician serve a similar purpose.

Applying Tools: Two Sets of Eyes

Earlier we reviewed the respective duties of pharmacists and pharmacy technicians. In today's pharmacy, with the increased demands on pharmacists' time, the jobs of receiving the prescription, entering the information into the computer, and filling the prescription have increasingly gravitated to the pharmacy technician. The pharmacists' job more and more is centered on checking the completed prescription, performing a prospective drug review on the prescription, and counseling the patient. Another reason for this division of labor is the advantage of using two sets of eyes. If the pharmacist both fills and checks a prescription, the two stations tend to blend into one, rather than remaining as two separate operations.

Applying Tools: "Show and Tell" Counseling

Every patient who leaves a pharmacy with a prescription is most likely to receive its best benefits if she or he knows certain things about the medication, for example, how to take it, what it was prescribed for, and what side effects may occur while she or he is taking it. With some prescriptions additional information will need to be provided to the patient. Physicians should have discussed these items with their patients and should have answered all of their questions before they left the office. The problem is this does not always happen. This is why pharmacist counseling is important. While counseling is a job only for the pharmacist, pharmacy technicians should understand the process if they are to assist the pharmacist's preparation.

A counseling technique taught in pharmacy schools is the Indian Health Service approach of asking questions of patients to determine what they know about their medication. This allows the pharmacist to "fill in the blanks." **Indian Health Service counseling** asks these three questions[3]:

1. What did your physician tell you this was for?

2. How did your physician tell you to take it?

3. What side effects did your physician tell you to expect while taking this medicine?

Counseling used in combination with a best practice called "Show and Tell" has also proven to be an effective way to catch mechanical medication errors. It involves a pharmacist removing the prescription bottle from the bag and showing it to the patient. The pharmacist may read part of the label to the patient at this time, particularly the name of the medication and the directions. This practice provides an extra check on two common errors: wrong patient and wrong directions. The pharmacist may open the cap of the bottle and show the tablets or capsules to the patient. While doing so, the pharmacist asks the Indian Health Service questions. Showing the drug to the patient provides an additional check for the pharmacist and allows the patient to connect the appearance of the drug with its purpose. While not all mechanical errors could be caught in this manner, many could.

Mrs. Franks' case provides a good example of the value of "Show and Tell" counseling. Right before Mrs. Franks received her prescription that contained warfarin 5 mg instead of the correct 1 mg, the pharmacist would have counseled the patient. If the pharmacist performed limited counseling and said only, "This is your warfarin, an anticoagulant (or a blood thinner); take one tablet a day," this error would probably not have been caught.

If the pharmacist used "Show and Tell" with Indian Health Service counseling, this error could have been caught. The pharmacist might have read the label to the patient: "Mrs. Franks, this is your warfarin 1 mg; it is a blood thinner (or anticoagulant). The directions are to take one tablet daily." The pharmacist might then have opened the lid, shown Mrs. Franks the tablets inside, and, at the same time, asked the three questions. Because most pharmacists would visually recognize the difference between a 5 mg warfarin tablet and a 1 mg warfarin tablet, there is a chance this error could have been caught.

Preparing for Counseling

Technicians can help the pharmacist by preparing for "Show and Tell" counseling. The technician can make sure all of the patient's prescriptions are in a basket. The basket could have a note on it indicating the number of prescriptions for this patient or family (although each family member should have a separate basket). The note could make sure all prescriptions are delivered at the same time. Depending on the pharmacy's workflow, the technician may be directed to avoid stapling the prescription bag shut when "Show and Tell" counseling is to be used.

The pharmacy may not use "Show and Tell" or Indian Health Service counseling for all new prescriptions. There may be a list of criteria the pharmacy uses to determine when these techniques are needed, and it may be the job of the pharmacy technician to recognize which prescriptions fit the criteria and to alert the pharmacist. The technician may affix a note to the basket or use a special colored basket so the pharmacist will be sure to see it during the quality check.

Applying Tools: Prospective Drug Review

Like counseling, prospective drug review is not within the job description of the technician, but the technician may be able to assist the pharmacist in preparation for this step in the workflow. Prospective drug review[4] looks at a prescription in relation to the other drugs the patient is taking, a patient's condition, and the patient's disease. The pharmacist may need additional information contained in the patient's profile that may already be in the computer. It is call "prospective" because it is performed before the prescription is dispensed to the patient.

> **Quality Note 6-C   DUR and Prospective Drug Review**
>
> The term drug utilization review (DUR) will frequently be used as a synonym for "prospective drug review" or "prospective drug utilization review." The terms are used interchangeably in this text.
>
> However, pharmacy technicians may hear pharmacists use the terms to refer to different acts. A DUR is sometimes considered a *retrospective* view at how drugs are being utilized by the patient. In this context, a DUR looks at how a drug or combination of drugs is working. The pharmacist's DUR takes place *after* the prescription has been dispensed to the patient and after the patient has taken at least some of the drug. A *prospective* drug review takes place *before* the prescription is dispensed.

Collecting Knowledge to Assist in the Prospective Drug Review

The prescription in Figure 6-3 uses Mrs. Franks' prescription as an example, showing both the front and the back. Compare Figures 6-2 and 6-3. Notice Mrs. Franks answered the receiving technician's questions differently when she presented the prescription, indicating to the technician that she had an allergy to aspirin. This may not have been an actual allergy as we generally think of that term. She may have misunderstood her physician's directions when told to avoid aspirin while taking warfarin.

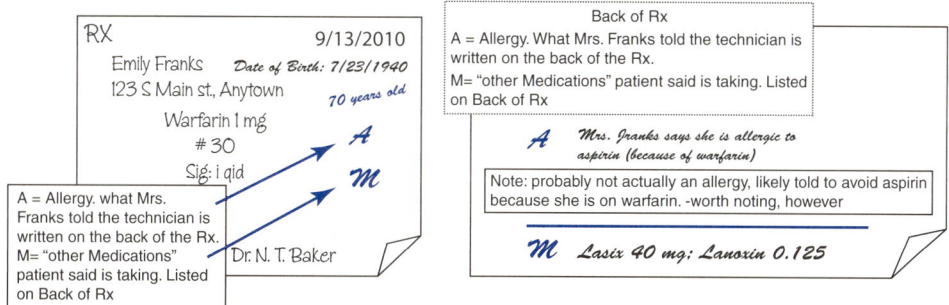

Figure 6-3 Rx with Best Practices—Collecting Information
© Cengage Learning 2013

It is common to tell warfarin patients to avoid aspirin. Aspirin also has an *anticoagulant effect* and the combination of aspirin and warfarin may result in increased anticoagulation. Mrs. Franks may have understood this as the combination "thinning" the blood too much. Note in Figure 6-3 that Mrs. Franks also told the technician she is taking other medications. Since Mrs. Franks had been getting all of her prescriptions at this pharmacy, these drugs may already have been in the computer. There should be a similar note on the back of each new prescription Mrs. Franks has presented to the pharmacy. The data-entry technician checks each time to be sure the information in the computer is correct. OTC drugs, vitamins, and herbals are also drugs and should be noted. Some of these may not have been in the computer on the day Mrs. Franks presented her warfarin prescription.

Figure 6-3 provides an illustration of information collected by a technician that could assist the pharmacist in preparing for a prospective drug review. By collecting selected information from the patient, the technician has made as certain as he or she can that allergy and other medication information in the computer is as up to date as possible.

Documentation—Protecting the Pharmacy

In Figures 6-2 and 6-3, there is also documentation of what the patients told the technician when the prescriptions were presented. The patient in Figure 6-2 told the technician she was not taking other medication and did not have any allergies. Mrs. Franks said she was.

For purposes of an illustration, presume Mrs. Franks had said she was not taking other medication because she did not want to tell the pharmacy technician she had filled a prescription for fluconazole, an anti-fungal drug, through a mail-order pharmacy. Since this prescription was filled at a different pharmacy, it was not in our pharmacy's records. Fluconazole can react with warfarin. In one case a woman who was well maintained on warfarin with a good INR of 2.3[5] saw her INR increase to 14, which is dangerously high, after she began taking fluconazole. Unaware of Mrs. Franks taking fluconazole, our pharmacist would be performing a prospective drug review with incomplete information.

The technician's notation of what Mrs. Franks said when she presented her prescription could protect the pharmacy from a lawsuit for failure to warn Mrs. Franks of the danger of taking these two drugs at the same time. The technician's documentation provides proof the pharmacist could not warn Mrs. Franks because she was not truthful. It is evidence that the pharmacist was not negligent. Proper documentation is important in pharmacy-risk management.

By adding the collected information to a patient's profile, the technician has made sure the information is up to date. The pharmacist will need to know what is in the profile during the prospective drug review. There may be a computer terminal at the final check and drug review stations, which are often combined into one. If there is a terminal at the DUR station, the technician can pull up the patient profile and the scanned prescription, if it is part of the pharmacy's resources, for the pharmacist. Some pharmacies do not have a computer terminal at the final check and drug review area. In those cases, some pharmacies may have the computer-entry technician print a copy of the patient's profile and any warnings given by the computer. These are put into the patient's basket and delivered to the pharmacist at the final check and drug review stations.

If there were to be any interactions with Mrs. Franks' medication or allergies, the computer should have provided an alarm that there was a potential problem. The pharmacy technician at the computer-entry station must call the pharmacist whenever there is such a warning. The case of Heidi Happel (*Happel v. Wal-Mart*) described in Chapter 2 provides an example of what can happen if this does not occur.

Applying Tools: "Take 5"

Apply "Take 5" to Mrs. Franks' case. As the prescription moves from one station to another, it should be checked by the person receiving it at each station so that a mistake can be caught. "Take 5" is the first step at each station. For example, the technician entering the prescription information into the computer first checks ("Take 5") information received from the prescription-receiving station. For a new prescription, the entry technician knows the prescription received should resemble the ones in Figures 6-2 and 6-3.

Similarly, the technician getting ready to fill the prescription at the assembly or filling station first checks ("Take 5") to see if the prescription label and receipt are correct. The filling technician is looking to see if the label contains:

1. the right patient (including address, phone number, etc.)
2. the right route of administration (e.g., otic, ophthalmic)
3. the right directions (e.g., one daily or one four times daily)[6]
4. the right drug
5. the right strength

By one account, up to 40 percent of all mistakes may be made at the computer-entry station.[7] Review the information in Figure 4–6 regarding computer-entry QREs recorded by a group of pharmacies using a PMC Quality Commitment, Inc. system to track near-misses and errors. The information is not statistically valid for all pharmacies, but it is useful for our purposes. Computer-entry QREs in these pharmacies accounted for 42 percent of all mistakes for this time period.

Figure 6-4 shows that mistakes can and do happen throughout the workflow. The advantage of "Take 5" is that it provides additional checks at several points. NASPA's Sentinel System™, a part of the Pharmacy Quantity Commitment® quality-assurance system, uses "Take 5" three times with every prescription.

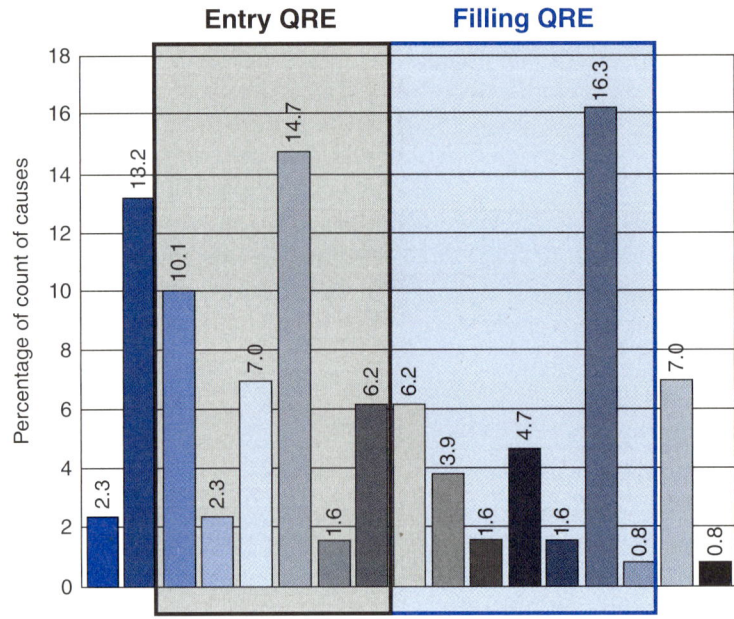

Figure 6-4 Ninety-Day Study of Causes of QREs in Selected Pharmacies
© Cengage Learning 2013

If a "Take 5" performed by the technician filling the prescription catches a mistake made during data entry, the information in the computer will need to be corrected and the label will need to be redone. Presume, for example, that instead of the correct 0.125 mg strength of a digoxin prescription being entered into the computer, the label checked by the filling technician during "Take 5" read "digoxin 0.25 mg." A potential error has been avoided, but now time is required to fix the mistake. Each time a quality-related event is found, time will be required to redo the prescription. Correcting mistakes takes time.

If, however, the error in this example was not caught until the pharmacist's final check, the entire prescription would have to be redone, rather than just the computer entry. For each near-miss, the pharmacy must, in essence, fill one more prescription for free. "Take 5," like all best practices, invests seconds to save minutes. Imagine that the prescription had reached the patient. According to the Auburn University College of Pharmacy observational study discussed earlier, this happens 3 million times a year.[8] Even if the patient discovered the mistake before taking it, loss of time dealing with the error is expanded greatly. Loss of time, however, is not the greatest concern when an error reaches a patient. The patient is the primary concern. Time and efficiency in a pharmacy are, nevertheless, important.

Everyone Corrects His or Her Own QRE

It seems mean to say, "It's your mistake. You fix it." It is, however, the best way to be certain everyone learns and improves. This best practice, perhaps, belongs in the chapter on training, but it is also a best practice that should be incorporated into the pharmacy's policies and procedures and thus into the workflow. For example, when performing "Take 5," a computer-entry technician notices from the birth date on the prescription that the patient is 73 years old, but the new prescription does not have an indication that this patient is over 60. Under the best practice of "Under 6 / Over 60," the patient's age should have been written in red or another distinctive color (review again the prescriptions in Figures 6-2 and 6-3).

The easiest and least time-consuming way to correct this problem is for the computer-entry technician to pick up a red pen and write "73 years old" on the prescription. While the immediate problem would be solved, an opportunity for the receiving technician to learn would be lost. Time would be saved this time, but more time will be lost in the future if the other technician is not given an opportunity to learn.

We all learn best when we learn of our mistakes and are required to take time to correct them. While it is not always possible, the best practice is to return the item to the person who made the mistake and allow him or her to correct it and learn. When doing so, it must be made clear this is not punishment or a way to chastise the person who made the mistake, but is a part of the pharmacy's training program.

Triple Check

"Triple check" means there are three checks made by the filling technician before the finished prescription is presented to the pharmacist for checking. As part of the workflow, the three checks are always made at the same time and place.

1. When pulling a stock bottle from the shelf, the filling technician checks the name on the new prescription with the name on the stock bottle. If the prescription order is a refill and

the original prescription is not available,[9] the check is made against the information on the printed receipt.

2. When the stock bottle is taken to the prescription counter, the technician checks again the name on the stock bottle against the name on the prescription.

3. After the bottle is filled, another name on the bottle versus the name on the prescription check is made.

Several additional checks will still be performed before the prescription is presented to the patient. At a point in the filling, according to the designed workflow, the technician makes a check of the NDC number on the label against the NDC number printed on the receipt, or the technician scans the bar code on each as a check. Figure 6-5 shows a simplified illustration of a name and NDC check.

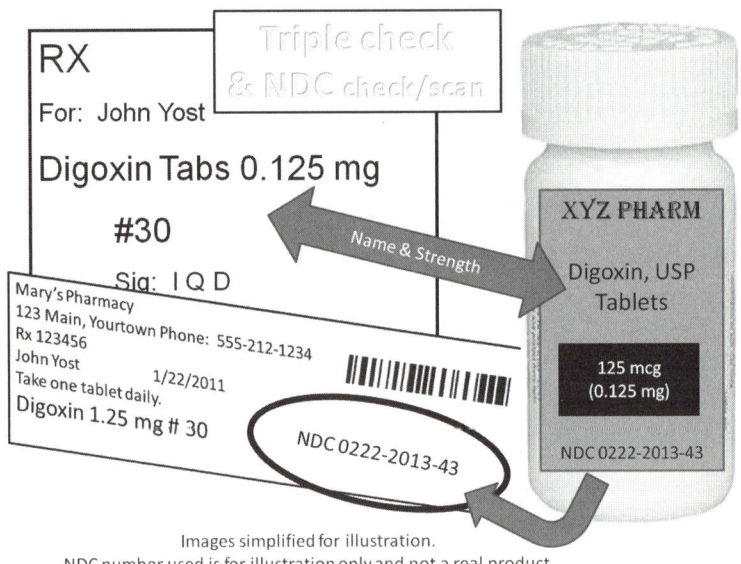

Images simplified for illustration.
NDC number used is for illustration only and not a real product

Figure 6-5 Triple Check and NDC Check or Scan
© Cengage Learning 2013

RxErcise 6-C   How Can Errors Still Be Made?

Note many redundancies are built into the workflow. If each check is made each time, it should be difficult for a mechanical medication-dispensing error to reach a patient.

But we know that, despite all of this, errors are made every day in pharmacies across the country. Be prepared to discuss why.

Placing Best Practices in the Workflow

In this chapter we have discussed several best practices. These are not the only best practices that can or should be introduced into a pharmacy's workflow. The purpose of studying them is not to learn a few tricks that can reduce the risk of medication errors. The purpose is to help technicians and pharmacists discover why and how best practices can be used in pharmacy.

Once the pharmacy has decided which best practices to include in its workflow, it must map the flow from the beginning to the end, train its staff in its use, and then determine if the plan is working. Are medication errors being prevented or are some still being made? This part of the program involves monitoring. When a pharmacy monitors, it looks for other mistakes that are still being made so that it can continue to make the system better. This is why CQI is called "continuous" quality improvement.

Cool Tools

The best practices studied thus far have mainly involved manual checks by human beings. Many of these checks can be done through the use of electronics and optical units. More and more of the functions of filling prescriptions can be accomplished using computers and machines. These tools do not make human errors. Machines can perform the same task over and over without becoming bored and without skipping steps. Machines do not feel pressured to work faster. They do their jobs in the same manner whether there are two people in line or 23.

As humans we build habits that help us resist the temptations to skip a step and leave something out of the process. Machines cannot doing many of the things human beings can, but they can perform repetitive, mechanical tasks and do them the same way each time.

In the next few years, more machines will be introduced into the practice of pharmacy. These can reduce the risks associated with certain errors, but they may also introduce other problems. In this section we will look at some of the machines, robots, electronics, and optical scanners that pharmacy technicians will see in practice. This is only a skimming of the topic and an introduction to the area. Many of the gadgets and gizmos that will be commonplace in a few years have not been built yet. Examples used do not constitute an endorsement of the products or assert that one is better than its competitors. Examples are used here only as examples.

Scanners

Bar code scanners have been in use in hospital and community pharmacies for many years. In essence they are bar code readers that verify the bar code on the stock package matches the bar code printed by the computer.

Several companies manufacture and sell pharmacy scanners. The example shown in Figure 6-6 is from the RxScan® family of products from Retail Management Products, Ltd. This company has been marketing scanners for pharmacy use for over a decade. Started by a pharmacist, it began with simple scanner applications and has recently introduced more sophisticated systems. The RxScan Plus Prescription Verifier®, shown in Figure 6-6, is described by the company as,

> ... a battery operated, handheld, portable computer with a built in laser bar code scanner. It is not tied to any other computer and with its self-contained programming, can be carried and used at any location during the Rx filling and and verifying process.[10]

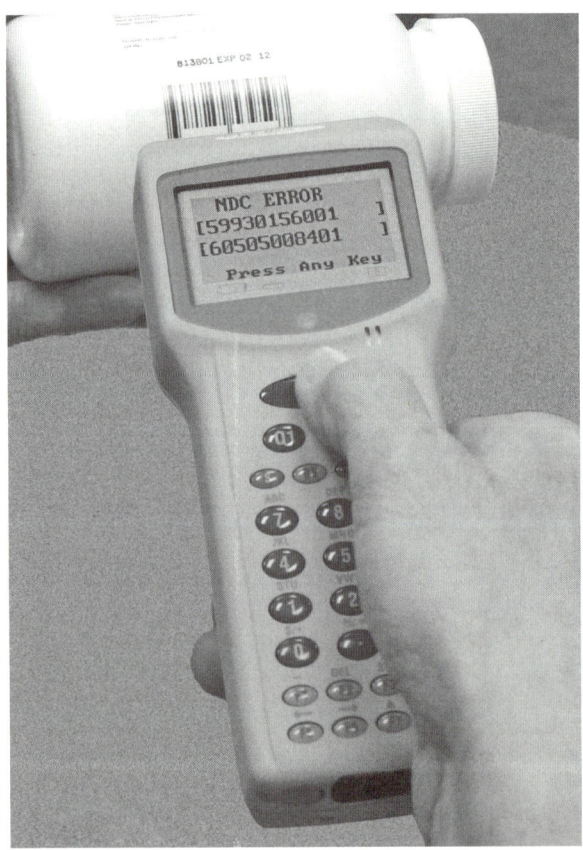

Figure 6-6 Rx Scan
Source: Retail Management Products, Ltd.

The field is changing rapidly. A later version of a scanning application from the same company, shown in Figure 6-7, describes a product that provides much more information. The company describes the later version as follows:

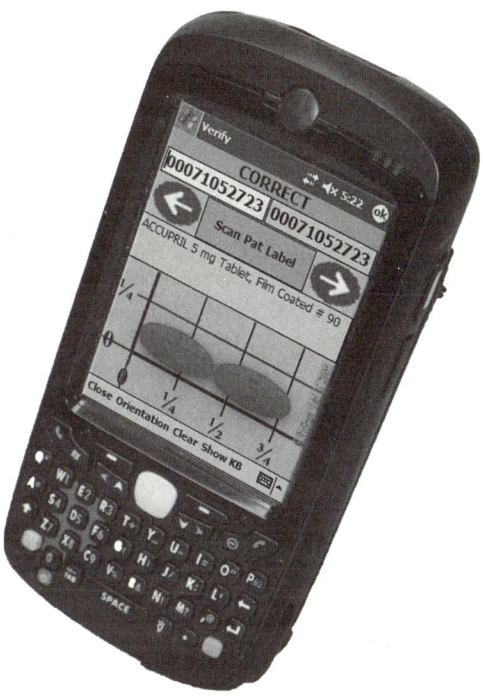

Figure 6-7 RxScan Ultra Prescription Verifier
Source: Retail Management Products, Ltd.

The RxScan Ultra Prescription Verifier *has been designed to save prescription-filling time and to reduce prescription errors caused by the prescription being filled with the wrong medication, strength, or dosage form.* The user scans a NDC number bar code on the patient label or receipt and then the NDC number bar code on the stock drug container from which the prescription is to be filled. Using a patented process the RxScan Ultra then compares the two NDC numbers and visually and audibly alerts the user as to whether the NDC numbers match. When the match is correct the display will show a picture of the correct product.

The color product display speeds up the final checking process. Without having to open the manufacturer's container, the pharmacist can match the content of the patient's bottle with a picture of the correct product on-screen.

There is little doubt that the use of scanners can reduce mechanical errors. In a November 2009 article in *Pharmacy News*, author Mark Gertskis quoted the Pharmacy Board of South Australia registrar, Peter Halstead, as crediting bar code scanners with reducing by half the number of "human selection" medication errors at the point of dispensing.[11]

Robots

Another advance in medication-error reduction in pharmacy has been the rise in the use of robotics. More and more, robots are being used for dispensing in both hospitals and retail pharmacies. They have grown in sophistication and will continue to evolve. Early models of robots merely counted tablets from individual, prefilled bins. While they added convenience and were more efficient, they were limited in their ability to reduce the risk of errors. Newer robots can fill the prescriptions, prepare the labels, and place the labels on the prescription bottle. Several companies have been important in the introduction of robots in the pharmacy market. As examples, we will look at two, ScriptPro, and Parata Systems.

ScriptPro, LLC

One of the leading manufacturers of prescription robotics in the United States is ScriptPro, LLC. The company makes several sizes of robots for hospital and community pharmacies. One of ScriptPro's products is called "SPUD," for SP Unit Dispenser, Robotic Pharmaceutical Dispensing System, shown in Figure 6-8. The company describes the benefits of this particular robot as follows[12]:

> SPUD is a prescription-dispensing system that automatically loads, stores, and delivers unit-of-use and prepacked products using bar code technology. The system holds up to 700 products in a small footprint, reducing pharmacy traffic and increasing filling accuracy.
>
> To dispense a product, SPUD verifies the requested product code sent from the pharmacy management system against products loaded in the SPUD. Once a match is made, SPUD quickly delivers the product at the rate of up to 225 prescriptions per hour. A user then scans the product bar code, prints the prescription label, and applies it to the product.
>
> Products are loaded into SPUD with one product bar code scan. Regardless of the order in which the products are placed on the loading conveyor, SPUD automatically stores like products together based on shelf availability.

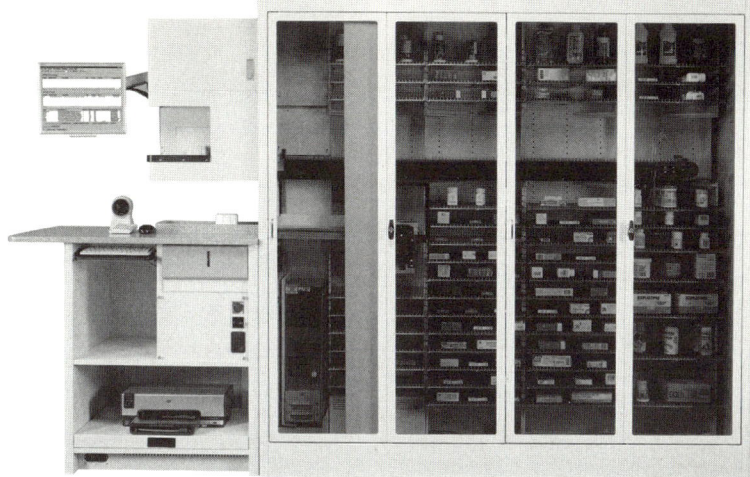

Figure 6-8 ScriptPro SPUD
Source: ScriptPro, LLC

For maximum throughput, SPUD interrupts the loading process to dispense medications, and during downtime, consolidates similar products on shelves.

SPUD assists with inventory management and cost control by displaying configurable inventory overage and shortage alerts. SPUD also manages product- and shelf-expiration dates.

Parata Systems, LLC

A second company that is competing for the pharmacy robot market in the United States is Parata Systems, LLC. As of 2011, Parata listed two products on its website: the Parata Max and the Parata Mini. The larger robot, the Parata Max (see Figure 6-9), indicates it "selects the correct cell for dispensing 100 percent of the time . . . when proper processes are followed by the pharmacy." It does this, the company says, by using "bar coding to verify a match between the inventory bottle NDC, unique to medication and strength, and the bar code on the dispensing cell."

Parata Systems touts its safety by listing several ways in which the Parata Max "improves the safety of your dispensing operations." The company, in making its claims of 100% accuracy, notes, "Parata automation uses bar-coding to verify a match between the inventory bottle NDC, unique to medication and strength, and the barcode on the dispensing cell. Parata automation selects the correct cell for dispensing 100 percent of the time, ensuring accurate drug and

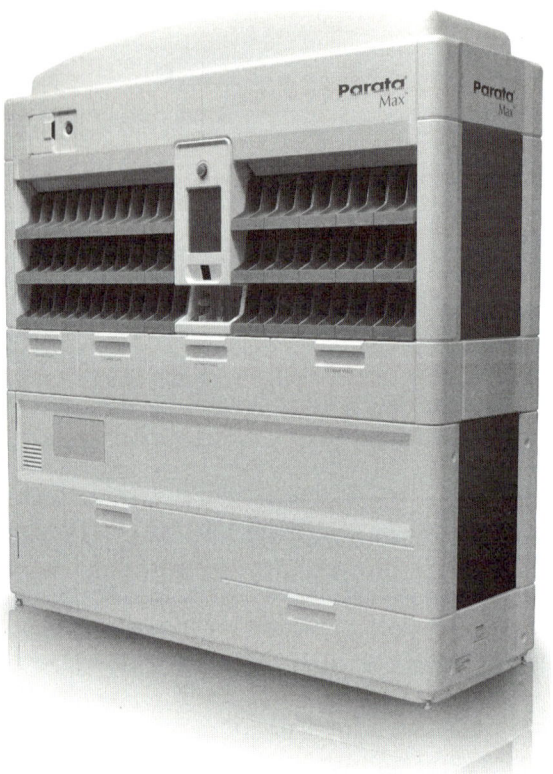

Figure 6-9 Parata Robot
Source: Parata Systems, LLC

total dosage when proper processes are followed by the pharmacy." Among the claims made are:

100 percent accuracte for drug and strength.

Parata Max® is 100 percent accurate for drug and strength. Scan the bar code on the stock bottle and then on the dispensing cell to confirm a match. Audible and visual warnings alert the technician to a potential error.

More time for specialty services.

When Max is dispensing up to 60 percent of your total prescription volume with 100 percent accuracy, your pharmacy team has more time to provide value-added services, such as medication therapy management, compounding, or vaccinations.

Increased time for DUR and counseling.

When you free time from dispensing activities, your team has more time to conduct thorough drug utilization reviews and provide patient counseling. The results are evidenced through improvements in error avoidance and patient adherence.

Highest counting accuracy.

Parata's cell counting accuracy is 10 times higher than the industry standard, ensuring your patients get the right medication in the right strength every time.

GREENGUARD certification.

Parata Max is GREENGUARD® certified for indoor air quality, having met the even more stringent Children and Schools^{SM} certification.

Both Parata and ScriptPro have been successful in marketing their robots to the pharmacy market. Eventually, additional companies will enter the market. The robots are very good at doing their programmed function the same way each time. The problems have usually arisen from human error.

A problem that has been seen with robots is that they can be taken for granted, when everyone assumes each prescription is correct and checking becomes lax. The robots fill only what they are instructed to fill. As we discussed earlier, a large percentage of the pharmacy mistakes occur at the computer-entry station. Since the information is inputted directly into the robot, the pharmacy may miss the "Take 5" check of the data-entry process, comparing the label and prescription information by the filling technician. The robot cannot perform this function, so the pharmacist's final check becomes more critical. If there is a tendency for the pharmacist to check output from the robot less strenuously, mistakes can be missed.

Another problem is the robots in many pharmacies are used for only about 60 percent of the drugs in the inventory. While this may allow pharmacy technicians to concentrate on prescriptions that call for less-used drug products, it may cause problems if pharmacy staff looks at these prescriptions as less important or as interruptions in the daily flow. Also, some technicians have complained that when the robots are not working, either because of maintenance or malfunctions, the workflow becomes confusing. Prescriptions that would normally be filled quickly by the robot now must be filled manually. Mistakes can be made in this stressed environment. Despite any faults robotics may have, however, they are here to stay and will become increasingly incorporated into pharmacy practice. The fact that they may create new problems is not surprising. Pharmacy technicians will need to develop newer best practices to accommodate them. There is no doubt they can reduce the number of medication errors when used properly and carefully.

Verifying Systems—Pass Rx

Among the newest electronic quality products are **verifiers**, prescription-verifying systems. There are several and in the future there will be more, but here we will discuss one, the Pass Rx® Verifier by Centice, LLC[13] (see Figure 6-10).

The Pass Rx® Verifier may be used by the pharmacy technician prior to delivering the completed prescription to the pharmacist for checking, or may be used by the pharmacist as part of the pharmacist's final check process. The Pass Rx® uses overlapping systems to verify that the drug in the finished prescription bottle is what was entered into the computer. One of the methods of verification is by a camera that uses, according to the company, "patented spectroscopy technology." It performs a spectrographic analysis of the medication

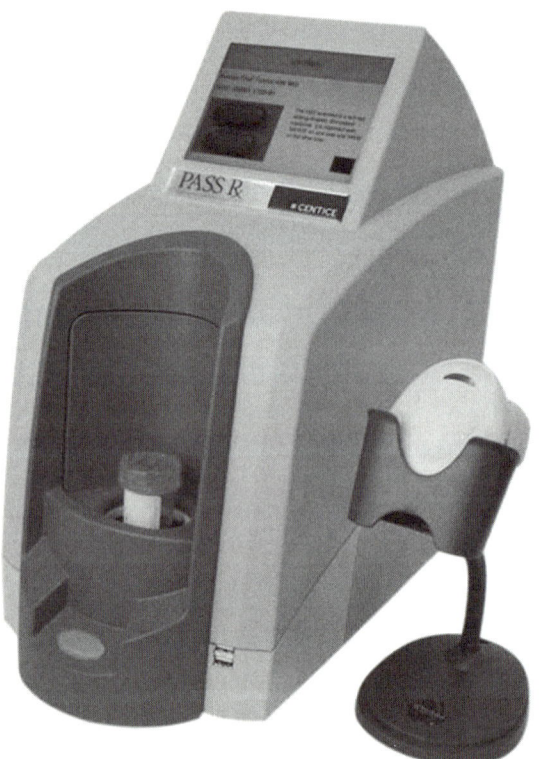

Figure 6-10 Pass Rx Verifier
Source: Centice Corporation

in the prescription bottle and compares it with a database of almost all commonly used drugs. It also provides the pharmacist with a picture of what the correct drug should look like by using a bar code scanner that is set next to the Pass Rx® Verifier. Along with the picture of the correct drug is a notice to the user, which appears on the LCD screen, that is part of the Pass Rx. These notices are visible at the top of the machine. Samples of the readings are shown in Figures 6-11, 6-12, and 6-13.

The Pass Rx® Verifier screen tells the reader when the prescription passes and when it fails. A failed reading means the drug in the prescription bottle does not match the one entered into the computer. The Pass Rx® Verifier can be used to scan new or refill prescriptions. The machine also provides a message when the count is too low for verification and when the Pass Rx® cannot determine if the drug is correct. This "cannot determine" message occurs if the drug in the prescription bottle is not in the database. The company says this does not happen often. It also occurs when the packaging is one that the machine cannot read such as a birth-control pack.

The verification reportedly takes about six seconds. During this time the reader can check the directions and patient information. Six seconds do not provide enough time to perform a drug review. Note in Figures 6-11, 6-12, and 6-13 that the Pass Rx® Verifier also has a camera that takes a picture of the contents of the bottle. All of the information can be downloaded to the company where it can be stored.

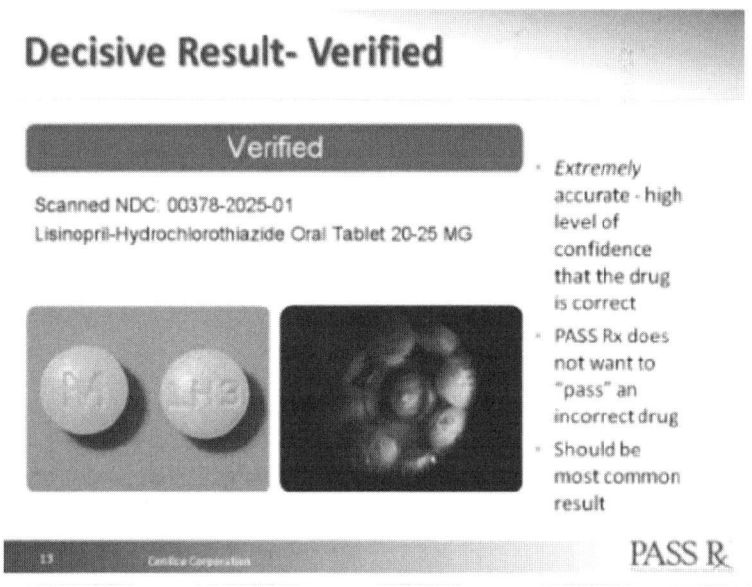

Figure 6-11 Rx Correct, Verified
Source: Centice Corporation

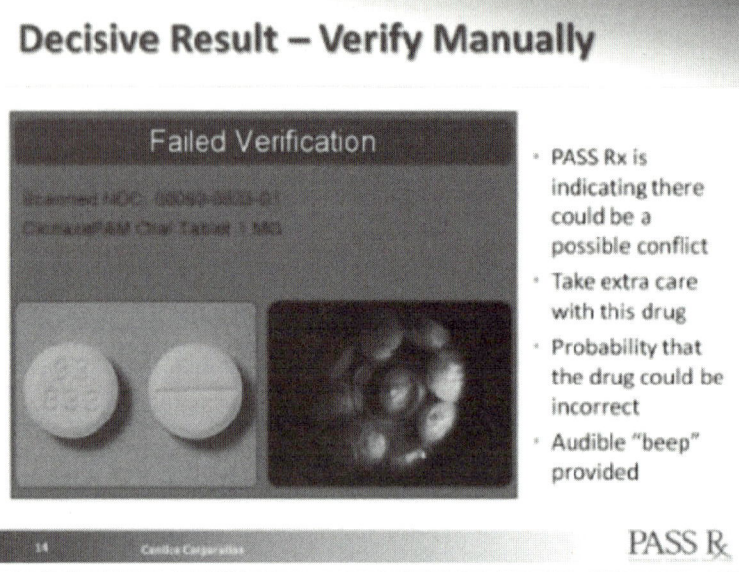

Figure 6-12 Rx Correct, Failed
Source: Centice Corporation

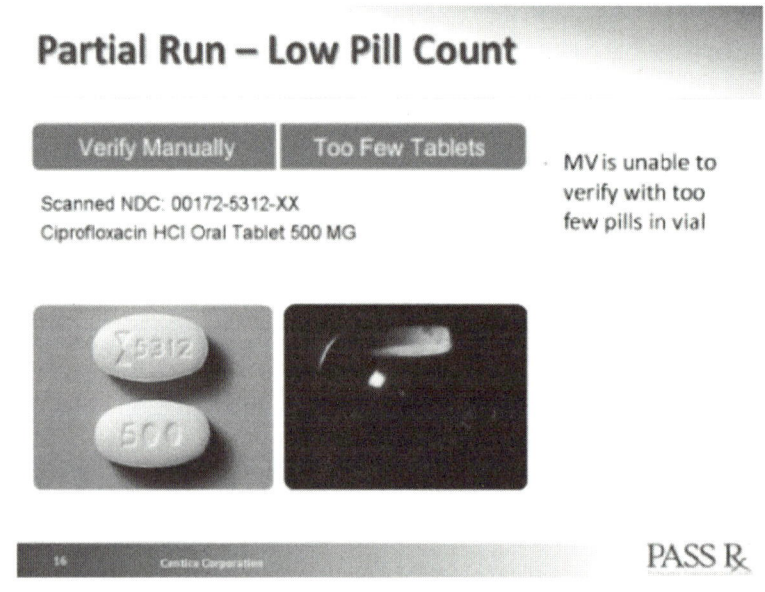

Figure 6-13 Rx Questioned
Source: Centice Corporation

The information can be retrieved if needed later. This documentation can provide proof that the prescription was correct at the time it was filled. The information can also be used to analyze the pharmacy's accuracy rate as part of the monitoring of the quality system.

E-Prescribing

The possibility of the widespread use and acceptance of **electronic prescribing** has been touted for years as promising fewer errors due to the ability for a prescriber to enter a drug order directly into a pharmacy's computer system. This would, it is claimed, reduce the number of wrong drug claims since, as its supporters presume, many errors are caused by the inability of pharmacists and pharmacy technicians to correctly read and interpret the physician's order. While physicians' handwriting is legendarily bad, it is unknown how many of the medication errors each year are caused by this factor.

The **Centers for Medicare and Medicaid Services (CMS)** believes that e-prescribing is an important element in patient safety. On its website it says: "A prescriber's ability to electronically send an accurate, error-free, and understandable prescription directly to a pharmacy from the point-of-care is an important element in improving the quality of patient care."

E-prescribing remains voluntary, but, under Medicare Part D, prescribers will be given incentives for adopting it. Soon those who do not use some form of e-prescribing will be penalized. Written prescriptions will eventually either cease to exist or be reduced to emergency situations. This may take several years to accomplish.

One of the leading networks providing e-prescribing is Sure-Scripts, which lists the following benefits of e-prescribing[14]:

"Cleaner" and more accurate prescriptions

Prescribers can confirm prescription-benefit information prior to sending an e-prescription; therefore there is no need for the pharmacist to verify these details.

Improved patient safety

Prescribers can check for harmful drug interactions by reviewing patient medication history at the point of care. And because there is no handwriting for the pharmacist to interpret, there is less potential for errors caused by similar-sounding drug names.

Lower health care costs for everyone involved

E-prescribing via the Surescripts network makes it easier for prescribers to select medications that are preferred by the patient's health plan, that meet therapeutic guidelines, and are cost effective for the patient. E-prescribing also helps drive down health care costs by reducing the potential for medication errors.

For pharmacies specifically, SureScripts says there will be "fewer callbacks, less keying and rework, and more time for pharmacy staff to do the things that matter."[15] Other professional organizations, including ISMP and AMA, also believe e-prescribing will reduce medication errors.

E-prescribing is more than the transmission of prescriptions. SureScripts provides a broader consideration of what it is, saying,

> E-prescribing occurs when a prescriber uses a computer or handheld device with software that enables a prescriber to:
>
> ***Electronically Access That Patient's Prescription Benefit:*** Electronically accessing a patient's prescription-benefit information—both formulary and eligibility—allows prescribers to choose medications that are on formulary and are covered by the patient's drug benefit. Prescribers can also choose lower-cost alternatives such as generic drugs. Dispensing pharmacies are less likely to receive prescriptions that require changes based on the patient's drug benefit, which, in turn, reduces unnecessary phone calls from pharmacy staff to physician practices regarding drug coverage.
>
> ***With a Patient's Consent, Electronically Access That Patient's Medication History:*** Electronically accessing a patient's medication history allows prescribers to receive critically important information on their patients' current and past prescriptions and to become better informed about potential medication issues with their patients (e.g., catching potentially harmful drug-to-drug and drug-allergy interactions). Prescribers can use this information to improve safety and quality. And—by understanding the cycle of dispensing related to a prescription—prescribers can gain insight into a patient's medication adherence.
>
> ***Electronically Route the Prescription to the Patient's Choice of Pharmacy:*** Exchanging prescription information electronically between prescribers and pharmacies improves the accuracy of the prescribing process and saves time. Time savings primarily result from reduced pharmacy phone calls and faxes related to prescription-renewal authorizations, as well as from a reduced need for pharmacy staff to key in prescription data.

There is little doubt, particularly considering the more complete definition of what the term includes, that certain errors will be avoided through the use of e-prescribing. Pharmacy technicians and pharmacists should keep in mind, however, that other mistakes may result from the electronic transmission of prescriptions directly into the pharmacy's computers. Physicians selecting the incorrect drug from a list on a handheld PDA will happen just as surely as a pharmacy technician selecting the wrong line in the pharmacy computer. Worse, there may be fewer ways to guard against such errors. As e-prescribing begins to dominate prescribing, pharmacy technicians and pharmacists will need to use greater caution to protect patients against newer risks.

More technology is making its way into pharmacy practice. In the future there will be many more machines that will assist in dispensing medication and reducing medication errors. Technology cannot replace pharmacy technicians or the pharmacists, but it can and will help to redefine the roles of each. Regardless of the technology used, it will remain the role of the humans in pharmacy practice to protect patients.

Summary

Every year, billions of prescriptions are filled by pharmacists and pharmacy technicians across the United States. Each is individually prescribed and filled, and some errors are inevitable. In order to prevent or reduce the risk of errors, pharmacies develop workflows. Within these workflows, best practices are incorporated that can possibly stop mistakes from being made, or catch mistakes that are made.

Best practices take many forms. Some are mechanical, such as triple check and NDC checks. Some serve as reminders to check one more time, such as "Mark-It." Some use the newest robots to perform mechanical functions. Some use electronics to verify the prescription is correct.

The best practices studied today will change over time. It is important that pharmacy technicians and pharmacists understand how best practices work. It is also important to understand how and when they can fail. Best practices are the steps in the CQI workflow. They will work only if used. That requires training and commitment.

Review Questions

1. Which of the following statements about best practices is or are true?
    A. Best practices are simple.
    B. They must be used every time.
    C. They are not complicated.
    D. All of the above.

2. Which of the following statements is or are true regarding the best practice called "Mark-It?"
    A. Mark the shelves of all dangerous drugs.
    B. Be selective and do not choose too many drugs for "Mark-It" treatment.
    C. Use only for tablets and capsules.
    D. All of the above.

3. A best practice similar to "Mark-It" is called:
    A. "Tall man lettering"
    B. "Show and tell"
    C. "Under 6 / over 60"
    D. "Two sets of eyes"

4. Indian Health Service counseling is most effective if used with what other best practice?

   A. "Show and tell"

   B. "Under 6 / over 60"

   C. "Two sets of eyes"

   D. None of the above; IHS counseling works best if used independently of other best practices

5. Indian Health Service counseling makes use of

   A. Open-ended questions.

   B. Med-guides.

   C. Patient-information leaflets.

   D. A series of scripted remarks unique to each classification of drug.

6. Unlike prospective drug review, a drug utilization review (DUR)

   A. Reviews all medication the patient is currently taking.

   B. Is a retrospective review.

   C. Occurs before the patient is admitted to the hospital.

   D. None of the above; the terms are interchangeable.

7. What action should be taken if a pharmacy technician notices the technician at the preceding station did not perform one of the best practices required by the workflow at that station?

   A. Immediately report the technician to avoid future mistakes.

   B. Correct the situation by completing the best practice and saying nothing.

   C. Return the prescription to the technician at the previous station to correct the oversight.

   D. Record the mistake and correct it.

8. When performing an NDC check on a new prescription, a technician should

   A. Check the middle three numbers only.

   B. Not use the stock bottle if the last two numbers are the only ones that do not match.

C. Check the NDC number in the computer against the NDC number that was printed on the receipt.

D. Verify that the first set of numbers and the second set of numbers are correct.

9. In simplest terms, how does a bar code scanner work?

   A. It checks the drug in the bottle against a set of codes in the computer.

   B. It uses spectrographic analysis to verify.

   C. It checks the bar code on the stock package against the bar code printed by the computer.

   D. It checks the name of the drug on the stock bottle against the computer information.

10. Which of the following statements is or are true concerning robots?

    A. Manufacturers claim they are 100% accurate when they perform the task they were manufactured to do.

    B. In the average pharmacy, they are used only to fill about 60% of the drugs in stock.

    C. When they are not working, either because of maintenance or malfunctions, the workflow becomes confusing and the staff can feel more stress.

    D. All of the above.

Endnotes

[1] Claim from files of Pharmacists Mutual Insurance Company. Names were changed and information modified to fit space and purpose.

[2] This claim is from the archives of Pharmacists Mutual Insurance Company. The drug and dosage is the same, except the original prescription was written for the brand name, instead of generically. Molly is not the real name of the patient. Names have been changed to protect privacy.

[3] Also called prime questions, you can find these explained on several websites including the website of Mercer University College of Pharmacy and Health Sciences: http://cophs.mercer.edu/P1SamplePortfolio.htm accessed March 15, 2001.

[4] For a discussion of prospective drug review as part of the pharmacist's duties, see Chapter 3.

[5] Optimum INR reading of a patient on warfarin is between 2 and 3. A reading of 14 is dangerous. This potentially could have made the result of the 5 mg erroneous dose even worse.

[6] This is an easy mistake to make because "one daily" is abbreviated as "i qd" and "four times a day" is "i qid".

[7] In an informal, unpublished study by Pharmacists Mutual Insurance Company of approximately 100 pharmacies that tracked their near-misses for at least one quarter, over 50% of QREs were committed at the computer-entry station. Fewer mistakes were made at the filling station, but more of the filling mistakes reached the patient. This was possibly because there were more opportunities to catch the earlier mistakes as opposed to those later in the workflow.

[8] Flynn, E. A., Barker, K. N., Carnahan, B. J., National Observational Study of Prescription Dispensing Accuracy and Safety in 50 Pharmacies, *JAPhA*, Vol. 43, No. 2, March/April 2003, pp. 191–200.

[9] In the state of Minnesota, the hard copy prescription is pulled on the first refill unless on the original fill it was double-checked at change of shift. With scanned prescriptions this is not as prevalent as earlier.

[10] http://www.rxscan.com/rxplus.shtml accessed March 16, 2011.

[11] Gertskis, M., Barcode Scanners Halving Errors, *Pharmacy News*, 11 November 2009, http://www.pharmacynews.com.au/news/barcode-scanners-halving-errors accessed March 20, 2011.

[12] ScriptPro, LLC. Product information quoted from website and used by permission of the company. http://www.scriptpro.com/Products/Robot-Dispensing/Package-Dispensing-Robots/SPUD/ accessed March 20, 2011.

[13] DISCLOSURE: The author of this text book prepared a White Paper for Centex on the use and benefits of the Pass Rx. Baker, K. R., Verifying Quality—The Keystone of a Quality-Assurance System: Parts 1 and 2, November 9, 2010, an overview of medication errors in pharmacies and an introduction to the PASS Rx Pharmaceutical Authentication Sensor System. The White Paper can be found on the company's website, http://www.centice.com/whitepapers/verifying-quality-part1 accessed March 20, 2011.

[14] http://www.surescripts.com/about-e-prescribing/benefits-of-e-prescribing_for-everyone.aspx accessed March 20, 2011.

[15] http://www.surescripts.com/about-e-prescribing/benefits-of-e-prescribing_for-pharmacies.aspx accessed March 20, 2011.

CHAPTER 7

Refining the Workflow

OBJECTIVES

Upon completion of this chapter, the reader should be able to:

1. Explain the need for a team in order for the pharmacy's quality system to succeed.
2. Understand the role of each individual station in achieving quality.
3. Describe how stations must work together as a total quality workflow.
4. Discuss the importance of the pharmacy technician in assisting the pharmacist to perform a prospective drug review.
5. Describe how developing quality habits is an important part of learning workflow.
6. Explain how pharmacy technicians can prepare material for pharmacists' counseling to take place.
7. Discuss how a system of best practices makes up an effective workflow.
8. List the various steps in a typical workflow.
9. Explain the concept of an algorithm in making decisions.
10. Discuss the role of each pharmacy technician in assisting others to develop pride in a quality job done well.

KEY TERMS

Algorithm: An algorithm is a list of criteria that form a decision tree. Its use allows a pharmacy to select individual patients or conditions that may most need a particular service such as in-depth counseling. A counseling algorithm may look for certain drugs that would be particularly dangerous because of their method of action or potential interactions. It may also look for disease states such as diabetes, or patient traits such as one who takes more than five drugs.

Internal customer: A term used to identify coworkers. The importance of the term is that it emphasizes the need to focus work, at least partly, on other members of the team. Each member of the team serves all others. The importance of customers, discussed in the following chapter, is not diminished by recognizing obligations to internal customers.

Process workflow: Just as the pharmacy has a workflow that begins with receiving a prescription and ending with the delivery of the completed order to the nursing floor or the patient, each station or process has its own workflow. An individual station's workflow should be mapped by steps beginning with receiving the order to delivery to the next station.

Sig code: A sig code is a software-provided shortcut designed to make entering directions into the computer easier and faster. For example, typing "1tqid" causes the directions, "Take one tablet four times a day" to appear.

Will call: A section of the pharmacy department, usually in a community pharmacy, that has been set aside for completed prescriptions that have not yet been picked up.

OUTLINE

The Workflow
Refining and Adding Detail to the Workflow
 Receiving the Prescription
 Computer Data Entry and Label Preparation
 Assembling the Drug/Container/Label/Receipt and Filling the Order/Prescription
 Pharmacist's Final Check
 Pharmacist's Prospective Drug Review

Pharmacist's Counseling of Patient
   The Case of the Scanned Prescription and the Improbable Error
   A Counseling Algorithm
Delivery of the Order/Prescription

Additional Considerations in Laying Out a Workflow
Teamwork and Internal Customers
Summary

The Workflow

In this chapter we will use much of the material studied in previous chapters. In preceding chapters we examined the basics of a workflow. We looked at a series of processes that moved the prescription from the place where it entered the pharmacy to where it was delivered to the nursing floor, the nursing home, or directly to the patient. We described the places along the line as a series of stations. The simplest workflow moves through the following stations:

- Receiving the prescription
- Computer data entry and label preparation
- Assembling the drug/container/label/receipt and filling the order/prescription
- Pharmacist's final check
- Pharmacist's prospective drug review
- Pharmacist's counseling of patient
- Delivery of the order/prescription

When the prescription is received in the pharmacy at station one, a number of best practices need to be used in collecting basic information about the patient, insurance billing information, and whatever other information is necessary to fill the prescription. We can then prepare a map for a detailed workflow using best practices studied earlier. Mapping a detailed workflow provides a training platform for the pharmacy staff. Training is integral to implementing the third stage in the risk-management process.

In this chapter we will begin a mapping that will later become an outline of the pharmacy's training program. The workflow developed here will purposefully be simpler than that used in most pharmacies because the purpose here is to demonstrate how a pharmacy workflow is designed, not to prepare a complete CQI system to be incorporated into a pharmacy. The exact workflow developed for a pharmacy will depend on several processes and procedures, some of which may be unique to that location or organization. For example, a hospital workflow will differ from that of a community pharmacy. The workflow in a pharmacy will also be dictated, to a large extent, by the CQI system the pharmacy has chosen.

The workflow we will design for the purpose of study in this chapter will be for a community pharmacy (a hospital pharmacy workflow would not differ dramatically). To simplify the discussion here, we will make certain presumptions that may not be valid in real life. For example, in our first station, Receiving the Prescription, we will presume that the only way we would receive a prescription is from a patient walking into the pharmacy and presenting the prescription to the technician at the pharmacy counter. Also in our simplified workflow, we will look only at new prescriptions, although we know that approximately half of the prescriptions in a typical community pharmacy would be refills of a previous order. Our pharmacy has no scanner to scan the new prescription into the computer, so the original prescription will be sent through the workflow almost to the very end.

The purpose of this chapter is to study how a workflow functions and how it is used as part of the training of the pharmacy technicians and pharmacists. At each station there will be a mini workflow for that process, ending with the materials being transferred to the next station.

Refining and Adding Detail to the Workflow

Receiving the Prescription

In our hypothetical pharmacy, a patient has presented to the pharmacy technician at the intake window, the first station along the path through the pharmacy, a new prescription. The steps the pharmacy technician takes will prepare the prescription for each subsequent station. Here we will expand the basic **process workflow** for this first station:

- Greet the patient and ask if he or she has other prescriptions to be picked up today.

- Check the new prescription and ask for the correct spelling of the name, including any prefixes (Dr., Mrs., Ms., etc.) and suffixes (Jr., Sr., III, etc.); circle a suffix that could indicate a different patient so the computer-entry clerk will be notified and select the correct patient.

- If the prescriber is in a group practice, make sure the prescription clearly indicates which physician wrote it; if not clear, ask the patient.

- Verify insurance information.
- Check the order for the date written; if the date is old, mark the Rx for the pharmacist to review. If the patient indicates the physician made a mistake when writing the date, mark this for the pharmacist's decision.
- Complete the patient address; make sure it is current; verify spelling.
- If not already on the Rx, write the patient's phone number on the Rx, checking to be sure it is current. (This may be used to verify the Rx is delivered to the correct person at the end when the prescription is picked up.)
- Verify and complete the patient birth date.
- If the patient is under 6 or over 60, use a red pen to write the age of the patient on the Rx (the pharmacy could choose to have the technician write "Over 60" or some other alert in red, but it should be consistent).
- Ask the patient if she or he has any allergies. *Note:* if the patient says that she or he was asked that last time, the pharmacy may authorize the technician to remind the patient, "We will ask with each new prescription because we think it is important to be sure your records are always up to date."
- If the patient indicates he or she has an allergy, place a capital "A" on the front and list what the patient said as an allergy on the back of the Rx. If the indication is there are no allergies, write "NKA" on the front of the Rx.
- Ask if the patient is taking any other meds including OTCs and herbals. If yes, write a large "M" on the front of the Rx and list the medications on the back. If the patient says that all of his or her medications are in the pharmacy's records, note that and ask about OTCs and herbals. If the patient says that he or she is not taking other meds, write "NOM" on the prescription.
- Circle any unusual dose (any dosage taken other than orally or more than two doses at a time). This alerts the pharmacist during drug review to check the total dose to be taken and to recheck the strength of the drug prescribed and given.
- Select a basket for the patient. *Note:* In some pharmacies the baskets will be color coded as to priority. For example, a green basket may mean the patient is not waiting while a white basket means the patient is waiting. A red basket may be used if the receiving pharmacy technician determines there is an emergency or priority and the Rx should be put in the front of the line.

- Place all new prescriptions and any refill bottles for this patient along with any necessary insurance cards into the basket and move the basket to the next station.

From this more detailed (although for our hypothetical pharmacy, simplified) workflow of this first station, the pharmacy now has a map and a script to use to train technicians and pharmacists who may work at this station. A real pharmacy would develop a similar process workflow for each other method of receiving a prescription: telephone, fax, electronic transmission, or PDA. Most steps would be the same. The pharmacy will now need to build a workflow for each of the other stations that will be used in the pharmacy's training program.

> **RxErcise 7-A   Identifying the Best Practices**
>
> Review best practices studied to date. For each of the station processes mapped in this chapter, underline the best practice. Make sure you know the purpose of each. What steps were left out that you think should be added?

Computer Data Entry and Label Preparation

The pharmacy must now determine which steps and best practices should be included in its second station. In designing the workflow for this pharmacy, we simplified it by limiting the process to new prescriptions received from a patient at the intake window. For the second station, we will further simplify the process by presuming the patient is already in our computer system. Once the pharmacy has prepared this, workflow modifications are relatively simple.

- As the baskets with the new prescriptions and any refill bottles are transferred from the receiving station, place them in order depending on how they are to be processed at this station.

- "Take 5"—Take a few seconds to review the Rx for the steps that should have been taken at receiving (e.g., patient under 6 years old not marked, address missing, etc.). If anything is incomplete, hand basket back to receiving clerk to correct.

- Enter the patient's name (if refill, enter Rx number to be refilled) into the computer.

- Check to be sure the correct patient has been selected.

- Check allergies on new Rx and make sure the computer profile for this patient is correct.

- Check other medications indicated on new Rx and make sure computer profile is up to date.

- Select the drug and strength of drug. (It depends on the software as to how this is done. In some pharmacies the stock bottle may be pulled and scanned in. In most pharmacies the drug is entered by typing the first few letters and then selecting from a list provided on the computer screen.)

- Double-check drug and strength.

- Type directions. Note: In most pharmacies the software provides a shortcut through the use of what are called **sig codes**. For example, typing "1tqid" causes the directions "Take one tablet four times a day" to appear. While this increases efficiency, it may lead to errors. The technician may mean "Take one teaspoonful four times a day" but get the "Take one tablet four times daily." Other examples have led to not just embarrassing, but dangerous directions such as "Take three teaspoonful," when the correct direction should have been "Take 3 mL," indicating a mark on the supplied dropper. The mother in that case gave the three teaspoonsful.

- Double-check directions.

- If the computer notifies of any warnings (e.g., allergies, drug interaction) call the pharmacist before it is cleared—a "pharmacist only question." If the software allows and procedures indicate, print out warnings and place them into the basket with the new Rx to go through the workflow to the pharmacist final check area. The pharmacist will need to know any other drugs the patient is taking for a drug review. If the pharmacist does not have a computer screen, the technician may print out a patient profile, if permitted by the software.

- Is an FDA med-guide required for this drug? If so, pull one from stock or print from software and place in the basket for the pharmacist to use during counseling and to be delivered to the patient.

- Print the label with receipt and patient-information leaflet and place them in the basket with the new Rx and deliver it to the filling technician.

Assembling the Drug/Container/Label/Receipt and Filling the Order/Prescription

Once the label has been printed, the pharmacy technician at the filling or assembly station can begin to work. At this station the technician will assemble all of the material needed to complete the prescription: the drug, the label, the receipt, printed material, and auxiliary labels. At the end of this station, the patient's prescription will be complete and ready for a final quality check by the pharmacist.

- As the baskets with the new prescriptions, labels, patient-information leaflets, and any required med-guides are transferred from the computer data entry station, they are placed in order depending on how they are to be processed.

- "Take 5"—Take a few seconds to review the Rx for the steps that should have been taken at the receiving and data-entry stations (e.g., right patient? right drug? right strength? right directions? med-guide required?). If anything is incomplete, hand the basket back to the receiving clerk or the data-entry technician to correct.

- Note if there are any red highlights on the new Rx: allergies, other medications, unusual doses, vulnerable patient (over 60, under 6).

- Using new Rx (not printed label unless refill), pull the stock bottle from the shelf. (This makes sure a computer-entry wrong drug or strength is not carried through to filling. Also it gives a second interpretation of the original Rx after the data-entry technician and before the third and definitive reading of the Rx by the pharmacist at the final quality check. If there is any question or difference, call the pharmacist to verify immediately.)

- Check drug name and strength on new Rx against drug name and strength on the stock bottle. (If shelf is marked as "problem drug," double-check.)

- If the Rx is for a vulnerable patient, over 60, under 6, check one more time before pulling from the shelf.

- Return new Rx and stock bottle to the pharmacy counter. Before counting out drugs, check name against name again.

- Before counting out drugs, do an NDC number check of the receipt (what was entered into the computer) and stock bottle. If a scanner is in use, scan NDC numbers as a check.

- Count out drug and put into prescription bottle. *Note:* A safety cap must be used unless specifically requested not to by the patient or physician, in which case patient should sign the back of the Rx.

- Place the label on the prescription bottle using "2-second" rule.

- Perform a final name versus name check between label and original Rx if new prescription ("triple check" rule).

- Place completed Rx with receipt, patient-information leaflet, warnings from computer, profile from computer, and any med-guides that are required in the basket for pharmacist's final quality check.

- Deliver the basket with all material to the pharmacist. (There may be alternatives such as having the technician pull up the scanned Rx image on the screen in the pharmacists' final check area if the pharmacy scans the images. The technician may attach the receipt to the bag, unstapled, so the pharmacist knows it is finished and ready for a check.)

- If the prescription is put into a "will call" area, meaning the patient is not waiting, the filling technician may put a sticker on the bag indicating a new prescription for counseling or a drug review may be warranted.

Pharmacist's Final Check

Once the prescription has been completely filled, it is delivered to the pharmacist who will perform a final quality check, a prospective drug review, and counseling. While this is not the pharmacy technicians' area, they should be familiar with these steps in order to understand how they can be of assistance.

Perhaps no part of the quality process is more important than the pharmacist's final quality check. Up to this point, the technician has done most of the work involved in preparing a prescription. It is the pharmacist, however, who will be held primarily responsible for any error that reaches the patient. This does not mean that the technician is absolved of all responsibility or liability for a misfilled prescription. If technicians are negligent in performing any of their duties, they may be sued along with the pharmacist. Most juries, lawyers, and judges up to now have concluded that the pharmacist, who has the superior training and education, should be held to the higher degree of scrutiny.

In a few states, usually in special circumstances only, boards of pharmacy have allowed a tech-check-tech procedure to replace mandatory pharmacist checks. This procedure is not generally accepted and pharmacist checks remain the standard. The boards of pharmacy and state legislatures remain reluctant to allow a procedure that bypasses active pharmacist involvement in the dispensing function.

It is thought that pharmacists, because of their education and training, need to be directly involved in all aspects of the delivery of dangerous, Rx only drugs in the United States. While boards have accepted that pharmacy technicians may relieve the pharmacist of much of the mechanical aspects of the workflow, they are unwilling to proceed further in the area of the final check. There are also professional reasons to maintain pharmacist involvement here. The final check provides an opportunity for pharmacists to familiarize themselves with the medication to be dispensed to the patient while certifying the prescription and seeing that the accompanying material is correct. Knowledge of the current medication and the opportunity to review what is being dispensed are necessary for the pharmacist to perform the duties of prospective drug review and counseling, which are the tasks performed in the next stations. The pharmacist's final-check workflow could be designed with the following steps:

- The pharmacist received the basket with the patient's completed prescription along with the other material added by the technician.

- If the prescription is new, the pharmacist reviews and interprets the new prescription as ordered by the prescriber. (If the new prescription has been scanned into the computer system, the prescription should be pulled up, either by the technician or the pharmacist so the image is available on the screen at the pharmacist's final check station.)

- "Take 5"—Review the work of receiving, data-entry, and filling technicians. If a mistake is found, allow them to fix it before proceeding.

- Check new prescription and label for
    - Patient
    - Address (is it the correct Dan Smith?)
    - Physician
    - Directions
    - Drug and strength

- Check for patient-information leaflets.

- Check if an FDA med-guide is required and, if so, is in the basket for delivery to the patient.

- Check name versus name on the stock bottle, label, and new prescription.

- Check NDC number (or scan).

- Check for any indication this patient requires special counseling (see the section "A Counseling Algorithm" below).

- Move to Drug Review Station or begin drug review here.

Pharmacist's Prospective Drug Review

Pharmacists' training and education uniquely qualify these professionals to review prescriptions for problems of health-related issues. Allergies, interactions, and overuse are only some of the medication errors that can be prevented when a pharmacist reviews the medication prescribed in light of other drugs and conditions associated with an individual patient. Pharmacy technicians collect important information and material needed by the pharmacists to perform a drug review, which might contain the following steps at a minimum:

- "Take 5."
- Review patient profile.
- Note, among other things,
  - allergies,
  - interactions with other drugs,
  - overuse, and
  - underuse.
- Prepare for counseling.

Pharmacist's Counseling of Patient

Pharmacists increasingly are responsible, legally and professionally, for counseling patients prior to the first use of a drug. For the past several years, every pharmacy school in the United States has taught the use of open-ended questions as a form of counseling. The advantage of this approach is that it allows the pharmacist to discover what information the patient already has and what additional knowledge of the drug the patient may need. As was noted in Chapter 6, this form of counseling was developed in the 1960s by the Indian Health Service and has become the most commonly preferred method. It is often used in combination with the best practice known as "Show and Tell" counseling.

The Case of the Scanned Prescription and the Improbable Error

No matter how well a workflow is laid out or how good the technology is, there will occasionally be unexpected results and problems. Scanning prescriptions into the computer system is a convenient advancement in pharmacy practice and can be credited with improving quality and increasing efficiency. The image is by definition an exact reproduction of the original prescription.

Once the prescription is scanned, it becomes part of the computer system and the original can be safely filed away.

After scanning and filling thousands of prescriptions, a pharmacy received notice of an error involving the mislabeling of a prescription. The prescription had been written by the physician as, "Take $1½$ tablets daily." The prescription called for 45 tablets, which was a 30-day supply.

The prescription was filled and dispensed to the patient. The directions on the bottle, however, were wrong. The label read "Take $½$ tablet daily." The prescription was written as a new prescription, but the patient had been taking the same medication, written by the same physician, with the same directions, for several months. Regardless of the incorrect directions on the new label, the patient took the medication as had been previously prescribed and as he had been taking it. He took one and a half tablets every day.

The error came to light when he called the pharmacy for a refill at the end of 30 days. When the pharmacy began filling the prescription, the patient's insurance company rejected the claim because the refill was too early. Forty-five tablets a day at a dose of a half tablet a day should have lasted 90 days. Confronted with the error, the pharmacy tried to determine what happened.

The original hypothesis was that the technician typed the directions wrong. The image of the scanned prescription, however, clearly showed that the technician typed the directions exactly as the prescription appeared on the screen: "Take $½$ tablet per day." The next hypothesis was the physician wrote the directions incorrectly, or had changed the dose the patient was to take. The original prescription was retrieved from the file where it had been placed immediately following the scan. The physician's original prescription clearly showed: "Sig: $1½$ q d." Somehow, when the prescription was scanned, the "1" failed to appear on the image.

The company had never seen this happen before. They tried to replicate the mistake by rescanning the original prescription, but every time the physician's directions clearly showed on the scanned image as "Sig: $1½$ q d." The final explanation that was that a piece of dust had gotten on the scanner or on the prescription in exactly the place necessary to cover the "1" and made the image appear as: "$½$ tablet daily."

Any time there is an error, the pharmacy staff will look for a best practice that could prevent a repeat of the incident in the future. Here there are two possibilities. First, the technician who scans a new prescription will need to recheck the scanned image against the original to verify it is correct. A problem with this approach is that a repeat of the exact problem is improbable and the fix of rechecking may be impractical.

The second possible solution is the use of Indian Health Service counseling with "Show and Tell." One of the Indian Health Service questions is, "How did your physician tell you to take this medication?" The answer and the label would not have agreed and may have started an inquiry before the patient left the pharmacy. Indian Health Service counseling with "Show and Tell" can catch many common errors.

In 2009 the Oregon State Board of Pharmacy appointed a select committee to study whether counseling could reduce the number of mechanical-type medication errors. The committee delivered its report in February 2010 at a meeting of the Oregon Pharmacists Association.[1] The committee found that Indian Health Service counseling with "Show and Tell" was more likely to catch errors than counseling that did not use these techniques.

In reaching its conclusion, the Oregon State Board of Pharmacy committee reviewed 99 medication-error complaints, of which 70 were mechanical errors:

28 wrong strength or dosage form

20 wrong drug

16 wrong patient

6 wrong directions

The committee found that if the Indian Health Service questions had been asked while the medication was shown to the patient, most, although not all, of the mechanical-type medication errors would have been prevented. The results for each category were:

- 14 percent of the wrong strength or dosage form errors could have been avoided;
- 65 percent of the wrong drug errors could have been avoided;
- 75 percent of the wrong patient errors could have been avoided; and
- 83 percent of the wrong direction errors could have been avoided.

A possible counseling-station workflow using the Indian Health Service prime questions[2] and "Show and Tell" would include the following steps:

- Speak to the patient in a place where others cannot overhear the conversation in accord with HIPAA requirements.
- Ask the patient "What is your birth date?" or "What is your address?" (If a new prescription, the birth date will be on the prescription. If the patient's birth date is not readily available, the address will be on the receipt.)
- Remove the prescription bottle(s) from the bag. (The technician makes sure the bag is not stapled and is accessible.)
- Read the patient name, drug name, and directions on the bottle.
- If the medication comes in tablet or capsule form, open the bottle and show the contents to the patient.
- Ask: "What did your physician tell you this was for?"
- If the patient knows the answer, go on; if not, go over the uses and ask, "What did you see the physician for today?" Do not go on until the patient knows why he or she is taking the medication.

- Ask "How did your physician tell you to take this medication?"
- Ask, "What did your physician tell you to expect?"
- When you have received satisfactory answers showing the patient is familiar with how, when, and why the medication is being taken, proceed.
- Review any possible side effects the patient should know to possibly expect.
- Consider other remarks particular to this drug, (e.g., "With warfarin it is important to have your blood tested regularly for clotting" or "An INR should always be between 2 and 3" or similar advice).
- Ask, "Do you have any other questions for me?"
- Make any special remarks regarding this medication (e.g., "Take until it is all gone" or "Use in the ear" or "Be sure you take it as directed").
- Proceed to delivery and collection of money. This may be done by the pharmacist or technician or a clerk, depending on the pharmacy's protocol.

A Counseling Algorithm

Sometimes, because of time or other constraints, a workflow must be other than ideal. Rather than disregarding a best practice completely, such as Indian Health Service counseling and "Show and Tell" counseling, a middle path may be appropriate. The perfect should not be the enemy of the good.

If the pharmacy decides its pharmacists cannot perform full Indian Health Service and "Show and Tell" counseling for all new prescriptions, the pharmacy may develop an **algorithm** to select those patients who would be most helped by the technique. A counseling algorithm is a problem-solving procedure using a series of questions or steps to identify an individual patient in need of a particular service.

The algorithm may identify certain drugs considered particularly dangerous due to their method of action or potential interactions, for example, warfarin, digoxin, or monoamine oxidase (MAO) inhibitors. There could be many others. The algorithm may also focus on elderly patients, diabetic patients, heart condition patients, or other patients who may be considered for inclusion. Patients who take a lot of medication, patients who take certain combinations of medication, and patients who have questions may all be considered. The elements of the algorithm might be written on a specially prepared checklist used to determine if selected conditions are met. The technician could check the areas that appear to be relevant for a particular patient and place the slip in the basket with this patient's prescriptions. When the basket arrives in the pharmacist's final check area, the pharmacist can review the checklist and consider spending additional time with this patient.

Such a list should not diminish the importance of all other patients. The list produced by use of a special algorithm should serve only to notify all staff working on these prescriptions that extra time may be required in a particular case.

> **Quality Note 7-A   An Algorithm—What Might Be Included?**
>
> Often pharmacists and technicians complain that patients do not want to be counseled. For some patients that may be true. It may be difficult to spend extra time with these patients. However, patients identified by the algorithm are more likely to consider their need worthy of additional time. The algorithm can be designed to select vulnerable patients by concentrating on factors that indicate a special need. An algorithm checklist may include the following factors (see Figure 7-1):
>
> - Disease:
>   - Diabetic
>   - Heart condition
>   - Advanced high blood pressure
>   - Cancer
>   - Extreme or chronic pain
>   - Others
> - Medication:
>   - Warfarin
>   - Insulin
>   - Methotrexate
>   - High blood pressure
>   - High doses of controlled substances
> - Patient:
>   - Lives alone
>   - Older, particularly those over 75 years
>   - Infirm
>   - On more than five medications

(continues)

> **Quality Note 7-A An Algorithm—What Might Be Included?** (continued)
>
> - Less literate
> - Refilling prescriptions too soon, particularly controlled substances
> - Refilling prescriptions too infrequently, particularly chronically used drugs, such as high blood pressure medications

If a counseling algorithm is to be used, some appropriate steps in the workflow would need to be added. One of the technician stations could be modified to direct the technician to mark and include the algorithm checklist in the basket for the pharmacist. Which station(s) is selected may depend on where the information is most accessible, usually the computer-entry station. The particulars of use of an algorithm will be determined by the pharmacy and pharmacists. Which items would be included within the factors used is also a pharmacist decision. An algorithm will usually be used only if all patients cannot be counseled.

In designing a workflow for our hypothetical pharmacy, we presume the pharmacy has decided on the use of a counseling algorithm and has decided to include the following items as factors that may trigger more intense counseling for a particular patient. The pharmacy has added the following steps to the computer-entry station workflow:

- Review algorithm checklist for this patient.
- Check items on algorithm that apply.
- Place algorithm checklist in basket if applicable.

An algorithm may be designed using the criteria discussed above and may appear similar to the form shown in Figure 7-1.

> **RxErcise 7-B Algorithms**
>
> Design an algorithm for your pharmacy.
>
> What additional items would you add to a counseling algorithm?
>
> Should the age of the patient be a factor? If so, why, how, and what?
>
> What are the arguments against adding too many factors to a counseling algorithm?

Delivery of the Order/Prescription

An additional mechanical error that can prove to be particularly dangerous is a prescription delivered to the wrong patient by the pharmacist or the pharmacy technician. The delivery part of the

> **Algorithm Checklist**
>
> Pharmacist: This patient meets the following criteria for your consideration.
>
> **Patient:** _____
>
> **Diseases**
> - ☐ Diabetic
> - ☐ Heart condition
> - ☐ Advanced high blood pressure
> - ☐ Cancer
> - ☐ Extreme or chronic pain
> - ☐ Others
>
> **Medications**
> - ☐ Warfarin
> - ☐ Insulin
> - ☐ Methotrexate
> - ☐ High blood pressure medications
> - ☐ High doses of controlled substances
>
> **Patient**
> - ☐ Lives alone
> - ☐ Over 75 years
> - ☐ Infirm
> - ☐ On more than five medications
> - ☐ Less health care literate
> - ☐ Refilling prescriptions too soon, particularly controlled substances
> - ☐ Refilling prescriptions too infrequently, particularly chronically used drugs, such as high blood pressure
>
> 2011, Ken Baker

Figure 7-1 Algorithm Checklist
© Cengage Learning 2013

workflow should contain a verification procedure designed to reduce the risk of giving a patient someone else's medication.

In the report to the Oregon State Board of Pharmacy by its select committee discussed earlier, 16 of the 99 total medication errors studied involved giving the prescription to the wrong patient. The committee reported that 100 percent of these claims could have been avoided if one of two open-ended questions had been asked of the patient at the time of delivery. Those questions are:

- What is your birth date?
- What is your address?

These questions can be asked on both new and refill prescriptions and may be asked by anyone who delivers the prescription to the patient. Interestingly, the committee concluded that only 75 percent of these errors would have been prevented by the use of Indian Health Service plus "Show and Tell" counseling alone.

ADDITIONAL CONSIDERATIONS IN LAYING OUT A WORKFLOW

When we consider designing and implementing a workflow, we think of the movement of a prescription and eventually a product from one physical place to another. A patient delivers her or his physician's order at one end of the counter and after a series of events along the pharmacy's counter, it is delivered at the other end to the patient in a bag with a receipt attached to the bag. There are several stops along the way where the pharmacy technician performs a job. A pharmacy technician receives a prescription and, after performing the required procedures, delivers it to a pharmacy technician who enters the information into the computer. It is then passed with the label to a filling station and from there to a pharmacist who checks the prescription and performs professional duties. It is easy to begin thinking of this as just a mechanical movement of product along an assembly line.

But think deeper about the process. Think of it as healthcare. Pharmacy technicians and pharmacists do not build automobiles or toaster ovens. They provide life saving medications that, if done wrong, can result in injury or death. The pharmacy workflow is not just the process of assembling a prescription. Think of the workflow as a place within which you practice your profession.

Each step within each station moves the physician's order closer to completion with the drug that will treat your patient. Some of the steps you take will be for the purpose of avoiding a mistake. Some of the steps have been designed to catch a mistake before the medication is delivered to the patient. They may be designed to catch a technician's mistake, or a physician's mistake, or a pharmacist's mistake, or even a patient's mistake. Consider every step as necessary every time.

Each prescription order is filled one at a time. While you are filling that order, all of the others do not matter. A pharmacy technician cannot skip steps because there are several people in line waiting for service on other prescriptions. A pharmacist once asked, "If the company does not provide us with enough help, are prescription errors the company's fault?" The answer is no. A lot of factors may be considered as causes of errors, but each prescription is filled one at a time. The failure to provide a sufficient number of workers to complete a job within a particular period of time is an economic problem. If a patient at the end of the line becomes tired of waiting, he or she may leave and go somewhere else. The company will lose that business. It should never be allowed to become a safety problem.

Teamwork and Internal Customers

Before finishing with the discussion of workflow, it will be valuable to give some thought to the part of the workflow that makes everything else work—the team. How well we treat our patients and customers may be dependent upon how well we treat our **internal customers**. Sick patients are not the pharmacists' and pharmacy technicians' only customers. Every organization operates as a team. This is particularly true of a pharmacy. In order to get things done, each person must interact with several other persons. The more smoothly these individuals work together, the better the team functions and the more efficiently the process works as a whole. A busy pharmacy may have three, four, or more technicians working at the same time, plus one, two, or three pharmacists. Each person is an internal supplier and each has an internal customer.

The hypothetical pharmacy for which we designed the workflow in this chapter serves as a good example of the importance of an internal customer. Assume there are four pharmacy technicians working with one pharmacist.[3] For simplicity, one technician is at the receiving station, one is at the computer-entry station, and one technician is at the filling station. The fourth takes care of the "**will call**" and receives payment at the cash register. The pharmacist performs the final quality check and a drug review on each prescription. In addition, the pharmacist counsels on each new prescription and some refills as necessary. The pharmacist may also take payment while counseling the patient.

The pharmacy technician at the receiving station performs his or her duties and then passes the material along to the technician at the computer-entry station. It is easy to begin thinking of the job as just performing those tasks at the station to which one is assigned at the time. If the team is to work to its highest level, however, each individual's thinking needs to be broader. Considering the others in the workflow as internal customers improves the atmosphere and final quality.

Deming stressed the importance of the internal customer. Just as the patient is a customer and is regarded as the most important element in success, so the internal customer is critical to quality. When a pharmacy technician completes the list of processes at his or her station and passes the basket on to another member of the team, that person is her or his customer. One job must be to satisfy that internal customer. Only if quality is delivered to the technician's internal customer does the technician have the right to expect quality from all other members of the staff. If the team focuses on satisfying each internal customer, quality improves.

Deming's 14 principles are lessons for management. Management's job is to provide the tools workers need to provide quality of workmanship. Some of these principles also apply to the jobs of the pharmacists and pharmacy technicians in the workflow. Consider the following restated principles directed to the pharmacy technicians and pharmacists as obligations to the team and internal customers:

- Every member of the quality team has an obligation to help the others do a better job. Each needs to react to the needs of those internal customers whom they serve. Immediate action is taken on any prescriptions returned that need correction. Every member of the team needs to rectify any conditions that may be detrimental to quality.

- Just as management has the obligation to encourage effective, two-way communication within the pharmacy, each member of the team has the same requirement.

- Quality does not function well in an atmosphere of fear. If any team member is fearful that she or he will be reported for minor infractions, she or he cannot be productive. Everyone must learn, but when possible in a constructive manner.

- Quality functions best when there is an atmosphere of cooperation. All members of the team must try to break down any barriers that exist between members of the team. This can be done by encouraging problem solving through teamwork, combining the efforts of all those who are a part of the workflow.

- Just as management has a duty to remove all barriers that "inhibit the worker's right to pride of workmanship," all members of the team should strive to help others build confidence in themselves and the pharmacy's quality system.

- It is management's responsibility to "institute a vigorous program of education and retraining." However, every member of the team has an obligation to assist everyone else to learn and succeed.

Teamwork is necessary for quality. Seldom do pharmacy technicians or pharmacists work alone. If the pharmacy is to have a sense of pride in quality well done, it will be because all members of the team function together, each supporting the other.

Summary

Each year over 80 percent of all claims against pharmacies, pharmacists, and pharmacy technicians result from mechanical errors—wrong drug, wrong strength, or wrong directions. Preventing mechanical errors is within the job description of each pharmacy technician. The technician is in a position to reduce the risk of such errors occurring because at least half of a typical pharmacy workflow is within the technician's scope of responsibility.

The workflow described in this chapter is general and is incomplete. Each pharmacy will devise its own and the best practices that are a part of it. A CQI workflow is not something that can be read, or even studied, and then put aside. It must become a part of the daily routine. The CQI steps must be practiced until each can be performed without checklists and without looking at instructions. Each station workflow must be practiced until, like an athlete, performance is done without conscious thought. In the next chapter we will discuss training, which is necessary if a workflow is to reduce the risk of medication errors.

Review Questions

1. At which stations would the pharmacy technician perform the best practice "Take 5?"
    A. Receiving
    B. Data entry
    C. Filling/assembly
    D. b and c, not a

2. A scanner is essentially an electronic way to perform what best practice?
    A. NDC check
    B. "Take 5"
    C. "Mark-it"
    D. "Triple check"

3. At what station should the pharmacy technician write the birth date of the patient on a new prescription?
    A. Receiving
    B. Data-entry

C. Filling/assembly

D. Delivery

4. At what station should the pharmacy technician perform a "triple check"?

   A. Receiving

   B. Data-entry

   C. Filling/assembly

   D. Delivery

5. At what station is the pharmacy technician directed to mark a prescription if there is an unusual dose?

   A. Receiving

   B. Data-entry

   C. Filling/assembly

   D. Delivery

6. At what station should the pharmacy technician adhere to the "2-second rule?"

   A. Receiving

   B. Data-entry

   C. Filling/assembly

   D. Delivery

7. At what station would the pharmacy technician first make use of the information on the back of a prescription marked with a red "M" on the front?

   A. Receiving

   B. Data-entry

   C. Filling/assembly

   D. Delivery

8. At what station need the pharmacy technician be concerned about the age of the patient?

   A. Receiving

   B. Data-entry

   C. Filling/assembly

   D. All of the above

9. What is the definition of "unusual dose" in relation to the marking of a new prescription?

   A. A dose directing "3 at bedtime"

   B. An otic preparation

   C. A rectal suppository

   D. All of the above

10. What is a sig code?

    A. It is the name given to a best practice to mark a prescription with the age of a senior citizen.

    B. It is a shortcut for entering prescription directions by which a few key strokes are translated into full directions.

    C. It is a term that stands for "significant dosage."

    D. It is a series of codes to direct the pharmacist to pay special attention to this prescription for a number of reasons pursuant to the code entered.

Endnotes

[1] "Medication Error Reduction," Meeting of OSPA at Lane County, Oregon, 28 February 2010, PowerPoint presentation by committee members. Points are from the Report to Oregon State Board of Pharmacy.

[2] See, for example, Mercer University College of Pharmacy, http://cophs.mercer.edu/P1SamplePortfolio.htm accessed March 25, 2010.

[3] The number of technicians per pharmacy may be limited by state law or board of pharmacy regulations.

CHAPTER 8

Training for Quality
Making CQI Work

OBJECTIVES

Upon completion of this chapter, the reader should be able to:

1. Explain the need for testing every member of the staff in the pharmacy's quality system.
2. Understand the need for a system of training for all members of the staff.
3. Describe a method of training in a quality-assurance system.
4. Discuss the importance of testing each member of the staff following training.
5. Describe one method of creating a training method in the form of a game.
6. Explain why a commitment to quality is necessary if a quality program is to be successful.
7. Discuss the importance of a culture of learning.
8. List 10 elements of a quality-training system.
9. Explain the role of mentors in quality training.
10. Discuss the role of shift experts in quality training.

KEY TERMS

Continuous Quality Improvement (CQI): A CQI program is a workflow process designed to reduce the number of errors in any system. CQI is the term most often used in pharmacy practice for systems implemented to reduce the risk of a medication error reaching a patient. Other names often used are total quality management (TQM), quality assurance (QA), and quality improvement (QI). CQI systems should be structured to constantly improve and not remain static. This implies there must be an element of monitoring a system to discover and correct any vulnerabilities in the system.

Culture of learning: An environment within the pharmacy where all members of staff, including managers and executives of the organization, accept that continuous improvement includes an organized workflow, regular training, quality tools, and an emphasis on the importance of the people who make up the quality team. Everybody is a part of the system and they commit themselves to those goals of quality, service, and continuous improvement.

Mentoring programs: Mentors are peers who assist new employees in acclimating to the pharmacy. Mentors are particularly helpful in training new hires to understand and use the pharmacy's CQI program. Mentors may not be the trainers, but they function as confidants to whom new employees may go with questions.

Shift expert: A person appointed to act as the quality expert on a shift. There should be at least one person on each shift who knows the quality system and can answer questions. Each shift expert needs to regularly communicate with others to be sure the messages to team members on that shift and throughout the pharmacy are consistent.

Training: Training is teaching. It includes guiding, educating, and testing members of the team to be assured that all employees know how the pharmacy's quality systems function, what an individual employee's role is in the CQI program, and why each step in the pharmacy's quality workflow is necessary.

OUTLINE

Training to Make Quality Work
The Goal of Training
   Consistency of Purpose
   Refusal to Accept Mistakes or Defective Workmanship
   Drive out Fear

Ten Steps to Effective Training
   Commitment
   Leadership
   Culture of Learning
   Lifelong Training

- Test Then Build
- Results Oriented
- Reward Accomplishments
- A Universal Program
- Build Quality Habits
- Make Training Fun

Begin the Training
- The Case of Teaching Your Kid to Buckle Up
- Checklist for Training

Techniques and Tools
- Checklists and NO Checklists
- *The Case of the Baby's IV*

Testing
- Written Test and Practical Exam

QRE Tracking as Training and Testing

Summary

Training to Make Quality Work

The best quality-assurance plan will not work if it is not fully implemented and used. In order to ensure that a plan is used, the staff must be trained. Pharmacy technicians need to understand the need for **training** and be cognizant of the pharmacy's quality goals because they are and must be a critical part of designing, introducing, implementing, and improving continuous quality improvement (CQI) systems. Technicians who begin working in a dispensing role in the pharmacy may become the trainers and managers of the future.

Few people can perform a job well the first time, but the more a particular task is performed, the more skilled a person becomes at that task. Since medication errors can occur at various points in the pharmacy workflow, best practices are developed and integrated into that workflow as part of a CQI system in order to reduce the risk of a mistake occurring that could lead to a medication error. Designing the system is an important step in assuring patients they will receive prescriptions that are correct and as prescribed, and receive the professional services of a prospective drug review and appropriate counseling.

Once the CQI system is designed and implemented, all members of the pharmacy staff must be trained in its use to be certain the system is employed to its fullest potential for every prescription. Testing must follow and continue as long as the system is in use. In this chapter we look at both training and testing as if each were part of one continuing process. The purpose in this chapter is not just to train a pharmacy technician, but also to prepare a future trainer and pharmacy manager.

The Goal of Training

A discussion of training begins with a review of Edward Deming's 14 principles of management. Following these principles is necessary if a pharmacy organization is to reach its goal of consistent quality, that is, efficiently dispensing prescriptions and services with the lowest possible level of medication errors. Three of the 14 principles are particularly relevant to our discussion of training.

Consistency of Purpose

Deming's first principle involves creating a consistency of purpose. A quality enterprise is consistent in always striving to improve its products and services. Deming warned against sacrificing long-range needs for short-term profitability. The goal in training is to achieve this consistency. In pharmacy this means aiming for zero QREs, which will lead to zero errors. Perfection may never be obtained, but zero errors remains the target. By improving each day, the pharmacy constantly moves slightly closer to that target.

Best practices are designed to prevent or catch mistakes before they become an error. Several best practices are aimed at preventing the same mistake. Thus, we saw that the workflow in filling a prescription required a triple check, an NDC check, a pharmacist's final check, and an added three "Take 5s." This redundancy was calculated to make it increasingly more difficult for an error to get all the way through the workflow to the patient. Omitting any one of those best practices would slightly increase the possibility of error. The goal of training is to ensure that each best practice in the CQI workflow is performed every time, that there is a consistency of purpose. The enemy in achieving this consistency is the short-term profit of time—hurrying to save one or two seconds.

Refusal to Accept Mistakes or Defective Workmanship

The second goal in training is akin to Deming's second point in his list of 14 principles. Training must instill in each member of the team a philosophy of refusing to accept any mistakes or defective workmanship. No matter how busy the pharmacy is or the amount of pressure being applied at the moment, no one is willing to sacrifice quality and the constant striving for perfection.

Since one of the goals in instituting a CQI program is to constantly improve each process, an important part of the training is to instill this concept. In order to do so, the training must do more than teach the steps to be followed; it must teach *why* each step is a part of the program. The best teaching methods are interactive. In order to build a refusal to accept mistakes into the consciousness of the trainee, trainees must see how the CQI workflow uses redundancies and multiple best practices to reduce medication errors. But when an error occurs, there must be a response; something must be done to prevent a repeat of the situation. Learning strict obedience to a series of steps may work in standard cases, but there will be times when an unusual situation will demand thinking outside the regular process. An understanding of the concepts and goals will be needed in those cases.

Since technology is constantly changing the way we practice pharmacy, there will always be newer and more innovative ways to train the staff. The best training uses a melody of methods, for example, computer programs, textbooks, learning sheets, and even interactive games. Trainers need to find ways of training suitable for each employee, including **mentoring programs**, **shift experts**, and others. While one person may serve as the trainer, the pharmacy's training program should make effective use of each member of the staff to be sure everyone is knowledgeable about the quality program.

Drive out Fear

Training should be positive and not a negative event. An otherwise good, well-intentioned training program can be defeated if it instills fear in those being trained. All employees must feel they can ask any questions and report any shortcomings they perceive regarding the workflow, pharmacy operations, and professional environment. The pharmacy may ask technicians for comments and observations. New employees can offer a fresh view compared to those who have worked within a system for a period of time. Not only will management be quickly alerted to potential problems, often before they lead to errors or injuries, but also each employee will feel a part of the system.

For training to be effective, it must encourage two-way communications. One of the principles of quality management is that the system must "drive out fear." It can do this by bringing all employees into the discussion of quality and CQI systems. Pharmacists, managers, and pharmacy technicians should all feel free to voice their opinions and thoughts.

Training can use some of the same techniques used in monitoring the results of the CQI program. The pharmacy can measure the results of its training program by using statistical methods to improve the training, and hence to improve its quality system that will reduce medication errors.

Training in quality should include emphasis on productivity and efficiency because training can increase productivity. The fewer number of prescriptions a pharmacy has to redo on a daily or weekly basis because of a QRE, the more productive the pharmacy will be. This is one test of success and profit.

A final goal of the training program must be to allow all members of the team to take pride in their work. Every work environment has barriers that inhibit the worker's pride. A good program of education, training, and retraining can constantly improve to produce a high level of pride.

In order to accomplish all of these lofty goals, the pharmacy must have a clearly articulated training and employee-development plan. Management, including management at the very top, must be committed to continuously improving quality, increased productivity, and efficiency. These result in superior service to the patient and to pride of workmanship throughout the staff.

Ten Steps to Effective Training

Effective training requires a plan. A plan begins with a set of goals outlining what is to be achieved and has a strategy for effectively realizing those goals. There are ten steps to effective training.

1. Commitment
2. Leadership
3. Culture of Learning
4. Lifelong Training
5. Test Then Build
6. Results Oriented
7. Reward Accomplishments
8. Universal Program
9. Build Quality Habits
10. Make Training Fun

Commitment

If the pharmacy is to have a consistency of purpose that will result in the least number of errors possible, all members of the team must be committed to that result. Commitment begins with allocating time for training. Pharmacies are busy and finding training time is not easy.

Initially, the pharmacist in charge of developing the training schedule may involve only the pharmacy technicians, but eventually pharmacists need to be included. Since over 80 percent of all claims involve mechanical errors, concentrating initial training on pharmacy technicians can prove effective. As they demonstrate their commitment to training and quality, pharmacists will be motivated to participate.

Since training will take time away from some other activity, everyone must understand that it is an investment that will save both time and money in the long run. If through training the pharmacy can reduce the number of near-misses, it can save the time spent on rework caused by QREs. The amount of time required for initial training in a new CQI system can be considerable, but once a system is in place and all members of the team have been trained, the benefits of greater efficiency and productivity will be evident.

A commitment to training does not end after the initial training. Regular refresher sessions should be scheduled. These sessions may be short and may occasionally be fun. A degree of competition may be added so long as it does not detract from the overall purpose. Regular training provides a way to reach the goal of efficiently filling prescriptions with the least possible number of errors and near-misses.

Deming taught that management's job is to provide the tools required to achieve quality. Pharmacy technicians and pharmacists must make the best use of the tools provided, including the CQI program.

Leadership

The road to quality requires effective leadership. In pharmacy there will be leaders at several levels, each with a specific responsibility. The CEO delivers the tools necessary and corporate commitment. The pharmacist-in-charge develops training schedules and leads the team in implementation of the program. And a person (a pharmacist or a pharmacist technician) should be designated to be the leader in charge of training, testing, and monitoring the pharmacy's CQI system; this person should be able to patiently assist all members of the team. Everyone in the pharmacy should recognize who is in charge of each of these important functions.

Culture of Learning

With everyone committed to excellence in quality and with the leader in place, the pharmacy is in a position to establish a **culture of learning**. Training should be made relevant to each member of the staff so that each understands the pharmacy's principles, ideals, and goals. Building a culture requires making everybody a part of the system and committed to the concept of quality. There are several ways in which the pharmacy and the quality leader can make training relevant. It may require imagination and creativity, but mainly it requires a desire to help everyone succeed. Training can then move to the mechanics of the workflow.

Learning is not a one-time lesson. It is an ongoing process. Scheduled lessons may be monthly, quarterly, or annually. A culture of learning can be spread by mentors assisting new employees.

Lifelong Training

Continuous training means continuous learning. Times change, as do needs and practices. There is a tendency to believe that what we do now is correct and there is no need to change. And so, once we have received training in a CQI system, we are reluctant to change. However, the commitment to constant training and learning must be a part of a company's policies and procedures. It begins with management and must spread to the leaders, all the staff, and all new employees. It is not just the understanding that training is necessary, but that the need for training never ends.

New employees benefit from training, but so do established employees. As part of a culture of learning, there must be instilled in each member of the team a desire to learn. Introduction to new concepts needs to be seen as an exciting opportunity, not a threat. This cannot be done by telling someone what they are to do, but rather by showing them how new concepts can benefit them.

Some pharmacists believe their time is best spent performing what are technician functions, such as computer data entry and filling prescriptions. They do not accept the proposition that if pharmacy technicians performed these mechanical functions, pharmacists would be released to spend time with counseling and drug review. For some pharmacists this reluctance may arise from a lack of feeling comfortable in these new roles. Likewise, pharmacy technicians who have practiced in the same manner at the same location for a period of time may find it difficult to accept a new workflow with different expectations. Developing a system of continuous learning can help overcome these fears of change.

Test Then Build

In order to train effectively, it is important that the training and the system itself be tested prior to introducing it on a large scale. Using the risk-management cycle, the techniques and steps in the system are first tested on a small scale, monitored, and then changed if necessary. With the changes in place, the system is tested again. The steps in building a training program follow the risk-management process.[1]

1. Identify the risks, problems, or inefficiencies in the proposed training system.

    a) To effectively train employees, the pharmacy must first establish the goals of the training program. Then it can develop a plan that will accomplish these goals.

    b) In developing the plan, the pharmacy asks:

        i) How will the training system be accepted by employees?

        ii) Is this plan the best use of time for each member of the team?

iii) Are there inefficiencies in the planned training system?

iv) Is the new plan easily understood by all members of the team?

2. Select the techniques to teach the program in the most efficient manner.

   a) Revise inefficient steps to perform the task in less time or with fewer movements, while maintaining the purpose of each step.

   b) Select teaching techniques that make the training effective and will maintain interest in learning.

3. Implement and perfect the training plan on a small scale as a trial before introducing it to the entire team.

   a) Before any system of training is completely implemented, test it on a small scale.

   b) Test it at one location, on a select number of staff, or on one shift.

   c) Involve others at the testing stage so the test has the benefit of input from the group.

4. Monitor and ask, "Did it work?"

   a) If the training worked in the test, implement it full scale in the pharmacy.

   b) If it did not work, or there were parts of the system that should be improved, make changes and retest.

   c) The ultimate question must be: Is the new training system effective?

Results Oriented

Without measurable results, training and the CQI system may be viewed as merely an expense. If training works, it should be quantifiable. Management needs to know that the pharmacy will obtain an acceptable rate of return on any investment, including the time and expense of training. The pharmacy and the team also need to know their time and training resulted in reasonable results. For both groups the primary measure is the reduction of medication errors. If management sees a beneficial return, the pharmacy's technicians and pharmacists will find it easier to request budgeted funds for future training.

Measurement of success of a CQI program designed to reduce medication errors begins by establishing a benchmark against which success may be compared. A benchmark is established by recording the number of QREs that happened in a selected period of time, such as 30 days. This number can be compared to the number of QREs that happened during an equal period of time after training has been implemented. Until a sufficient amount of data can be collected, the pharmacy will have only anecdotal evidence that the system is working. But within a relatively short period of time, sufficient real numbers will be collected to establish a benchmark and later to provide statistically valid evidence for comparison.

Results-oriented training also requires testing each person who works in the pharmacy's CQI workflow. The pharmacy needs to know how effective its training is for each employee. It can develop a testing system that will grade the employee on what each employee has learned. Individual testing also provides a method of rewarding those who succeed.

Reward Accomplishments

The largest investment most companies make is in their employees. If a company is to maximize its investment, employees must be able to work to their maximum potential. To do so, they must be trained to perform their job. This is particularly true when it comes to a system of continuous quality improvement.

A CQI program should allow everyone to succeed. It should be a source of pride. Nothing provides more pride in employees than knowing they are doing something important and doing it well. Employees must feel they are a part of the CQI system, not merely workers doing a job.

Training should emphasize the necessity of a particular job and why employees' work is important to overall success. Each employee should have a realistic set of goals and a way of knowing when he or she has succeeded. Not only should an employee know, but everyone else should also know when a member of the team has reached a goal. Reorganization among peers is a way of instilling pride and motivating each employee to strive for the next level of excellence.

Rewards may be as simple as a gold star on their uniform or a certificate proclaiming they have met a goal. While programs should be uniform for all, they should also be tailored as to the amount of effort it takes an individual to attain a certain level. Employees should be expected to continue their training to maintain their level of accomplishment. To prove continued proficiency, there should be a system of periodic testing with recognitions and rewards.

A Universal Program

CQI will require the pharmacy to establish one system that can be replicated throughout the enterprise. This means that each pharmacist and pharmacy technician will be trained in the same system.

This is particularly important in a pharmacy chain or a hospital with more than one location or pharmacy worksite. All members of the team should be able to move from one location to another without jeopardizing the system or a patient.

All people become creatures of habit and find it difficult to change. Problems come when established habits differ from new steps being taught as part of a CQI program. Pharmacies should adopt a universal training with no member of the staff outside the program. This may prove difficult with a few pharmacists and pharmacy technicians who have been in the same position for a long time. If, however, the pharmacy is to employ a system of CQI to the greatest extent possible, all employees, pharmacists, and pharmacy technicians need to be part of the same system.

One problem in achieving optimum success from a pharmacy quality system is if each individual has been able to use his or her own method of preparing a prescription. Pharmacy technicians may have been told to use a certain set of best practices, but were allowed to perform each in whatever manner and order they chose. Some of these individual methods may have been very good; some were less effective. Although everyone said they used all of the steps and best practices, there was no way to verify that. Only when an error was reported would it be discovered that an NDC check or a name check or some other practice was left out by a particular employee.

The problem with individualistic approaches is they do not develop a uniform system, without which the pharmacy cannot be certain that each best practice and step in the workflow is used each time. Under pressures of time, long lines, people waiting, or other events common in daily pharmacy practice, steps can be omitted. Individual, nonuniform application of a system does not allow efficient, periodic testing that can be done using an enforced uniform workflow.

Some employees believe their methods of workflow are superior to the ones taught by the organization. The truth is some of them may be, and that possibility needs to be open for discovery. New ideas should be considered and some other ways may warrant a trial. If, after testing, the new idea proves superior, it may be introduced into the system. This is consistent with the concept of continuous quality improvement. If a pharmacy technician or pharmacist has a better way to work a process, it should be shared with the team.

There are occasionally problems with uniformity (at first there will be a resistance to change), but there are many more advantages. A uniform system results in more best practices being used more often, leading to fewer mistakes, less rework, and a smaller number of errors. The purpose of a CQI system is to make errors increasingly difficult to reach the patient. Requiring all to use a uniform, proven system reduces the risk of an injured patient. Eventually new habits will replace old ones. This requires patience and leadership.

Build Quality Habits

An advantage of everyone using a standardized workflow is it allows the development of uniform quality habits that can be tested. Quality habits make it more difficult for a person to skip a best practice at times of stress or pressure. One of the purposes of training is to ensure the use of each best practice every time.

The Auburn University College of Pharmacy observational report concludes there are over 3 million potentially serious medication errors delivered to patients from community pharmacies each year.[2] The Pharmacists Mutual Insurance Company Study of Claims suggests that over three quarters of all claims against pharmacies, pharmacists, and pharmacy technicians are a result of placing the wrong drug or wrong strength of the correct drug in the bottle.[3] From our review of NDC numbers and how they work, it is obvious that if an NDC or scanner check is performed each time, these errors could not be made.

In the case of the 4-year-old child with pink eye that we studied in Chapter 2, the child received the otic instead of the prescribed ophthalmic form of his medication. In that case the pharmacist who made the mistake was asked if he ever used an NDC check. He replied, "Yes, every time." Because the NDC numbers of the ophthalmic and otic are different, it is obvious he did not. This pharmacist is not alone in thinking he checked the NDC number every time.

If we were to poll a group of pharmacy technicians and ask if they use NDC checks when filling prescriptions, almost all would say yes. And they would tell us they "always" use an NDC check. The problem is not to convince technicians they should use an NDC check, or other best practices. The problem is developing a method to ensure they use it each time they fill a prescription. A quality habit is itself a best practice. The entire workflow must become a habit, with each step in each process performed in the same manner and in the same sequence. Eventually, the process is engrained into the manner of work so that it becomes difficult to skip a step or best practice.

Make Training Fun

Training is a part of work. Anything that can make training more interesting is likely to be more effective than training that is boring and dull. Making work of any kind fun requires innovation and carries the risk of going too far and lessening the value of the training.

Training must be professional and include various methods of instruction and education. CQI instruction can include lectures and classroom situations. It can also involve role playing, such as how to handle a situation when an error occurs or when a patient calls to announce, "This is wrong." Simulated experiences such as talking to a patient who is wrong and one who is right can be valuable. They lead to better outcomes when the real thing occurs in the pharmacy.

A valuable method of learning may be roundtable discussions involving pharmacists and pharmacy technicians. For example, it could be a 60-second discussion at the prescription counter regarding a mistake that was caught.

Some fun ways of learning may take time to set up, for example, inventing a game that can instill important ideas. Consider the popular TV game show Jeopardy®. Most people will know how Jeopardy® is played. The contestant selects a position on the board out of 25 positions that are displayed. Each position has a topic and a dollar value, or in the following example, a point value. When a contestant selects a square on the board, the host causes the square to change to show an answer. The contestant must come up with the question to match that answer. If the contestant is correct, he or she gets the points. If not, the host shows the correct answer and then returns to the board.

A training game using questions and answers may be created using Microsoft® PowerPoint®. The process is fairly simple. The steps in creating the game are in RxErcise 8–A.

RxErcise 8-A   Create a "Jeopardy" Game (Individual or Group Exercise)

To make a "Jeopardy" game, you will need a computer with the PowerPoint program installed on it. The staff can play the game throughout the day or during a timed period. The instructions are below. The squares can contain either questions or answers.

1. Open PowerPoint and, using the table formatting, make a table with five columns across and six down, similar to the one in Figure 8-1.
2. Make headings across the top five squares to define your categories
3. In the first set of rows, place a value, increasing in each successive row.
   - Create 25 new pages—one for each answer (e.g., "Take 5"; see Figure 8-2). This is the page that will come up when you click on the square you select for this answer.
   - Now create 25 additional new pages, one for the correct question for each answer; if the contestant gets it wrong, you can hyperlink over to this page for the correct question (see Figure 8-3).
4. Now you need to hyperlink the answers and questions. In each square with a value, highlight the value (e.g., "5 points") and right click. Select "hyperlink" and "inside this document", and click on the page for the answer (see Figure 8-4).
5. At the bottom of each question page and each answer page, place a symbol; right click on the symbol you choose and hyperlink it back to the board so after each answer you can return to the board for the next contestant.
6. You will need two symbols on the answer pages since you will need two alternatives—one to return to the board if the contestant gets the answer correct, and one to hyperlink to the correct question if the contestant gets it wrong.

Best Practices	Theory	Words	Steps	testing
<u>5 points</u>	5 points	5 points	5 points	5 points
10 Points	10 Points	10 Points	10 Points	10 Points
20 Points	20 Points	20 Points	20 Points	20 Points
50 Points	50 Points	50 Points	50 Points	50 Points
100 Points	100 Points	100 Points	100 Points	100 Points

Figure 8-1 "Jeopardy" Game
© Cengage Learning 2013

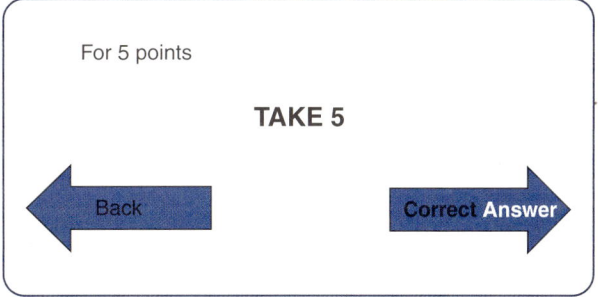

Figure 8-2 Answer to Question in the Training Game
© Cengage Learning 2013

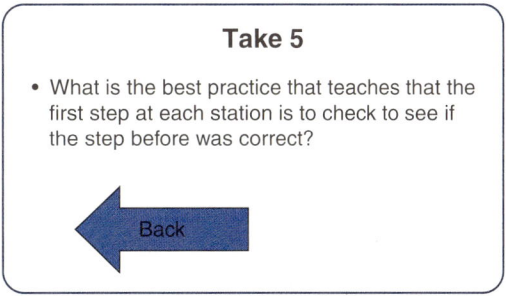

Figure 8-3 Correct question to the Answer for Take 5
© Cengage Learning 2013

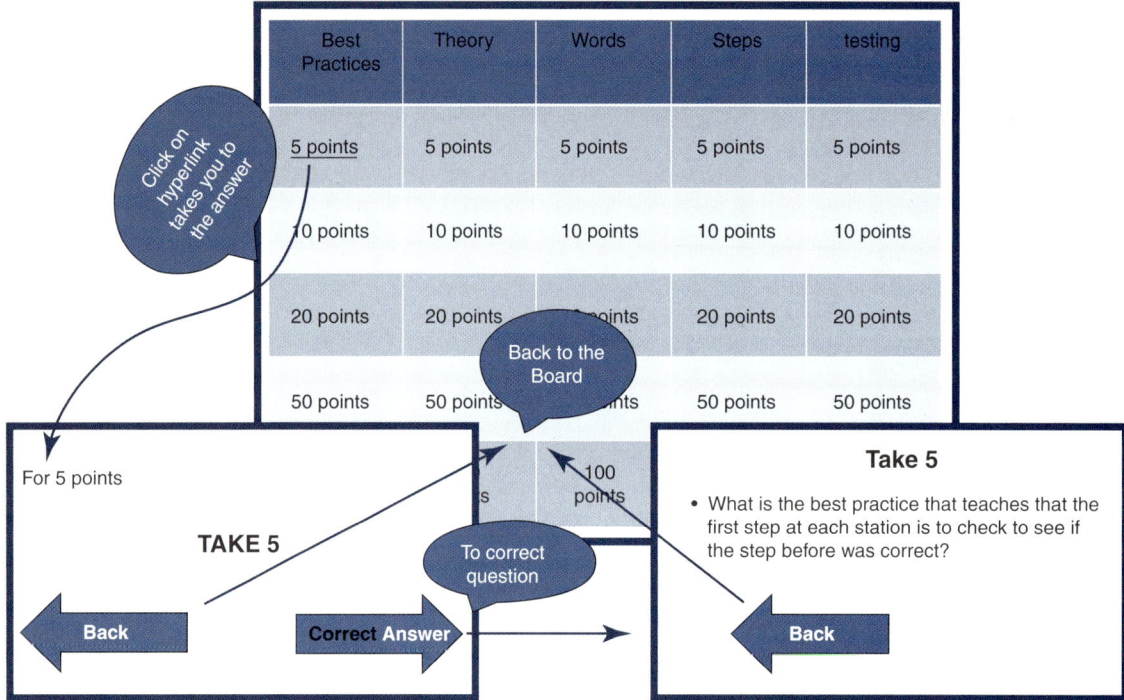

Figure 8-4 Making your own training game using questions and answers along the line of the TV show "Jeopardy®". The trainee chooses a question with a point value under a category. Using PowerPoint® link takes the trainee to an Answer. They provide the question. To check the answer they clink on the link to correct answer.
© Cengage Learning 2013

Begin the Training

A way to begin CQI training is by establishing a uniform workflow though which the staff can build quality habits. In most pharmacies a CQI workflow will already exist. In a typical workflow there are six stations, each with a mini workflow of detailed steps and best practices (see the sample in Chapter 7). Three stations will generally be the workstations of the pharmacy technician: receiving the prescription, entering the data into the computer, and filling the prescription.

One goal of the pharmacy's training program is for each pharmacy technician to learn to follow each step in exactly the order presented in each workstation. The pharmacy technician practices the steps until he or she can perform each step in order without a checklist. This develops quality habits.

The Case of Teaching Your Kid to Buckle Up

Let us look outside the pharmacy for an example of quality habits and training. Imagine you have a sixteen-year-old son or daughter and you are teaching him or her to drive a car for the first time. One of your concerns is that someday he or she may be in an accident. An important part of your training, therefore, is to make sure that you train your son or daughter to drive safely as well as to master the technical skills involved in operating a motor vehicle. You know one safety measure in driving an automobile is the use of seatbelts.

First, you want to impress upon your child the importance of wearing seatbelts. James Madison University in Virginia has developed several programs in public safety, including one for automobile safety. The university publishes a list of statistics regarding the use of seatbelts[4] that you can use to convince your child of the need to develop a quality habit of always using a seatbelt while driving:

- One out of every five drivers will be involved in a traffic crash this year.
- Motor vehicle crashes are the leading cause of death among people age 44 and younger and the number one cause of head and spinal cord injury.
- Approximately 35,000 people die in motor vehicle crashes each year. About 50 percent (17,000) of these people could have been saved if they had worn their safety belts.
- More than 90 percent of all motorists believe safety belts are a good idea, but less than 14 percent actually use them.
- For every 1 percent increase in safety belt use, 172 lives and close to $100 million in annual injury and death costs could be saved.
- Safety belts, when used properly, reduce the number of serious traffic injuries by 50 percent and fatalities by 60–70 percent.
- For maximum protection safety belts should be fastened before traveling any distance or speed. Seventy-five percent of crash deaths and injuries occur within 25 miles of home. More than half of all injury-producing motor vehicle crashes involve low speeds under 40 mph.
- Motorists are 25 times are more likely to be killed or seriously injured when they are "thrown clear" than when they remain inside their vehicle.
- In a 30-mph collision, an unbelted 160-pound person can strike another passenger, crash through a windshield, and/or slam into the vehicle's interior with a 4,800-pound force.
- Motorists can increase safety belt usage by example and verbal reminders. Nine out of 10 people buckle up when asked.
- Safety belt use is one of the best defenses against the unpredictable actions of the drunk driver.
- Today over 25 countries around the world have some type of mandatory safety belt law. Results of these laws were measured; usage rate went from 20–25 percent before passage to 60–90 percent after passage.
- A common cause of death and injury to children in motor vehicles is being crushed by adults who are not wearing safety belts. One out of four serious injuries to passengers is caused by occupants being thrown into each other.

- About 80 percent of all injuries to children in car crashes are injuries to the head, causing brain damage, permanent disfigurement, epilepsy, or death.
- Of every 100 children who die in motor vehicle crashes, at least 80 would have survived if they were properly secured in an approved child safety seat or in safety belts.
- Three out of four families with child safety seats fail to use them correctly. Adults need to follow manufacturer's instructions and secure seats properly before every trip.
- An estimated 80 percent of American children are immunized against contagious diseases, but less than 10 percent are properly restrained when riding in a motor vehicle.

James Mason University's statistics are convincing. Just as a study of medication errors will, hopefully, convince pharmacy technicians of the importance of a working quality-assurance program, statistics might also motivate your child to use a seatbelt each and every time he or she gets into a car. The best way for you to ensure that is to develop in your child a quality habit. When you begin your training you tell your child, "Fasten your seatbelt." You tell him or her the same thing every time he or she gets in the car as part of their training. You and your child develop a regular process:

1. get in car;
2. fasten seatbelt;
3. start car.

You insist that this happen in the same order every time your child gets ready to drive the car. After a few weeks, your child will have developed a habit and it will become difficult for him or her to start the car without fastening his or her seatbelt. Hopefully you have built a quality habit. We can do the same thing in a pharmacy workflow with best practices.

There are a lot of theories about how habits are created and how long it takes. Common wisdom says it takes 21 days to develop a habit. Some experts say it may take as many as 66 days.[5] Whatever the number may be, in order to create a habit, the same thing must be done over and over in the same sequence. A pharmacy workflow contains steps for each station. These steps incorporate best practices. A goal of training is to teach all members of the staff to use the outlined steps in the same sequence each time. After a period of time the training should have created quality habits. It should become more difficult for any member of the staff to skip or forget to use any best practices he or she has been trained to use.

Apply the lessons from The Case of Teaching Your Kid to Buckle Up to training staff to use the pharmacy's CQI program. We can train the pharmacy workflow in the same manner. Consider the NDC number check as an example. If all technicians are taught to use an NDC check immediately before they open the stock bottle and are taught to do it at this same time repeatedly, they should eventually form a habit. Once the habit is formed the technician will have a difficult time opening the stock bottle without having first checked the NDC number.

Each technician is told to review each step and understand why each is necessary. This is an important part of the training. The steps for the filling process are repeated below. After each is an explanation that may be a part of the training regarding that step. The trainer may also use examples of claims, such as the ones in this book. Training is more effective if the trainees know why they are taking each step. The following Chinese proverb exemplifies the difference between just instructing and actually training:

Tell me, I'll forget;
Show me, I'll remember;
Involve me, I'll understand.

☐ As the baskets with the new prescriptions, labels, patient-information leaflets, and any required med-guides are transferred from the computer data-entry station, they are placed in order depending on how they are to be processed.

One of the reasons for the basket system is to guard against prescriptions for one patient becoming confused with another patient. If we can develop a habit of placing work to be done in an organized manner, we can further protect against creating problems when we take one patient's prescription out of order. If the pharmacy uses colored baskets to cause one order to be put ahead of another, we train the technician to recognize this and act accordingly. It also impresses upon everyone the need for all items to be assembled at the beginning of the process.

☐ "Take 5"—take a few seconds to review the Rx against the steps that should have been taken at the receiving and computer data entry stations (e.g., Right patient? Right drug? Right strength? Right directions? Med-guide required?). If anything is incomplete, hand the basket back to the receiving clerk to make necessary corrections.

Each pharmacy technician must begin each station with a "Take 5" review for any mistakes or omissions that may have been made up to that point. While this step takes a matter of seconds, it is an important step in quality review. A testing question for each pharmacy technician is, "What is the first job at this station?" The answer is always, "Take 5." If this step is automatically performed at the beginning of each process, the risk of an error going all the way through the workflow to a patient is reduced.

☐ Note if there are any highlights on the new Rx from the receiving technician—allergies, other medications, unusual doses, vulnerable patient (over 60, under 6).

This step is to look and note. It is important because it emphasizes the special nature of certain prescriptions: those with an "A" (allergy); "M" (other medications); age in red (under 6 / over 60—vulnerable patient); and any dosage form that could be out of the norm. The action a pharmacy technician should take at this point is a pause while thinking: "special patient" followed by "one more check."

☐ Using the new Rx (not the printed label unless a refill), pull the stock bottle from the shelf. This makes sure a computer-entry QRE of wrong drug or strength is not carried through to filling. It causes a second interpretation of the original Rx, after the data-entry technician and before the third and definitive reading of the Rx by the pharmacist at the final quality check. If any question or difference is noted, the pharmacy technician must call the pharmacist to verify immediately.

Physician's written prescriptions account for a number of the drug orders received in pharmacies. Many are illegible, and mistakes in reading or entering them can be made with every computer entry. Pharmacy technicians need to be trained to pull the stock bottle based upon the prescription itself, not the label or receipt. If a mistake is made by the entry technician, using the label would reinforce that incorrect entry. Eight to 9 percent of the claims against pharmacies are caused by incorrect directions typed on the label. Once a mistake is made, it may be repeated with each refill. On its website, Pharmacists Mutual gives a description of these types of claims and cites the following:[6]

> *"Wrong Directions" are a significant number of the claims reported in the Pharmacists Mutual Study. These cases involve incorrectly entering the directions into the computer on new prescriptions. In one claim the pharmacist entered a new prescription for birth control tablets into the computer and inadvertently typed "Take two tablets daily." For nine months this patient refilled her birth control prescription every 15 days, apparently without anyone at the pharmacy noticing.*

☐ Check drug name and strength on new Rx against drug name and strength on stock bottle (if shelf is marked as "problem drug," double-check).

There are four main checks of right drug and strength during filling. As a best practice we call these "triple check + NDC." This is the first of three name versus name checks. By training the technician to make this check at the same place each time, a quality habit is created. This is check ONE.

☐ If this is a vulnerable patient (over 60, under 6), check one more time before pulling from shelf.

This Rx deserves one more look; if a mistake is made here, it could be more consequential. The message is: vulnerable patient, check again.

☐ Return new Rx and stock bottle to pharmacy counter. Before counting out drugs, check name against name again.

This is check TWO—same place, each time.

☐ Before counting out drugs, do an NDC number check of receipt (what was entered into computer) and stock bottle. If a scanner is used, scan NDC numbers as check.

This is check + NDC—same place, each time.

☐ Count out drug and put into prescription bottle. *Note:* a safety cap must be used unless specifically requested not to by patient or physician (as documentation, the patient should sign the back of Rx if patient requested no safety cap).

When the prescription is for a controlled substance, the count is repeated to be certain the amount given is correct. An audit is taken of the number of all controlled substances at regular intervals. This audit goes to the DEA.

Safety caps are ALWAYS used unless the pharmacy has proof that (1) the patient requested otherwise; (2) the physician ordered no safety cap; or (3) it is one of a very limited number of drugs, such as nitroglycerine sublingual tablets, which are exempted by law. Should a child be injured after getting into a prescription bottle, the patient will often not remember giving oral instructions for no safety cap.

☐ Place label on prescription bottle using "2-second rule."

No bottle with medication inside it is left without a label for longer than two seconds. This best practice is used because occasionally there will be an interruption resulting in an unlabeled bottle being left on the counter.

☐ Perform a final name versus name check between label and, if new prescription, the original Rx (triple check).

This is check THREE—same place, each time. After three checks plus an NDC check, the risk of a mechanical error is reduced greatly. Note: if a technician has missed a mistake after making three checks, it is less likely that adding more checks of the same nature will be valuable.

☐ Place completed Rx with receipt, patient-information leaflet, warnings from computer, profile from computer, and medguide, if required, in basket for pharmacist's final quality check.

One final check to be certain the pharmacy technician is delivering everything to the pharmacist.

- ☐ Deliver basket with all material to the pharmacist. Alternatives may be added, such as having the technician pull up the scanned Rx image on the screen in the pharmacist's final check area. The technician may attach the receipt to the bag, unstapled, so the pharmacist knows it is finished and ready for a check.

While each step of the workflow is almost choreographed so that each step is taken in the same place at the same time, some pharmacists and pharmacy technicians have individual preferences. A pharmacist may want the technician to assist in small ways, such as have the patient profile ready for the pharmacist on the terminal; others will not. It is important to communicate these interactions and wants among the staff.

- ☐ If the prescription is put into a "will call" area, meaning the patient is not waiting, the filling technician may put a sticker on the bag indicating a new prescription or counseling may be warranted.

Consider the purpose of the sticker indicating "counsel this patient" and what other additions may be added at this part of the workflow. This will vary by pharmacy.

TECHNIQUES AND TOOLS

There are many ways and techniques for teaching. Here we will explore one that breaks a long series of steps into a set of simpler processes so the trainee can learn small, manageable bits at one time.

Once the pharmacy has set up its workflow, break it into a series of stations. This is the approach taken in Chapter 7 and in the example above. It is difficult to learn an entire pharmacy workflow in one setting; it is easier to master the steps one station at a time. The trainer/teacher should consider how he or she would like to be taught, and then choose one of the three stations that are mainly the technician's area, and begin. A training plan may follow a process such as the following:

- Introduce the theory. Use stories and claims to illustrate points. The trainee should be able to answer the following questions:
  - Why is reducing medication errors important?
  - How is a workflow necessary in reducing the risk of medication errors occurring?
  - What are best practices and what is their value in a workflow?
  - Why is it important that everyone use the same workflow?

- Explain the steps in the overall workflow and within each station.
  - Use printed material the student can study alone.
  - Begin training for one station.
  - Practice on that station until the trainee is familiar with each step.
- Test the trainee's knowledge.
  - Before declaring the training of any station complete, have the trainee demonstrate each step in the correct order without the use of notes or a checklist.
  - Ask questions to determine if the trainee is familiar with the workflow in this station.
- Following initial training, have the trainee join the regular workflow and fill prescriptions at the station for which he or she has been trained.
  - Use checklists until the student demonstrates knowledge of each step.
  - Without the checklist or any written material, have the student fill prescriptions in this station, completing the steps in the process by memory.
- Test again.
  - When the trainee feels comfortable, test again his or her proficiency with the steps in each station that the trainee has completed.
- Hold a roundtable discussion with the trainee regarding the workflow and answer any questions.
- Discuss any suggestions for change, remembering that a system must be uniform.
- Begin training in a second station and then at successive stations' workflows until all are mastered.
- Retest each member of the staff on a regular basis.

Checklists and NO Checklists

When an airline pilot prepares for takeoff, she or he and the copilot systematically go over each item in a long list of preflight items that must be completed before they can lift off. The pilots perform this ritual each time, always in the same order. They must be certain that each step has been checked.

If pilots use checklists, why not have technicians use a checklist to mark each step while filling all prescriptions? The answer is partly because it would be very inefficient. Using a checklist involving several steps as part of a high-volume operation would take too much time; that fact alone would probably cause it to fail. Pharmacies fill 200 or more prescriptions a day. After a period of time, marking the checklist could become a focus rather than performing each step. Pilots use checklists only three to four times a day. Because of the volume, checklists in the pharmacy would not be useful as part of a daily routine for each prescription order filled.

In his book, *The Checklist Manifesto, How to Get Things Right*[7] (2009), Dr. Atul Gawande articulates the importance of checklists in order to guarantee that each step is taken each time in the right order. He points out that in some complex operations such as flying an airplane and surgery, checklists are absolutely necessary. In such pursuits the job is done only a few times a day and a checklist is an acceptable and desirable practice.

Checklists are just as necessary in a pharmacy workflow, but they are used in a different manner. Pharmacy workflows are not generally complex (with some exceptions as we will discuss later); they are relatively simple. Each task is replicated hundreds of times a day. A pharmacy-station checklist can be, with practice, committed to memory. Pharmacists and technicians can develop quality habits, reinforced with testing and constant use, which can become more valuable than a physical checklist for each prescription.

> **Quality Note 8-A** **Checklist of Special Exceptions: Compounding and IV Preparation**
>
> There are exceptions within pharmacy practice for the use of checklists. There are some prescriptions that are complex, require very exacting actions, and are performed a relatively few times a day. In these cases, a written checklist may be considered not only desirable, but also necessary. Among these exceptions are compounded prescriptions and prepared IV solutions. Generally, these prescriptions cannot be checked in the same way that a commercially available product would be checked. When an exact formula is required, it should be accompanied by a checklist detailing what is to be done and in what order. This is particularly the case if these orders are partly or wholly prepared by a pharmacy technician to be checked by a pharmacist. The checklist becomes a necessary part of the pharmacist's quality check.

The Case of the Baby's IV

In an Ohio hospital, a pharmacy technician was mixing an IV solution for a young patient. The formula called for the addition of a normal saline solution to bring the IV to full volume. Normal saline solution is 0.9 percent salt, which matches the human body's saline concentration. The pharmacy technician could have used a commercially available normal saline solution that was premixed to equal 0.9 percent saline. She also had the option of using a stronger saline solution and weakening it with sterile water to get it to the 0.9 percent concentration of normal saline. She chose to use the stronger saline solution and to dilute it. It was not diluted as she intended. She accidently used the higher concentration of saline solution full strength to make the IV, resulting in a dangerously high saline concentration in the final IV mixture. The pharmacist checked the technician's work without realizing she had used the stronger solution. While checking, it was reported later, he saw an empty, commercially available 0.9 percent bag, which he mistakenly believed had been used in this IV. Under that belief, he approved the IV solution as prepared and it was sent to the treatment room. The baby died.[8]

RxErcise 8-B   The Eric Cropp/Baby Jessica Case

The case in Ohio is described by the Institute for Safe Medication Practices on its website. Read the events as described by ISMP following a conversation with Eric Cropp, the pharmacist involved.

> The error happened on a Sunday morning, with typical weekend staffing. Eric was busy and had taken no breaks and had not eaten any meals during his shift. Routine maintenance had been performed on the computer the night before, and the pharmacy system was not available until mid-morning. The labels for IV admixtures, which typically printed around 7 a.m., printed later that morning, causing a delay in preparing solutions. Eric received a call to dispense Emily's chemotherapy right away, although it was not needed until hours later (unknown by Eric at the time). After the technician mixed the solution, he felt rushed to check the chemotherapy, which was among many other solutions, vials, and syringes in a very small, crowded checking area. Eric saw an empty 250 mL bag of 0.9 percent sodium chloride near the bag of chemotherapy and assumed the technician had used it to prepare the base solution.
>
> Eric states that the technician later testified that she had told him something seemed "weird" about the solution. Eric does not recall this conversation. He only recalls asking the technician whether she had used sodium chloride, which she answered affirmatively. Eric also saw a vial of 23.4 percent sodium chloride on the crowded table and assumed the technician had used this vial to prepare the prior chemotherapy order, which required the use of an automated compounder. The chemotherapy Eric was checking had been prepared by an experienced technician, but instead of premixed 0.9 percent sodium chloride, she had used three vials of 23.4 percent sodium chloride. Eric failed to detect the error and dispensed the solution. In this case, the confluence of system and human errors led to tragedy.

What do you think? Discuss what lessons can be learned from this tragic case. No one can be certain that training or the use of a checklist would have prevented this tragic series of mistakes from happening.
How might training have helped in this case?
What were the results of this case?
Was it a fair result?

Checklists for Training

A way to use checklists in pharmacy is as part of training. The trainer may have the trainee technician fill 25 prescriptions at one station using a detailed checklist. As the technician fills each of these 25 prescriptions, he or she marks off the steps on the checklist. The trainee stops using the checklist when the trainer determines it is no longer needed. See Figure 8-5 for an example of a training checklist.

> ☑ Take 5—take a few seconds to review the Rx for the steps that should have been taken at receiving (e.g., patient under 6 years old not marked; address missing, etc.). If anything is incomplete, hand basket back to receiving clerk to correct.
>
> ☑ Enter the patient's name (if refill, enter Rx number to be refilled) into the computer.
>
> ☑ Check to be sure.
>
> ☑ Check allergies on new Rx and make sure the computer profile for this patient is correct.
>
> ☑ Check other medications indicated on new Rx and make sure computer profile is up to date.
>
> **Training Checklist Used by Trainee**

Figure 8-5 Checklist by trainee (all boxes checked)
© Cengage Learning 2013

The trainer then watches as one or two additional prescriptions are filled. Silently the observer marks each step as the trainee completes them. Any missed or out of place step on the checklist is noted as "missed" and the rest as "passed" by using a checkmark (see Figure 8-6). The trainee is allowed to retake the test until he or she can pass it without mistake.

> ☑ Take 5—take a few seconds to review the Rx for the steps that should have been taken at receiving (e.g., patient under 6 years old not marked; address missing, etc.). If anything is incomplete, hand basket back to receiving clerk to correct.
>
> ☑ Enter the patient's name (if refill, enter Rx number to be refilled) into the computer.
>
> ☑ Check to be sure.
>
> Missed → ☐ Check allergies on new Rx and make sure the computer profile for this patient is correct.
>
> ☑ Check other medications indicated on new Rx and make sure computer profile is up to date.
>
> **Training Checklist as Used by Observer (Monitor)**

Figure 8-6 Checklist by observer (circle for missed box)
© Cengage Learning 2013

The entire workflow for all stations should be written with each step detailed. For new technicians, training can begin by their reading a copy of this written workflow. The trainee is then trained at one station at a time, but each technician should have a copy of the entire workflow so it can be referred to at anytime as a refresher.

As the technician is shown to be proficient in each process, there should be some tangible recognition of the accomplishment. This reward may be small, such as a printed certificate or a name on a board citing this training has been successfully completed. Recognition should be placed where all of the staff can see it because recognition of one person may motivate others.

Testing

If the pharmacy is to make its training results meaningful, there must be a way of testing to show the person has absorbed the lessons. This goes further than merely being able to answer questions covering the training material, although that is a first step. The purpose of testing is to measure the value of the training and the employee's ability to use the workflow and the CQI system.

Written Test and Practical Exam

Written tests for simple workflows need not be long or complicated. The most important test for the trainee will be a practical exam, such as demonstrated in Figure 8-6 above. The observer is the tester. If a written test is used to see if the technician understands the basic principles of the pharmacy's CQI system, it may be given before or after the practical. It may also test theory and ask questions such as why? The "written" test may be in the form of a game loosely based on the "Jeopardy" example discussed above.

One question on each test, oral or written, may be as simple as: What is the first step to be taken at this station? The answer is "Take 5." Four or five questions such as this from different parts of the workflow may be sufficient. Much will depend on the trainees and how well they do with the practical exam. If training is lifelong, so is testing. A similar test or set of tests should be used periodically to demonstrate that each technician has maintained efficiency.

QRE Tracking as Training and Testing

The best proof of effective training and an efficient CQI workflow is the number of errors made. Even better is the number of QREs that happened that could lead to an error. One of Deming's principles is: "We will no longer accept mistakes as a part of the system." Without mistakes or QREs, there can be no errors. To know whether the pharmacy's workflow and training plan is effective, the pharmacy must establish a benchmark against which to compare before and after training.

Summary

Most pharmacies have a quality-assurance program. Many are very good. No program of quality assurance can be proven successful, however, unless it can demonstrate that it works. There are two ways to prove a system is working. One is to monitor the system over a sufficiently long period of time to show a reduction in mistakes and ultimately errors. The other is to be able to demonstrate that all employees are proficient in its operation. The former is the subject of the next chapter; the latter has been the subject of this chapter: an organized system of training and testing.

Review Questions

1. What is the first step taken at the filling station?
    A. "Take 5"
    B. "Triple check"
    C. "NDC check"
    D. Any step may be taken first, so long as all steps are taken at some point during the filling process.

2. What is the first step taken at the computer entry station?
    A. "Take 5"
    B. Entering the patient's name into the computer
    C. Checking the directions typed into the computer
    D. Any step may be taken first, so long as all steps are taken at some point during the filling process.

3. What is the first step taken at the pharmacist's final quality check station?
    A. "Take 5"
    B. Prospective drug review
    C. "NDC check"
    D. Any step may be taken first, so long as all steps are taken at some point during the filling process.

4. The difference between a good quality-assurance system and a great one can be said to be two elements. Name one of these elements.
    A. A quality checklist for each part of the workflow
    B. A system of monitoring the occurrence of QREs

C. A pharmacist quality final check area

D. The use of best practices

5. The difference between a good quality-assurance system and a great one can be said to be two elements. Name the other one of these elements.

   A. Pharmacist drug review performed on each prescription

   B. A system of rewards for technicians who have worked within the system for a defined period of time

   C. A system of testing and training

   D. A system by which technicians who make frequent errors are relieved of duty

6. According to studies of claims, mechanical errors account for over what percent of all claims?

   A. 25%

   B. 50%

   C. 80%

   D. 100%

7. A good training system coupled with a good quality-assurance system can result in reduced errors. Name an additional benefit.

   A. A more efficient workflow

   B. Less complaints by pharmacy staff

   C. Increased financial rewards for the staff

   D. Less productivity, but balanced with job satisfaction

8. What is a leader of the quality system in a pharmacy in charge of?

   A. Training

   B. Testing

   C. Monitoring

   D. All of the above

9. From management's point of view, it is almost impossible to view training as anything but an expense without what?

   A. measurable results

   B. approval by staff

   C. positive customer surveys

   D. a record of long-time employee retention

10. What is an advantage of having everyone using a uniform workflow?

    A. It allows all within the system to develop quality habits.

    B. It reduces expenses from using multiple systems.

    C. It increases job satisfaction.

    D. None of the above; a uniform workflow has proven to be disruptive.

Endnotes

[1] Review the risk-management process in Chapter 1.

[2] Flynn, E. A., Barker, K. N., Carnahan, B. J., National Observational Study of Prescription Dispensing Accuracy and Safety in 50 Pharmacies, *JAPhA*, Vol. 43, No. 2, March/April 2003, pp. 191–200.

[3] The latest published Pharmacists Mutual Claims Study is available at the company's website: http://www.phmic.com/phmc/services/RM/profliab/claimsstudy/Pages/TheStoryBehindthePharmacistsMutualClaimStudy.aspx accessed August 2, 2010. Also see discussion, Chapter 1.

[4] James Madison University, http://www.jmu.edu/safetyplan/vehicle/generaldriver/safetybelt.shtml accessed February 1, 2011.

[5] Burkeman, O., This column will change your life: How long does it really take to change a habit? "Self-help culture clings to the fiction of the 28-day rule." *The Guardian News and Media Limited*, 2011, http://www.guardian.co.uk/lifeandstyle/2009/oct/10/change-your-life-habit-28-day-rule accessed February 1, 2011.

[6] See Pharmacists Mutual Claims Study, http://www.phmic.com/phmc/services/RM/profliab/claimsstudy/Pages/TheMechanicalErrors.aspx accessed March 26, 2011.

[7] Gawande, A., 2010. *The Checklist Manifesto, How to Get Things Right*, New York: Picador Holt and Co.

[8] The Eric Cropp case. For a more complete description of this case, see Ohio State Board of Pharmacy. http://www.ismp.org/Newsletters/acutecare/articles/20091203.asp

CHAPTER 9

Monitoring and Learning from Mistakes

The Last Step in Quality

OBJECTIVES

Upon completion of this chapter, the reader should be able to:

1. Explain the need for monitoring in a quality system.
2. Understand the causes of medication errors.
3. Describe the term "variability" as it relates to risk management.
4. Discuss the use of tools to determine causes of errors.
5. Describe how recording information during monitoring can be used to reduce the risks of medication errors.
6. Explain the term "normal variation" and how it relates to monitoring.
7. Discuss the use of statistical controls in a quality system.
8. List ways in which a pharmacy may monitor its quality-assurance program.
9. Explain the importance of root-cause analysis in determining the causes of medication errors.
10. Discuss the importance of monitoring in order to make changes in the risk-management process aimed at reducing the risks of medication errors.

KEY TERMS

Benchmark: A benchmark is a standard that can be used to measure changes that occur subsequently in a particular area. A benchmark will allow a person to know if improvement has been made. In pharmacy if we measure the number of errors per 1000 prescriptions filled, we can use that figure to compare whether we improved when we filled the next 1000 and each thousand after that. The number we compare each thousand against is the benchmark.

Fishbone diagram: A tool for analyzing the causes of risk-management problems or effects. The fishbone diagram provides a way to examine the effects of Person, Machine, Method, Material, and Environment.

Incident reports: Usually a company-designed report that documents facts and information regarding the events surrounding a QRE that reached a patient. The report summarizes information identifying the patient involved, the medications concerned, and store personnel with information regarding the events. Most pharmacy operations require an incident report to be filed with management. In some states, the law requires such a report to be maintained.

Normal variation: A change where none of the factors or causes that work on or influence a system has changed. A normal variation is a change without a cause. It is a change that can be considered as caused by luck only.

Patient Safety and Quality Improvement Act of 2005: A federal law that protects all records collected for the purpose of improving quality in health care, so long as certain conditions are met that are set forth in the regulations. Two primary requirements are (1) the information must be collected for quality purposes, and (2) it must be sent to a patient safety organization (PSO) hired by the health care provider.

Patient Safety Organization (PSO): A quality organization recognized and certified by the federal department of Health and Human Services to collect and analyze data pursuant to the Patient Safety and Quality Improvement Act of 2005.

Root-cause analysis: An analysis that looks for the one or more causes that, if done differently, would have changed the results. It is not merely one of a number of best practices that would have prevented the error. In a root-cause analysis the cause is looked for, not a solution.

Sentinel event: A medical or medication error that resulted in serious injury or death. When a sentinel event is reported in a hospital, it must be analyzed by a peer-review committee. The committee will look for what and who caused the error and what measures may be taken to prevent a repeat.

Special deviation: Unlike a normal variation, a special deviation is a change caused by one of the factors or causes that influence. A special deviation (variation) is a change that was caused to occur. For example, if the pharmacy made a change in its CQI workflow and the number of QREs decreased, the result would be a special variation.

OUTLINE

When Something Goes Wrong
Imperfect Systems
    Recording Mechanical Errors
    Statistical Analysis
    Variation—A Measure of Quality
    Normal Variation
Recording Data
A Non-Punitive System
Analyzing Causes
    What Mistakes (Variations) to Track?
    Is It Working?
    A Possible Solution
Peer Review and Root-Cause Analysis
    The Case of the Wrong Drug in the Bottle
When to Worry
Can You Trust the Data?
A Problem with Collecting Data
    Patient Safety and Quality Improvement Act of 2005
Summary

WHEN SOMETHING GOES WRONG

Sometimes, no matter what we do or how good our system is, there will be errors and perhaps even injured patients. Pharmacy technicians and pharmacists have an important job to perform when something does go wrong. Consider the hypothetical in RxErcise 9-A.

RxErcise 9-A   *What to Do When Tommy's Mom Says, "This Is Wrong."*

Tommy Johnson is a six-year-old child. Tommy's physician prescribed an antibiotic for his sore throat. The antibiotic was amoxicillin 125 mg to be given three times a day. The prescription was filled and Tommy's mother picked it up at the pharmacy. When Tommy's mother got home, she looked at the prescription and immediately called the pharmacy. The pharmacy technician answered the telephone and Tommy's mother told her the prescription did not look right. She said, "This prescription is a capsule and I thought it was supposed to be a liquid. Tommy can't take this. Tommy needs a liquid."

Tommy's mom was correct. The prescription was for 150 cc of a liquid to be given one teaspoonful three times a day. The prescription was filled for a capsule of the right medication and the right dose, and the label indicated Tommy should take one capsule three times a day.

To have a well functioning quality-assurance plan, everybody on the staff needs to know immediately what needs to be done as soon as Tommy's mom says, "This doesn't look right."

Everyone on the staff needs to know beforehand how to react when the telephone call comes in.

In this hypothetical, how should the pharmacy technician who answered the telephone and the pharmacist who was on duty have handled the situation?

1. Prepare a script (dialogue) for future pharmacy technicians in the above hypothetical situation. What should they say if this happens again?

2. Outline the steps that the pharmacist should take in a future case.

3. Discuss what steps you think should be taken to make sure this error does not occur again.

Imperfect Systems

The success of a good, well-managed CQI system is proven by the facts that it reduces medication errors and that it is constantly improving. A program may never attain perfection, but each year it can be a little better than the year before. This does not happen automatically. It requires a continued commitment to the goals of the program, one of which is to monitor the system to discover what works and what does not.

So far in this text, we have studied the first three elements of the risk-management process. First, we identified the risks of medication errors occurring and looked at near-misses, mistakes, and QREs. Second, we looked at the placement of best practices in a workflow to reduce near-misses that could lead to errors. Third, we studied the implementation of CQI programs and the training of staff, especially pharmacy technicians. If you look at Figure 9-1, you see that two steps in the risk-management process remain to be covered: monitoring the system and then improving it by making changes in the workflow to further reduce medication errors.

The pharmacy needs to ask three questions:

1. Is the system working?
2. Have we reduced the risk of medication errors from reaching our patients?
3. Can we do better?

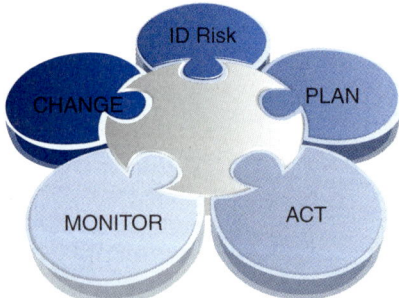

Figure 9-1 The Risk-Management Process
© Cengage Learning 2013

Monitoring means to observe and take measurements in the workflow. The pharmacy needs to know what, how many, and where QREs are occurring under the CQI system in place. Monitoring can be done in two ways: 1) Errors are analyzed individually in detail and 2) near-misses are analyzed collectively as part of a statistical analysis. Under the best practice approach, a combination of the two has proven effective for pharmacy.

Recording Mechanical Errors

Regarding the first way of monitoring, most pharmacies record mechanical errors, defined as mistakes in which the wrong drug, wrong strength of the drug, or the wrong directions get through the workflow to the patient, regardless of whether or not the patient takes any of the medication. They are usually recorded on company **incident reports**. This method involves documentation of errors of which the pharmacy is aware, followed often by an internal company or pharmacy analysis to find what factors led to the error, and then a determination of changes that could be made to the workflow to reduce the risk of a repeat of the situation.

The analysis is sometimes called a "peer-review" or a "root-cause" analysis. There are advantages to this approach. Since incident reports look only at QREs that reach a patient, there are fewer occurrences to be analyzed. The ones that are analyzed tend to be the most relevant since they are the ones that actually reached a patient. However, this error/incident reporting system has limitations, especially if this is the sole or primary method of monitoring. Error reports are retrospective; to analyze problems the pharmacy must wait until an error occurs. Another limitation is the small number of mistakes studied. Since the pharmacy analyzes only those QREs that reach a patient, the picture of the workflow's vulnerabilities is limited. A retrospective review is extremely useful, but it provides an incomplete monitoring system. Peer-review and root-cause analysis will be discussed later in this chapter.

Statistical Analysis

The second way of monitoring a pharmacy's quality-assurance plan is through statistical analysis and control. This method is more complete and is proactive. It does not require an actual error to occur. Because all near-misses as well as all errors are studied as a group, statistical analysis can give a more accurate picture of what is happening within the pharmacy workflow. Larger sets of numbers allow viewing and studying by graphs and charts, rather than looking at each occurrence individually.[1] The exact method of statistical analysis will depend on the amount of information collected.

The study of statistics and statistical control can be a complicated and daunting subject. In this book, however, we will look at statistical control and analysis only in the simplest of forms. One need not understand how statistics work or the intricacies of statistical analysis in order to implement a pharmacy CQI monitoring program. If the pharmacy finds it needs an expert in the subject, it can hire one. Almost all pharmacies and hospitals employ a **patient safety organization (PSO)**, whose job will include more detailed analysis of both types of information. A pharmacy technician and a pharmacist should understand the subject well enough to know how to spot a problem and decide where to concentrate their efforts in order to reduce the risks of medication errors.

Dr. Edwards Deming, whom we discussed in Chapter 1, was an expert in statistics. He was a PhD mathematician. As Deming began working on theories of management and quality, he realized that the best test of quality was looking at large numbers of products and seeing how they functioned. Much of Dr. Deming's early work was in the automobile industry. For example, if one car a company manufactured had a flat tire after driving it for a week, little would be revealed about which tires the company should choose. If, however, 5 percent of all of the cars manufactured in a month had flat tires within a week, the company might decide to examine the tires it was purchasing from its present source.

Apply a similar situation to pharmacy. Presume the following facts regarding prescriptions filled in this pharmacy last month:

- The pharmacy received a total of three complaints from patients.
- One prescription had incorrect directions on the label.
- Two prescriptions were filled with the wrong drug.

With only that information, the pharmacy may not know if a wrong label or a wrong drug represents the more significant problem in terms of which errors may happen next month. Since it does not know that, it cannot know which problem to address first. What if, however, the pharmacy had additional information:

- The pharmacy filled a total of 5,238 prescriptions.
- Two percent {104} had the wrong directions typed on the label.
- All but one of the wrong-directions mistakes were caught before they reached patients (i.e., most {103} were near-misses; one was an error).
- One percent {52} of the prescriptions was filled with the wrong drug, but the drug printed on the label was correct.
- Of the wrong-drug mistakes with the correct label, only one reached a patient (i.e., most {51} were near-misses; one was an error).
- Three percent {157} of the prescriptions contained the wrong drug, and the wrong drug name was printed on the label.
- Of the wrong-drug mistakes with the incorrect drug on the label, only one reached a patient (i.e., most {156} were near-misses; one was not, so one error).

The pharmacy now has more information on which to make a decision about how to proceed in improving the system. To make the analysis easier, it can convert the information into a spreadsheet, such as in Figure 9-2.

Analysis of Entry Versus Filling Errors

	Total	Percent	Near-miss	Error
Wrong directions	104	2%	103	1
Wrong drug: label wrong	157	3%	156	1
Total Entry QRE	261	5%	259	2
Wrong drug: label correct	52	1%	51	1
Total Filling QRE	52	1%	51	1
Total # Rx filled for period	5238	100%	310	3

Figure 9-2 Spreadsheet Analysis of Entry Versus Filling Errors
© Cengage Learning 2013

The data from the spreadsheet can be placed into a chart.

From the chart in Figure 9-3, it appears the pharmacy's biggest problem is in the number of QREs occurring at the data-entry station. Wrong directions and wrong drug on the label would have been mistakes at computer entry. Therefore out of 5,238 prescriptions filled, 261 QREs (5 percent) were from computer entry. In 1 percent of the cases, the label was correct but the drug was wrong, indicating these QREs were during filling.

RxErcise 9-A   Rework for Free

If, in the hypothetical above, the pharmacy had to retype the label in each of these wrong-directions cases, calculate how many additional labels the pharmacy staff had to retype. How much extra time do you estimate the technicians in this pharmacy would spend in typing these additional labels?

Medication Safety: Dispensing Drugs Without Error

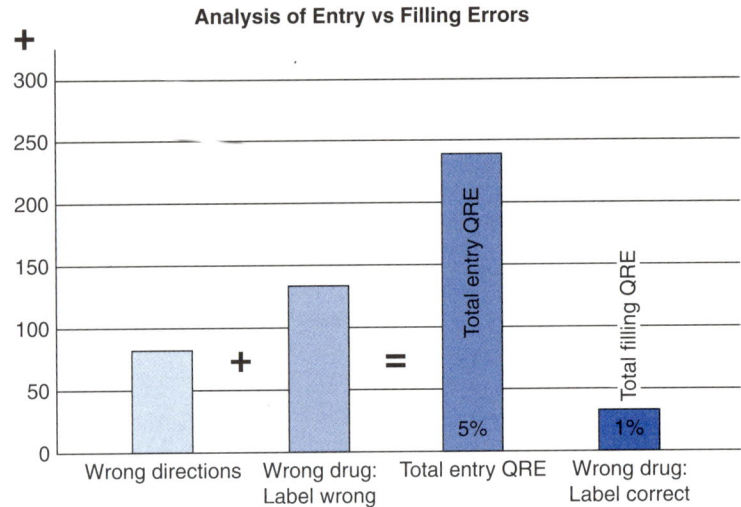

Figure 9-3 Chart Analysis of Entry vs. Filling Errors
© Cengage Learning 2013

Next month the pharmacy could have more errors unless it addresses the problem of computer entry. This is not to diminish the wrong drug cases, but the pharmacy should analyze which of the two situations needs addressing first. The pharmacy can prioritize improvement steps to be taken by attacking computer-entry problems first, and any changes needed at the filling station second.

In order to be able to use statistics such as those analyzed in the hypothetical pharmacy above, pharmacy staff must document all near-misses and errors that occur each day. This information becomes an important part of the analysis (study Quality Note 9-A).

> **Quality Note 9-A   It Takes a Lot of Mistakes to Make an Error**
>
> Note the other problems that become apparent when analyzing this pharmacy's data. Three QREs were not caught by the pharmacy's workflow. With the number of checks in a typical CQI workflow, there had to be several mistakes made. The system worked 310 times—the number of QREs caught. But the system failed three times—the number of QREs that were missed in order for these errors to reach a patient.

Variation—A Measure of Quality

There are several ways to measure quality. The Deming philosophy is that the true issue in quality is variation within the system. By variation, Deming meant any change in measurable output. "Output" may be the prescriptions filled in a month. The "variation" would be the number of QREs in that number of prescriptions.

A QRE is a variation from the norm. The "norm" is the number of QREs that could be expected each month.

For example, our goal each month is zero QRE. But since we are not perfect, each month we would expect to make a certain number of mistakes (QRE), what we would call a normal variation. If each month we make one error per 1000 prescriptions, that can be said to be our normal variation. This does not mean this many mistakes are acceptable; it means that this is what we can expect. This is the benchmark and the normal variation. If in a month we had two QRE per 1000 prescriptions, we recognize we may have a special problem. This is a special variation. It was probably caused by some new factor that we need to identify so we can correct for it.

In order to identify any change or variation, there needs to be at least two measurements. The first measurement establishes a **benchmark**, something to compare the second measurement to. To begin, decide what is to be measured, and then take a measurement of it to establish the benchmark.

As a starting place, measure how many QREs are made each month. Define a QRE as any mistake made anywhere in the workflow that gets from the station in which it is made to at least the next station. For example, assume a mistake is made by the technician at the receiving station, such as he forgot to ask about allergies. This is evident because he did not place a red "A" or "NKA" on the original prescription at the intake window. Before the prescription is passed to the next station, however, he realizes his mistake and corrects the problem. Under the definition of QRE given above, the mistake is not a QRE because it did not get to the next station before it was corrected.

With the next new prescription presented at the window, the technician again forgets to ask about allergies. This time it is the technician at the computer-entry station who catches the mistake, so it is a QRE and needs to be recorded. The technician who catches the QRE marks it on a sheet or notepad. So far there is one QRE for the day. The example works the same if there is only one technician on duty at the time. Even though the technician caught his own mistake, it is still a QRE because it was not caught until it reached the next station.

Normal Variation

At the end of one week, a hypothetical pharmacy filled 1,000 prescriptions. On the sheet for that week there are 40 QREs recorded. This can be the pharmacy's benchmark. The pharmacy for one week had a QRE rate of 4 percent of the prescriptions filled. For the second week, the pharmacy again recorded the number of QREs and compared that number with the number of prescriptions filled.

Assume for the second week there were also 1,000 prescriptions filled. In the second week, no changes were made in the workflow and everything remained constant. The same technicians worked the same number of hours and the same pharmacist was on duty. No new equipment was added and no actions were taken to reduce the number of QREs. This second week there are only 38 QREs recorded for a QRE rate of 3.8 percent. Was the difference significant? Perhaps not.

Since no quality system is perfect, there will always be some QREs. From week to week there will be some **normal variation**. A normal variation is a change where no factors that work on or influence a system changed. A normal variation is a change without a cause. It is a change that may be considered as caused by luck only. There are five factors or causes that Deming says will influence a process and cause a variation. The five factors (causes) are:

Person

Machine

Method

Material

Environment

Since in the example just given no factors changed and the change in the number of QREs was very small, this is probably just a normal variation. If any of these factors had changed, however, it would be a **special deviation**.

In the example above, presume that at the end of the second week a change was made in the CQI workflow. In week three, the same people worked the same number of hours and filled the same number of prescriptions (1,000), but the pharmacy introduced a change in the workflow. Since there was a change in at least one of the factors, a change in the number of QREs will be considered a special deviation. The factor changed was the "Method" by which prescriptions are filled. In this case, it would not be surprising if the QRE rate was reduced significantly. Presume that after the change was introduced into the CQI system, the number of QREs decreased to 15 QREs per 1,000 prescriptions filled, making the QRE rate 1.5 percent in week three.

RECORDING DATA

From this simple recording of data, the pharmacy can draw a graph showing the change in quality over a three-week period of time. See the graph in Figure 9-4.[2] From this graph, which could be posted in

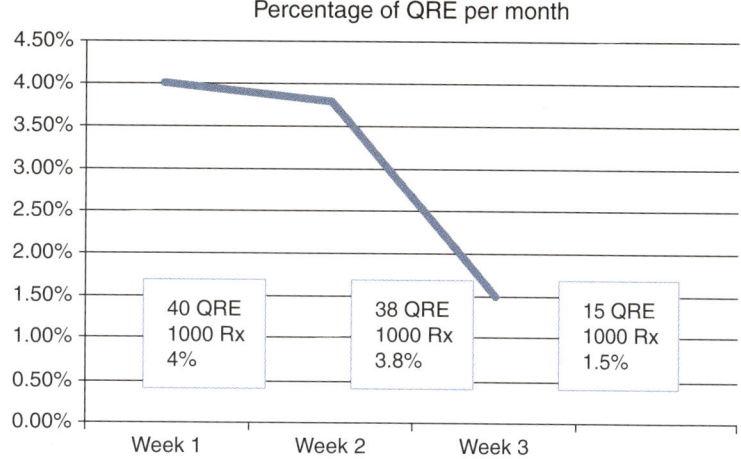

Figure 9-4 QRE Rate
© Cengage Learning 2013

the pharmacy, the staff members can see that they have increased the quality level in their pharmacy. This can provide good motivation.

The problem with the graph is the data collected does not provide any information that might be useful in determining what the problems are. The information cannot be used to make changes in the system that will lead to improvement. More information is needed and that will require time: time required to write down the information; time needed to make graphs or charts. If it takes too much time, people may soon tire of the exercise and the amount of information collected may become too little to be of value. It is best to reach some medium—enough information to be useful, but not so much as to jeopardize the system completely. One program[3] is designed so that each QRE can be recorded in 30 seconds or less. This still allows for a considerable amount of data to be collected.[4]

The problem of preparing graphs can be solved by using software that makes the graphs. Once the data is entered into a pharmacy's password-protected, secure database, the program automatically graphs the data according to the dictates chosen by the pharmacy. Most pharmacies will prepare one to four graphs or charts each month. While a lot of information and analysis is available, pharmacies are generally cautioned against trying to do too much at one time. A week's worth of data is probably not sufficient to see real trends in an actual pharmacy. A month-by-month comparison is more likely to be usable.

Consider what information may be useful. If the data includes the day of the week, the pharmacy can see if one day (e.g., Monday) is more likely to result in more problems than another day. Other items that could be tracked and recorded may include:

- Where or at which station did the QRE happen?
- Where was the QRE caught (including by a patient)?
- What QRE happened, such as a wrong drug, wrong directions?
- What was the name of the drug involved?
- At what time of the day did the QRE happen?
- Did the QRE reach the patient?

By recording the name of the drug, the pharmacy can determine if certain drugs cause more problems than others and therefore their shelves should be specially marked with colored tape as a warning to the technicians.[5] A simple chart may be designed that makes recording the data and transferring it into a database as easy as possible.

A Non-Punitive System

Most experts agree that a continuous quality improvement system must be non-punitive in nature.[6] If pharmacy staff members are disciplined for making mistakes, then eventually everyone will be reluctant to record any QRE and will begin to resent the CQI system itself. A punitive system will usually become self-defeating. The National Alliance of State Pharmacy Associations (NASPA) Pharmacy Quality Commitment® system purposefully does not ask for any identification of the person who made a mistake so that those using the program will not be concerned that they will be blamed or fired for making mistakes. In a non-punitive program the concept is that people do not fail; systems fail. In other words, if the system were working better, the mistake would not have been made.

There are, however, reasons for collecting and recording the names of pharmacists and pharmacy technicians who made the QRE. If done correctly, it can still be a non-punitive system. If the names of the people involved in a QRE were collected, the pharmacy could know which staff members may require additional training. It may also provide information as to which staff members work better or make less QREs at particular times or in a different environment. For example, some people may work better in a very busy pharmacy, while others require a slower pace.

Some mistakes are not just human errors, but may reflect an inability to follow the requirements of a quality system. Worse, some mistakes demonstrate a reckless disregard for the safety of the pharmacy's patients. In these cases, the person must be removed until the attitude changes. The collection of names would be beneficial in this circumstance.

> **RxErcise 9-B   You Design the Pharmacy's QRE Monitoring System**
>
> You have been asked to design a system to collect information on each QRE that happened in the pharmacy. Would your system collect the names of the people who were involved in filling the prescription? Discuss why or why not.

ANALYZING CAUSES

By considering each of the five causes mentioned previously (Person, Machine, Method, Material, and Environment) that may act individually or in combination to change the outcome of any process or workflow, it is possible to determine what created a particular result and then to decide how to correct a problem if one exists. Every effect, whether it is negative or positive, can be accounted for by one of these causes.

If, for instance, a patient receives the wrong drug in a prescription, the pharmacy must ask what caused the error. It can use an analytical tool often referred to as a **fishbone diagram**, shown in Figure 9-5, to help organize the pharmacy's analysis. The effect (problem) being analyzed is at the top of the diagram. Leading to the top are five potential causes of the problem or effect.

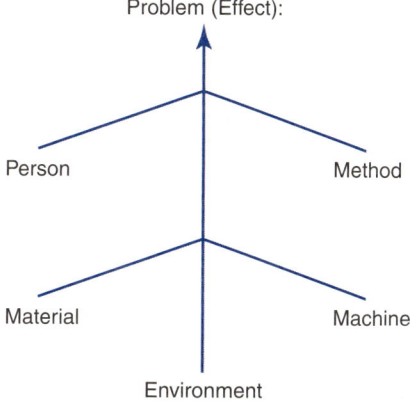

Figure 9-5 Fishbone Diagram
© Cengage Learning 2013

The pharmacy staff considers which of these causes or combination of causes led to the effect. At first, the items listed under each factor are possibilities to be considered and then eliminated or confirmed. Later, confirmed causes will form the basis for finding possible solutions to the problem.

Consider an example of an error involving a wrong drug dispensed. The primary confirmed cause (*root cause*) is that the pharmacy technician at the entry station selected the wrong drug from a list of drugs displayed on the computer screen by clicking on the drug above the correct drug. The investigation is also likely to find other failures in the system, each of which failed to catch the initial mistake. Each of these other causes will be noted on the fishbone diagram. In addition, the staff may prepare a chart that can be used to fill in the diagram (see Figure 9-6).

Cause	Factors leading to filling the Rx with wrong drug	Solutions and possible changes in system to consider
PERSON	Computer entry tech Filling tech Final check Pharm Counseling pharmacist	Institute retraining of all staff in use of best practices throughout workflow and need to follow each step in each process
METHOD	Entry: failed to recheck Filling: take 5; fill from original Rx rather than label or receipt	Workflow system failure. Need to emphasize system. Use incident as example of need. Each member of staff must review this incident. Retraining—see person
MATERIAL	Material not primary cause	
MACHINE	Computer software may have led to tech's confusion at entry	Contact software supplier. Work on solution
ENVIRONMENT	Busy, but not extraordinary; counter clear and neat	

Figure 9-6 Cause Chart
© *Cengage Learning 2013*

Both the chart and the fishbone diagram are tools to assist the investigator. Either tool or both can be considered as "thinking tools" to organize the search for a solution. They are also useful in considering whether the effect is a normal variation or is a special deviation.

What Mistakes (Variations) to Track?

Many mistakes may be made during a day in a typical hospital or community pharmacy workflow, but most of these need not be recorded or tracked for the purposes of reducing medication errors. The pharmacy needs to determine which items are significant. In the Auburn University College of Pharmacy Observational Study of Errors in Community Pharmacies, the observers found 77 errors (any deviation from the prescriber's order) out of 4,481 prescriptions. Of these errors, 93.5 percent were not judged to be clinically important. In other words, the vast majority of these errors would not have resulted in injury.

In this textbook we are concerned only with medication errors and therefore only with variability that may result in a potentially serious injury to the patient. There may be reasons, however, that a pharmacy may wish to cast a wider net and include more items to be tracked, for example, names spelled incorrectly and labels smudged, that might reflect on the pharmacy's reputation. If a pharmacy does not record such items, correction of this type of mistakes may not be addressed.

> **Quality Note 9-B   If You Really Want to Make a Patient Mad**
>
> A pharmacy brought together for a roundtable discussion some of its pharmacists and pharmacy technicians to discuss implementation of the company's CQI program. One question was: What types of mistakes should be recorded as near-misses? When one pharmacist suggested tracking instances where the pharmacy had typed the wrong number of refills on the label, another pharmacist said he thought that was trivial. "It is not trivial," the first pharmacist answered. "If you really want to make a patient mad, put on the label the wrong number of refills remaining." In the end, the vote was unanimous to track as a recordable mistake the wrong number of refills printed on the label.

The pharmacy will decide which QREs should be recorded. Those deemed significant for its purposes will be entered into a database so they can be tracked and later used to modify the CQI workflow. Consider such a list, keeping in mind that recording too many items may become overly burdensome and could lead to the system not being used at all. The following list may not be complete, but could be a reasonable starting place:

- The date the prescription was filled
- The time the prescription was filled
- New (N) or refill (R) prescription

- Did prescription get to the patient?
- In which process did the QRE happen?
    1. Receiving the prescription
    2. Computer data entry and label preparation
    3. Assembling and filling the order/prescription
    4. Pharmacist's final check
    5. Pharmacist's prospective drug review
    6. Pharmacist's counseling of patient
    7. Delivery of the order/prescription
- In which process was the QRE discovered?
    1. Receiving the prescription
    2. Computer data entry and label preparation
    3. Assembling and filling the order/prescription
    4. Pharmacist's final check
    5. Pharmacist's prospective drug review
    6. Pharmacist's counseling of patient
    7. Delivery of the order/prescription
    8. Discovered by patient
- What QRE happened?
    1. Wrong drug
    2. Wrong strength
    3. Wrong patient
    4. Wrong directions
    5. Incorrect refill information (question?)
    6. Receiving information incomplete
        a) Birth date
        b) Under 6 / over 60 age
        c) Address
        d) Allergy
        e) Other meds
        f) Other (explain)

7. Safety cap
    a) Not used when should have been
    b) Safety cap used when patient requested it not be used
8. Counseling
    a) Failure to counsel
    b) Inadequate counseling
9. Written patient information
    a) Printed patient information not given
    b) Required med-guide not given
10. Drug review
    a) Failure to perform
    b) Mistake in drug review
    c) Controlled substance
    d) Question validity
    e) Refilled too early
    f) Excessive refill
    g) Refilled without authority
    h) Prescription refilled without authority
11. Patient name spelled wrong (question?)
12. Physician name spelled wrong (question?)
13. Confidentiality or HIPAA problem (must explain)
14. Other (must explain)

- Prescribed drug (generic) and strength
- Dispensed drug (generic) and strength

By recording and tracking such information for each prescription that contained a QRE, the pharmacy could begin to analyze its system for a given period of time, such as a month, and could determine which parts of the workflow need the most immediate attention. If the pharmacy were using a commercially available system, such as the NASPA system, these decisions may have already been made. An advantage with this approach is that the forms, graphs, and charts are ready to use.[7]

By way of example, presume there is a pharmacy using the above list for recording and tracking QREs. On one day during which the pharmacy filled 100 prescriptions, there were 3 QREs. A chart made for the purpose of recording these at the end of the day could look like the one in Figure 9-7.

Time	N/R	To Patient	Where QRE Happened	Where QRE Discovered	QRE	Drug Prescribed	Drug Dispensed	Explain or Note if Needed
9:45 a	N	No	1	2	6 (b)	HTZ 50 mg	HTZ 50 mg	Patient 68 years old
1:15 p	N	Yes	2	8	1	Propranolol 40 mg	Paroxetine 20 mg	Called, did not take any
2:15 p	R	No	3	4	2	Warfarin 1 mg	Warfarin 5 mg	Tech corrected

Figure 9-7 Chart of QREs for Sept. 15
© Cengage Learning 2013

Having collected one day's information, it is placed into the pharmacy's database along with all other prescription QREs for the month and year. To make the information easier to use for analysis, the data can be put into a series of graphs, each selected to display the information in a format that will assist the pharmacists and pharmacy technicians to understand potential problems and possible solutions. Also, spreadsheets can assist the user in making simple graphs from the data entered. Designing a database that will provide graphs and charts is beyond the scope of this book, but there are several programs available that will perform this task.[8]

Is It Working?

When a sufficient amount of information has been collected, usually at least one month of entries, it can be analyzed. Often the information does not provide direct answers, but shows areas that should be further explored. From the information collected, the pharmacy should be able to produce a number of graphs and charts.

The graphs in Figures 9-8 through 9-11 are samples from the files of PMC Quality Commitment, Inc. While based on representative data, the graphs are considered hypothetical and do not represent the results of any pharmacy. Figure 9-8 shows the percentage of QREs entered for each day of the week. One question that this graph may raise is how many prescriptions are filled on these

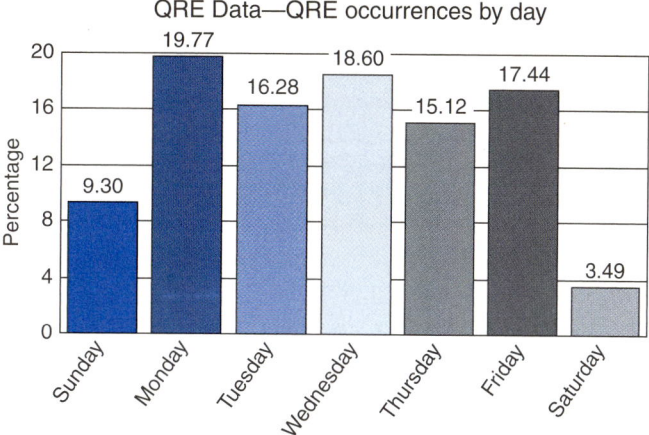

Figure 9-8 QREs by Days
© Cengage Learning 2013

days on average? One would suspect that the greater number of QREs by percentage would be on the busiest days. Why is Wednesday, typically a slow day, higher than Friday, typically a busier day? The answers could show which people in the pharmacy are better at entering data. If that were the case, it may provide an opportunity for the pharmacy to emphasize to those working on Fridays the importance of entering *all* QREs.

Of particular import would be for a pharmacy to know at which station most QREs happened and what they were. With this information the pharmacy could prioritize where to begin working on changes in the workflow. It may also indicate if new best practices should be added or which current ones should be emphasized. Figures 9-9, 9-10, and 9-11[9] represent the same data, but in Figures 9-10 and 9-11 one station, computer entry, is highlighted and isolated. Note that 42 percent of the QREs for the time selected come from the computer-entry station. Since a pharmacy should be reluctant to modify the workflow in more than one station at a time, it could use this data to set a priority for what it may work on for the coming month.

Figure 9-11 isolates the causes associated with the computer-entry process. To simplify changes in the workflow, the pharmacy could decide to work on only one cause for the next month. In this case it might be "wrong directions," as 14 percent of all QREs in the total workflow had this one cause—wrong directions typed (selected) during computer entry. Because an error in the directions could result in significant risk to patients, this may be an appropriate decision. The other areas cannot be ignored and the staff should

Medication Safety: Dispensing Drugs Without Error

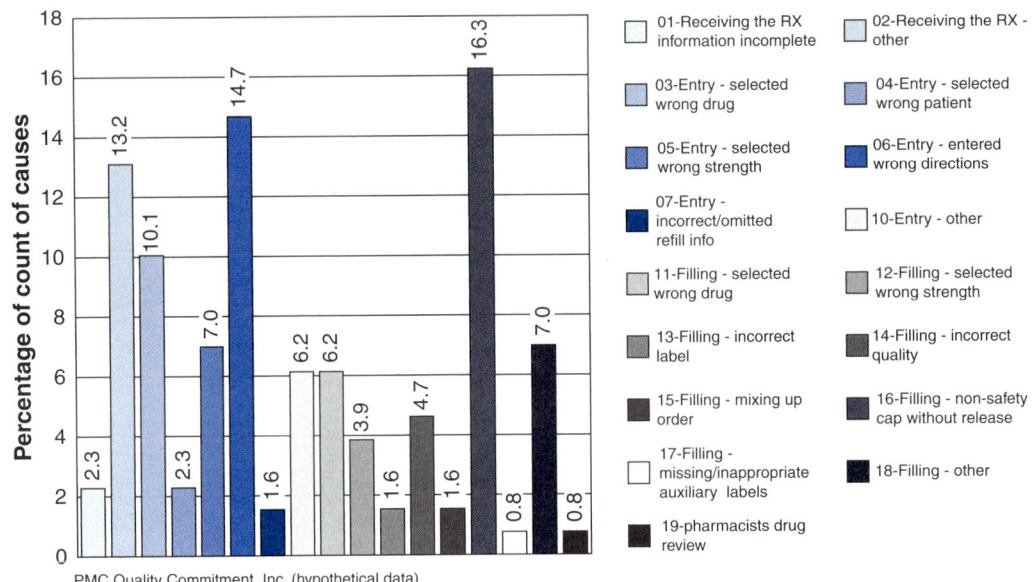

Figure 9-9 Where QREs Happened—All Stations
© Cengage Learning 2013

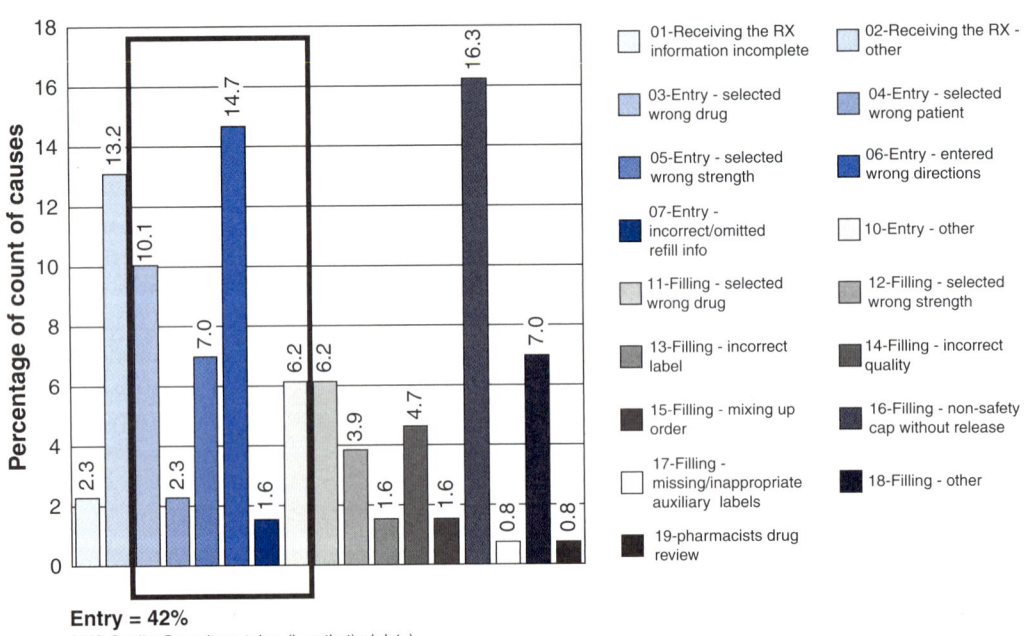

Figure 9-10 Total QREs—Entry Noted
© Cengage Learning 2013

CHAPTER 9 • Monitoring and Learning from Mistakes

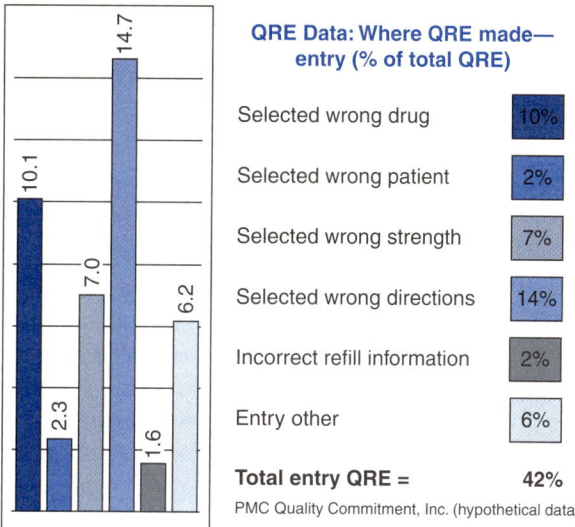

Figure 9-11 Entry % of Total QREs
© Cengage Learning 2013

be made aware of all the results found. Quality, however, is a marathon, not a sprint. Trying to fix too many problems at one time may result in a decrease in overall progress and possibly more errors.

A Possible Solution

Following monitoring in the risk-management process, a pharmacy moves to change the CQI workflow based upon its findings. A change decision for the pharmacy in the examples represented in Figures 9-9, 9-10, and 9-11 may be to simply concentrate on QREs at the entry station and emphasize the best practice "Take 5" at the beginning of the filling-station process. The pharmacy could also add an emphasis on checking the label at the pharmacist's quality-check station. At the end of the next month, a similar graph would again be printed and staff members would assess how successful their steps were in reducing these QREs. A different concentration, such as selecting the wrong

---

RxErcise 9-C *Statistical Control and Analysis*

Discuss as a group the relative advantages and disadvantages of using statistical control and analysis. Consider the following:

1. Time required to collect the data each day. How long would it take you to fill in three lines on a chart similar to the one in Figure 9-4? If the pharmacy had three QREs per day, how much total time would it take?

2. How much time would it take to analyze the data, using Figures 9-8, 9-9, and 9-10?

drug in computer entry, may be selected for the following month's area of concentration if the wrong directions solutions were successful. Each month there should be an emphasis on one or two problems. This is the concept of continuous quality improvement.

PEER REVIEW AND ROOT-CAUSE ANALYSIS

Much can be learned by analyzing individual errors that reach a patient. Recording and analyzing errors is mandated by the laws of several states, including Florida, California, Massachusetts, and Iowa. In most hospitals, each error that results in a sentinel event, a mistake that caused serious injury or death, must be analyzed by a peer-review committee. This committee will usually be made up of people from the areas involved. Others, such as the director of nurses, the pharmacist-in-charge, the chief of staff, or their designees, may be added. Because of the seriousness of the event, a high priority is given to these meetings. Peer review means the error or incident is being reviewed by professional colleagues (peers) of the people involved.

Typically in the states that require pharmacies to record each error, an analysis of those errors considered by the pharmacist-in-charge to be most relevant are presented as a summary at a pharmacy meeting, which may be quarterly or semi-annually. Examine the following analysis of an error.[10]

The Case of the Wrong Drug in the Bottle

Judy, a 62-year-old single woman, was newly diagnosed with high blood pressure. Her physician prescribed medication. Judy took the prescription to a pharmacy that she had not used before; she had taken very few prescription drugs in her life. They made a mistake on Judy's prescription. Instead of her high blood pressure medication, Judy was given testosterone tablets.

After three weeks Judy's blood pressure got worse and she was admitted to the hospital. She did not bring her prescription bottle with her, but she was able to tell the hospital staff what she (thought she) was taking for her high blood pressure. She was, of course, wrong because the pharmacy had made a mistake.

While in the hospital Judy was given the drug that her physician had originally prescribed. The tablets she took in the hospital came from the hospital pharmacy and they were the right drug. Judy noticed the difference in the looks of the tablets, but the nurse at the hospital told her it was just a different generic brand. After a few days in the hospital on the correct medication, Judy's blood pressure was under control. She was released from the hospital and told to continue taking her medicine.

When Judy was home, she again started taking the testosterone that had been mistakenly given to her by the community pharmacy. Again her blood pressure went up and again she was admitted to the hospital. This time she took her prescription bottle with her and the error was discovered.

When confronted with the error, the pharmacist at first denied making a mistake and later accused Judy of placing the testosterone in the pharmacy's prescription bottle. Eventually, after a series of regrettable encounters, the pharmacy admitted its error and an investigation was started to establish what had happened.

As a result of the investigation, the following facts were established:

1. The prescription filled immediately before Judy's was for a male patient and was for testosterone tablets.
2. The day after both prescriptions were filled, the male patient returned to the pharmacy complaining that the tablets he was given were wrong.
3. The male patient's bottle contained high blood pressure medication.
4. The male patient's prescription was corrected and he was given the correct testosterone tablets according to his prescription.
5. Judy was not counseled, but in accordance with state law, she was offered counseling, which she refused as noted by a log she signed when she picked up her prescription.
6. The label on Judy's prescription bottle was correct.
7. The pharmacy's technician had entered the information into the computer.
8. The pharmacist had filled (filling station) both prescriptions, Judy's and the male patient's.
9. It was a busy time in the pharmacy when each of these prescriptions was filled.
10. The pharmacist and the pharmacy technician both indicated they felt stressed at the time.
11. The pharmacist may have been filling several prescriptions at the same time by lining up several labels and receipts with stock bottles sitting on top of each.
12. The pharmacist's habit was to line up several prescriptions, pull the stock bottles for all at one time, and then count out all of the prescriptions and apply the labels to each filled bottle after all prescriptions had been counted. The pharmacist denied he did this on this day. The pharmacy technician could not recall that day but indicated this was a common practice in this pharmacy.
13. During the investigation, after the event, it was noticed that the prescription counter was cluttered with papers, magazines, and stock bottles. Many stock bottles that were not being used at the time were stacked up close to the filling area. It was explained that these stock bottles had been used earlier and they would be reshelved when it was not busy.

RxErcise 9-D   Analysis: The Case of the Wrong Drug in the Bottle

Analyze this case and discuss the following questions:

- How was the error on Judy's prescription probably made?
- What should have happened when the male patient returned?
- What best practices would you put into the workflow specifically to address Judy's case?
- Read the root-cause analysis section below. Name one root cause that, if it were removed from the facts, the mistake that led to the error would not have occurred.

When a suspected error is reported to the pharmacy, the staff must know how to handle it. This is as important a part of training as the workflow training discussed earlier. Because an error may result in a significant injury and will affect the pharmacy's reputation, errors provide powerful lessons for the staff. When a pharmacy analyzes an error, such as the one in Judy's case, it performs a **root-cause analysis**. A root-cause analysis looks for one or more causes that, if they had been corrected or eliminated, the problem would not have occurred. It is not merely one of a number of best practices that would have prevented the error. In a root-cause analysis we look for the cause, not a solution. Only rarely is a person the root cause. In the past, a pharmacy might have blamed the last person who had control of the erroneous prescription. The problem with this is that, even if that person were gone, the root cause of the error would not have been isolated or corrected, and eventually someone else would make the same mistake.

WHEN TO WORRY

One of the advantages of statistical control is it can answer the question of when to worry about the quality system. Recording and addressing near-misses by an analysis of graphs illustrating where mistakes have been made can show where vulnerabilities exist in the workflow system. By studying and correcting vulnerabilities before they occur, errors can be avoided at the source.

By graphing the number of near-misses, such as in Figure 9-1, the pharmacy can get a more accurate read of how the system is working and improving. If the number of QREs steadily declines, accounting for normal variance, the pharmacy can take comfort in the fact that risks of medication errors are decreasing and likely to continue to decrease. Other measurements are the pharmacy's success rate and its error rate.[11]

The statistical control method can answer the question of when to worry; just recording and analyzing errors cannot. Even if there were no errors this month, the presence of near-misses shows that eventually errors will occur. With error analysis the pharmacy must wait for an error to occur before it can address the cause. Even if a pharmacy's system is working well, but there is no documentable evidence, luck may be a factor in success. Failure, however, can usually be explained by an analysis of the system.

CAN YOU TRUST THE DATA?

As valuable as the collection and recording of QRE information is, it needs to be recorded regularly if it is to give a true picture of the pharmacy's quality system. One person, a pharmacist or a pharmacy technician, should be given the authority to coordinate all quality activities, including recording data. This person cannot be present at all times in order to ensure that all near-misses and errors are captured and entered into the database. The pharmacist-in-charge and the pharmacy's quality coordinator need some way to determine if everyone is using the system. One way to do this is to know the pharmacy's QRE rate.

The QRE rate is the number of QREs divided by the number of prescriptions filled for a certain period of time. This result multiplied by 100 gives the percent QRE rate. Most shifts should have a comparable QRE rate. For example, presume the pharmacy coordinator calculated the QRE rate for a pharmacy after one week, with the following results.

MONDAY:

    Filled: 370 prescriptions

    QREs recorded: 6

    QRE rate: 6 / 370 = 0.016 × 100 = 1.6% QRE rate

TUESDAY:

    Filled: 312 prescriptions

    QREs recorded: 7

    QRE rate: 7 / 312 = 0.022 × 100 = 2.2% QRE rate

WEDNESDAY:

    Filled: 200 prescriptions

    QREs recorded: 2

    QRE rate: 2 / 200 = 0.01 × 100 = 1% QRE rate

THURSDAY:

    Filled: 250 prescriptions

    QREs recorded: 0

    QRE rate: 0 / 250 = 0.0000 × 100 = 0.0% QRE rate

FRIDAY:

    Filled: 297 prescriptions

    QREs recorded: 4

    QRE rate: 4 / 297 = 0.013 × 100 = 1.3% QRE rate

SATURDAY:
- Filled: 326 prescriptions
- QREs recorded: 1
- QRE rate: 1 / 326 = 0.0030 × 100 = 0.3% QRE rate

SUNDAY:
- Filled: 97 prescriptions
- QREs recorded: 6
- QRE rate: 6 / 97 = 0.060 × 100 = 6% QRE rate

The pharmacy quality coordinator analyzes the data for this hypothetical pharmacy. In this example, the coordinator is looking for any percentages that are not in the normal range. Four of the days have a QRE rate of between 1 percent and 2.2 percent. The day with 1 percent was a relatively slow day and the day with the 2.2 percent was the busiest day of the week studied. While one week is probably too short to establish a normal range, it provides a reasonable starting place. Each week, as more data is added, a normal range will become clearer.

Three of the days are out of the range by a sizable amount. Wednesday had only one QRE recorded for the day. Thursday did not have any QREs recorded for the day. It is possible that these numbers are within a normal variable curve, but each deserves more study. A question that may be asked is, "Did any of the five causes (factors) change?" The most likely causes to change in this case would be people, method, and environment.

- For the environment: was that day busier than other days or was the environment much better than normal?
- For the method: was there a different workflow, or were there more prescriptions of a particular type such as nursing home prescriptions, which may be filled according to a different procedure, than other days?
- For the people: were there different people working on a particular day?

Presume that the only factor or cause that was different on these days was the pharmacist working behind the dispensing counter. Since most QREs would be caught at the pharmacist's final-check station, this cause may be relevant. The quality coordinator may decide to check to see if this pharmacist is properly recording each QRE he or she discovers. When one person on a shift is not following a procedure, it is possible others on the same shift may become lax in the same area.

Sunday was a particularly slow day in this pharmacy; there were only 97 prescriptions filled. It is significant to note that there were six QREs recorded on that day. This number is not likely to be within normal variation, so the coordinator may wish to examine other factors or causes. It may be there was only a pharmacist working on Sunday without a pharmacy technician. This may cause more mistakes and could lead, unless corrected, to more errors. The coordinator may wish to pay particular attention to Sundays for a period of time to look for trends. It could be there were new people on duty on Sunday, working without experienced staff. It is also possible the people working this Sunday have an incorrect definition of what is a QRE that should be recorded. Since there needs to be uniformity throughout the pharmacy in what is recordable, the coordinator may wish to examine such questions.

Generally, the quality coordinator will want to look for two results when examining recording accuracy. First, look for the days that are too good, meaning days that have too few QREs recorded. This may indicate the staff on these days is not recording all of the QREs. It may also mean that the staff that day was just very good and had few QREs. Second, look for the days that are worse than others, with more QREs than would be expected for the number of prescriptions filled. There are no perfect methods, but the numbers themselves, particularly the QRE rate, are a good place to start to answer the question, "How reliable are the numbers?"

A Problem with Collecting Data

We have discussed the advantages of collecting and recording data on medication errors and near-miss mistakes. Each error should be recorded and analyzed because these represent the most serious breaches in the pharmacy's quality system. Generally speaking, a pharmacy with a working quality system should catch 90 percent of all mistakes before they reach a patient and become an error. If that is the case, there should be ten times the number of near-misses as there are errors. Recording and analyzing near-misses allows the pharmacy to correct vulnerabilities before they become errors.

There are, however, potential disadvantages with collecting and recording near-miss and error data. Most recorded information of any kind can be subpoenaed by a lawyer and used in a lawsuit against the company possessing the information. This is one reason many pharmacies, physicians, and others in health care were, until recently, reluctant to record this type of information.

In 1995 the Alabama Supreme Court issued a ruling in a pharmacy malpractice case against a regional chain called "Harco Drugs."[12]

Harco's pharmacist had made a mistake filling a prescription for a cancer patient. The prescription was filled with medication for a heart condition. The plaintiffs (Holloway) were allowed to submit evidence of 233 prior incidents, error reports maintained by the pharmacy chain. Based partly upon those reports, the jury awarded additional damages, called "punitive damages," against Harco Drugs, Inc., despite the fact that the incident reports covered multiple years and Harco had over 150 pharmacies.

Fortunately, since 1995 the laws have changed to protect much, but not all, collected information. In Alabama, the same incident reports would today be sheltered from the plaintiff lawyer's subpoena.[13] The same is not true in all states, however. While most states protect hospital peer-review records, the same laws do not generally exclude such reports from community pharmacies. Many states that have passed laws requiring CQI pharmacy programs do today provide some protection from discovery. What was needed was a uniform federal statute.

Patient Safety and Quality Improvement Act of 2005

In 2005 the federal government passed a law to correct this situation for all health care quality records at both state and federal levels. The **Patient Safety and Quality Improvement Act of 2005**[14] protected all records collected for the purpose of improving quality in health care, so long as certain conditions were met that are set forth in the regulations. Two primary requirements are: (1) the information must be collected for quality purposes, and (2) it must be sent to a **patient safety organization**[15] **(PSO)** hired by the health care provider.

A PSO must be qualified and approved by the United States Department of HHS. Any organization can become a PSO, with only a few exceptions such as health insurance companies and accrediting bodies. A PSO is to assist the health care provider with the analysis and collection of quality data. The federal Agency for Healthcare Research and Quality (AHRQ) maintains a list of qualified PSOs. Two organizations familiar in pharmacy that are PSOs, or have affiliated companies that are PSOs, are ISMP and NASPA. ISMP is a quality organization this is itself listed as a PSO. The NASPA is an organization of state pharmacy associations that provides the Pharmacy Quality Commitment® quality-assurance program and maintains an affiliation with the Alliance for Patient Medication Safety (APMS), a PSO. Information submitted through the Pharmacy Quality Commitment® online database is automatically submitted to APMS. The passage of the Patient Safety and Quality Improvement Act of 2005 has alleviated much of the fear of collecting and using quality data.

Summary

The collection and recording of near-miss mistakes and errors, as well as the resultant analysis of what went wrong and what worked, require investments of time and money. If management or the pharmacy staff consider these investments as expensive, its quality system is likely to become marginalized over time.

In truth, quality is free, as explained by Philip Crosby in his book by the same name.[16] A program of continuous quality improvement results in less rework, less work for which the pharmacy will not be reimbursed, increased efficiency, and higher productivity. It begins with a good CQI system, effectively implemented and a well trained staff. To remain a good system it must be monitored and, when necessary, changed. Constant improvement is the key to quality. A CQI program protects the pharmacy, pharmacists, pharmacy technicians and most importantly, the patient.

Review Questions

1. What does "NKA" marked in red on the face of a new prescription mean?
   A. Diabetic patient
   B. No known allergy
   C. Patient without insurance
   D. Elderly patient requiring additional assistance

2. If an "A" is marked on the front of the prescription, what is on the back?
   A. Additional information regarding OTC drugs used
   B. List of controlled-substance drugs taken—"A List"
   C. A list of allergies the patient who presented the prescription has
   D. Nothing; this is not an indication additional information would be on the back.

3. The advantage of tracking errors is
   A. It allows for a root-cause analysis.
   B. Finding the most serious of the QREs.
   C. Allowing for a more detailed analysis of an individual QRE.
   D. All of the above

4. As Deming used the term, a "variation" is
   A. Any change in measurable output.
   B. A medication error.
   C. A QRE.
   D. Any mistake.

5. What word is used to describe a change where none of the factors or causes that work on or influence a system has changed?
   A. A normal variation
   B. A QRE
   C. A mistake
   D. All of the above

6. A problem that may be associated with recording the names of people who make mistakes is:
   A. A punitive system will usually become self-defeating.
   B. Less information may be collected.
   C. Fear may be instilled among the pharmacy staff.
   D. All of the above

7. There may be advantages in collecting the names of people who make mistakes, including:
   A. The pharmacy would know which staff members may require additional training.
   B. Some errors demonstrate reckless behavior and those people may need to be discharged.
   C. The pharmacy may discover which people work better in different environments.
   D. All of the above

8. Name a tool that can be used to analyze which causes may have led to a problem or effect.
   A. Fishbone diagram
   B. QRE analyzer
   C. QRE-rate graph
   D. Data-entry graph

9. A disadvantage of collecting only error information is:

   A. It may not be used to find the vulnerabilities in a system until after a mistake has actually reached a patient.

   B. Too much information may be collected.

   C. It could not allow for a root-cause analysis.

   D. It does not allow for individual analysis of a specific mistake.

10. What is the name commonly given to an error that resulted in serious injury or death?

    A. QRE

    B. Error

    C. Sentinel event

    D. Preventable adverse medical event

Endnotes

[1] Some near-misses and all errors will actually be studied individually, as in a 6-second consult best practice that will be discussed later in this chapter. Statistical control does not eliminate peer review and root cause analysis in pharmacy, although in some industries it is relied upon solely for monitoring.

[2] Note this graph is similar to the one illustrated in Chapter 1, except the numbers are different as they now represent another pharmacy with different information presumed.

[3] Pharmacy Quality Commitment® is a CQI program from the National Alliance of State Pharmacy Associations. It consists of a quality workflow [Quality Manager™] and a tracking/monitoring system [Sentinel System™]. See www.pcq.net.

[4] See www.pcq.net

[5] See the discussion of the best practice "Mark It" in Chapter 6.

[6] See Decker, S., 2007. *Just Culture, Balancing Safety and Accountability*. Farnham, Surrey, United Kingdom: Ashgate Publishing, Ltd.; also see the writings of Michael Cohen, President, ISMP at http://www.ismp.org

[7] The NASPA system of Pharmacy Quality Commitment® provides for on-line entry of all near-misses and errors into a preset data

base. Once the information has been entered the pharmacy may study, analyze and print a set of pre-designed graphs and/or charts. For example, the pharmacy can enter a "PQC™ Charting System" using a secure Internet program with its pharmacy data. After setting a date range to examine, the pharmacy can choose eleven data sets and a graph type or chart type. The graphs includes "QRE % by Day of week" and "QRE Success Rate." Figure 6-4 in Chapter 6 and Figure 9-8 in Chapter 9 are examples of an early version of a PQC™ chart of "Where QRE were made" and "Day of week," respectively, for a given period of time (generally any length of time up to one year).

[8] As noted in Endnote 7, in some systems such as the NASPA Pharmacy Quality Commitment® system the programming and database design has already been done and is user-ready. The cost of such a system may be less than the cost of a good database computer program.

[9] Figures 9-8 and 9-9 were also presented in Chapter 4.

[10] From the files of Pharmacists Mutual Insurance Company. All identifying information redacted or changed.

[11] Review Figures 1-2, 1-3, and 1-4 in Chapter 1.

[12] *Harco Drugs, Inc. v. Holloway*, 669 So.2d 878, 881 (Ala.1995)

[13] ALA. CODE § 6–5-551 (Supp. 2000).

[14] The Patient Safety and Quality Improvement Act is administered by AHRQ and HHS; the requirements and text can be found at: http://www.ahrq.gov/qual/psoact.htm accessed March 30, 2011.

[15] See the PSO website at http://www.pso.ahrq.gov/ accessed March 30, 2011.

[16] Crosby, P. B., 1980. *Quality Is Free: The Art of Making Quality Certain*. New York: Penguin Books.

CHAPTER 10

The Role of the Patient in Preventing Medication Errors

OBJECTIVES

Upon completion of this chapter, the reader should be able to:

1. Explain the value of apology laws in the states.
2. Understand the value of considering a patient as also a customer in relation to quality-assurance programs.
3. Describe problems associated with pharmacies admitting to patients that they make errors.
4. Discuss the Ryan Haight Online Pharmacy Consumer Protection Act.
5. Describe the problems associated with illegal prescriptions in relation to quality.
6. Explain how pharmacies can provide elements in a quality workflow to protect patients who do not take their medication as prescribed.
7. Discuss the use of statistical controls in a quality system.
8. List ways in which physician errors can be accommodated in the pharmacy's quality program.
9. Explain the importance of prescription-monitoring program legislation.
10. Discuss problems arising when patients abuse controlled substances in relation to the pharmacy's CQI program.

KEY TERMS

Apology laws: Laws passed in several states that provide for immunity for health care professionals who issue an apology when there has been an error. Physicians and health care providers can apologize and offer expressions of grief without concern that their words may be used against them in court. Pharmacists and pharmacies are covered only if they are included in the language of the statute or are defined as health care providers in that state.

Prescription-monitoring program: A database created by state law of all controlled-substance prescriptions filled or written in the state. All pharmacies and prescribers in the state are required to submit information on all controlled-substance prescriptions dispensed or written. Pharmacies and prescribers who submit information have access only for the purposes allowed under the statute.

OUTLINE

The Patient as Part of the Quality System
The Patient—Also a Customer
    The Patient and CQI
    Erasing the Fear of Using the Patient
Mechanical Errors
    The Case of the High Blood Pressure Patient and the Cancer Drug
Other Types of Errors
    Physician Mistakes
    The Case of Someone Made a Mistake

Patient Mistakes
    The Case of the Medication That Was Too Expensive
    The Case of the Lumberjack
    Prescription-Monitoring Program
Summary

THE PATIENT AS PART OF THE QUALITY SYSTEM

Quality assurance does not stop upon delivery of the medication to the patient. No system is perfect. Occasionally, a mistake will go through the pharmacy's workflow and will be delivered to the patient. The patient should be made a member of the quality team. How willing patients may be to think of themselves in this capacity depends on their attitude toward the pharmacy and its staff. It may also depend on how well the patient has been educated in medication safety. The pharmacy staff is in the best position to serve as the patient's educator in this area. Patients should feel they are a part of the pharmacy's quality team and they have a role in continuous quality improvement.

The obvious advantage of including the patient in the quality workflow is that it can protect the patient from medication errors. There is a side effect of this, too. Protecting the patient protects the pharmacy, pharmacist, and pharmacy technician from complaint, claims, and lawsuits. Even if there is an error, people who feel they have been treated fairly and honestly are less anxious to file. Many times such errors can be satisfactorily settled between the pharmacy and the patient, even if injury is involved. There is a maxim among trial lawyers, "People tend not to sue people they like." While the maxim may be overstated, there is truth in it. Patients, like all people, reflect the attitude of those they deal with, including their pharmacy staff.

THE PATIENT—ALSO A CUSTOMER

In pharmacy today it is considered less professional to refer to those who depend on pharmacy's professional services as "customers." They are "patients." When pharmacists took on more professional duties and increased their exposure to professional liability, the profession discarded the term "customer" for this more professional term. In many ways this is wise and represents a forward-thinking trend. A patient is a person who needs medical services, including those of pharmacists and pharmacy technicians. By using the term "patient," the sense of obligation to the person served is elevated. Unlike the barber or the hardware store proprietor whose first priority must be to make a profit while providing a service, pharmacists and technicians provide medical services while secondarily making a profit.

A leading medical ethicist, Edmund D. Pellegrino, MD, observed that health care professionals have a special obligation to those they serve. They have a contract, he noted, with "sick people." This means health care professionals must make a public and professional "commitment to work for the good of the patient." "Health care," Dr. Pellegrino said, "[is] an inherently moral enterprise rooted in [a] covenant with the patient."[1] Every pharmacy has a contract (covenant) with its customers. In essence, the agreement is a promise by the pharmacy to provide quality service to the patient in exchange for which the patient brings his or her prescription business to the pharmacy.

In some ways, however, whether serving in a hospital or a community pharmacy, it is worth remembering that these patients are also customers. When people who use a pharmacy's services are referred to as "customers," pharmacy professionals are reminded of other obligations. In 1890, Mahatma Gandhi observed:

> *A customer is the most important visitor on our premises.*
>
> *He is not dependent on us. We are dependent on him.*
>
> *He is not an interruption in our work—he is the purpose of it.*
>
> *We are not doing him a favour by serving him. He is doing us a favour by giving us the opportunity to serve him.*

Perhaps the highest service pharmacists and pharmacy technicians can provide to their customers and patients is covered by the medical adage, "First, do no harm." Above all, in pharmacy this means a duty to dispense the right drug in the right strength to the right patient with the right directions on the label.

Today professional pharmacists have more obligations than that. They have a professional duty to use their knowledge and education to assist their patients in using their medication for its greatest benefit. Pharmacists and pharmacy technicians also serve as part of a safety net guarding against errors by other members of the health care team. They do this through drug review, education, and in other, less obvious ways. As merchants, pharmacy staff can serve with a smile and with patience, even when the customer's demeanor would not warrant it. As Dr. Pellegrino reminds us, pharmacy's customers are often sick people.

In this chapter we will explore how the patient can assist pharmacists and pharmacy technicians to meet their need to deliver quality health care. We will also discuss how pharmacists and pharmacy technicians can help patients recognize when they should ask for help. Medication errors are more than mechanical mistakes. They involve using medication in the wrong way or at the wrong time. Medication errors may result from physicians' mistakes, pharmacies' mistakes, and even (and perhaps more often) patients' mistakes. The pharmacy's customer needs to assist pharmacies in all of these circumstances.

Here we will talk about more than legal duties. Professional and ethical duties are higher but often harder to recognize and meet. First, we will discuss pharmacy errors for which we need to enlist the services of the patient. In order to ask for such assistance, we may have to admit what no professional wants to say: we are human; we are not perfect; we make mistakes.

> **Quality Note 10-A Can I Say I'm Sorry?**
>
> Several states have passed **apology laws** that provide for immunity for health care professionals who issue an apology when there has been an error. Physicians and health care providers can apologize and offer expressions of grief without concern that their words may be used against them in court.
>
> Many times, all a patient wants is to have someone say, "I am sorry" and "We will learn from this experience."
>
> Visit the Internet to see if your state has an apology law. Go to http://www.sorryworks.net/laws.phtml
>
> *Careful:* in some states, pharmacists and pharmacies are not covered under the definition of "health care provider."
>
> *Also:* know if your professional liability insurance company has a clause in the policy prohibiting apologies.[2]

The Patient and CQI

Pharmacy is not alone in the quest for improved patient care. The medical profession faces even more daunting problems dealing with medical errors. Physicians have by necessity begun enlisting their patients as part of their quality systems. By studying medicine's attempts to bring patients into quality, pharmacy can learn valuable lessons. Perhaps the most glaring medical examples have come from surgery. Patients have been put on notice that they need to be part of the solution in avoiding surgical mistakes.

What worse event can one imagine than for a surgeon to cut on the wrong body part? In 2007 a *New York Times* reporter offered examples of just such happenings in her online health blog:

> Concerns about surgeons operating on the wrong part of the body made headlines this week after The Providence Journal reported that on three separate occasions this year, surgeons at Rhode Island Hospital operated on the wrong side of a patient's head. The most recent case happened last Friday, when the chief resident started to cut on the head of an 82-year-old patient.

The problem was not isolated to one hospital in Rhode Island. The reporter continued:

> On a percentage basis, surgery on the wrong side or area of the body is considered rare. But nonetheless, it affects hundreds of people a year, and hundreds more cases likely go unreported. This month, the Archives of Surgery ran a letter from The Joint Commission, the primary accrediting agency for hospitals in the United States, noting that it receives about nine voluntary reports per month of so-called "wrong-site adverse events" to

its Sentinel Event Database. Last September, the same medical journal reported that wrong-site surgery may be underreported by a factor of 20. That study concluded that there are 1,300 to 2,700 wrong-site procedures annually in the United States.

In response to this type of errors, the Joint Commission provides a brochure for patients called "Speak Up." In it, patients are warned:

Mistakes can happen during surgery. Surgeons can do the wrong surgery. They can operate on the wrong part of your body. Or they can operate on the wrong person. Hospitals and other medical facilities that are accredited by The Joint Commission must follow a procedure that helps surgeons avoid these mistakes.

There are several such brochures published by the Joint Commission, including one on medication errors in which it says, "Medicine mistakes happen every day . . . You can get the wrong medicine." It then recommends that patients ask questions and take an active part in preventing medication errors. Surgeons today often have the patient draw a large "X" on the leg to be treated, and ophthalmologists will place a piece of tape over the eye to be cared for, having explained to the patient exactly why they are doing so.

Erasing the Fear of Using the Patient

Pharmacies, especially those outside hospitals and medical clinics, have been reluctant to issue similar calls to their patients for help. The reason may be that pharmacy executives do not want to be the first to tell their patients that the pharmacy's pharmacists and technicians make medication errors. Perhaps a better answer is for a brochure to be printed on a broader basis, such as by the state pharmacy association. The profession as a whole would be speaking to patients on behalf of all pharmacies in the state. In this way no one pharmacy need be the first to say, "We are humans, too, and we can make mistakes." The time has come for pharmacy to enlist the help of the patient in reducing the risk of a medication error. The patient needs to be a part of the pharmacy's CQI system. Individual pharmacies should not wait for associations to act.

MECHANICAL ERRORS

Eighty percent of pharmacy claims are for mechanical errors: wrong drug, wrong strength, or wrong directions. One place the help of patients can be enlisted is at the time of counseling. ISMP suggests that counseling may be one of the most effective ways of preventing mechanical medication errors.[3] If a pharmacy is to make patients a part of its CQI, this is the natural place to start. In the best practice discussed earlier called "Show and Tell" counseling, the pharmacist shows the contents of the prescription to the patient and asks the Indian Health Service prime questions. The first is, "What did your physician tell you this is for?" The pharmacist could add: "This will not change unless we tell you. If we use a different generic, we will let you know. If it ever looks different, do not take it, but call us immediately."

With pharmacists providing this message to each patient, pharmacy technicians can be aware of it and be trained to react appropriately. When a different generic is used, the NDC number will change because the brand changed. The technician can alert the pharmacist to this fact so he or she can tell the patient. The pharmacy can develop its own best practice by providing a special sticker to place on the patient's prescription bag or by using a special, distinctive mark on the bag or receipt when the brand has changed.

Should a patient call in saying, "This looks different," technicians need to recognize this as a "pharmacist only question." (see "Establishing Pharmacist Only Questions," Chapter 3) The rule in the pharmacy becomes: It is a mistake until it is proven it is not a mistake. Several times an injury could have been avoided had a technician not answered a patient's question with, "It's probably just a generic—it's OK."[4]

Review the best practices discussed in earlier chapters and ask what was their purpose. Some of these best practices can be used to guide the present discussion of how to enlist patients in preventing medication errors.

Training pharmacy technicians in the use of the pharmacy's CQI program should include making them cognizant of the need to identify and engage vulnerable patients at the beginning of the process. Hospitals will do this differently, but let us experiment with how a community pharmacy may do so.

Patients still do not often appreciate the value of discussing their medication with the pharmacist. The following steps could be added to the receiving-station process workflow to encourage at least these special patients to take advantage of the education available.

- ☐ If the patient appears to meet the criteria of "vulnerable patient," make a note or pull an algorithm checklist and prepare it for the pharmacist by marking the item that may apply.

- ☐ Say to the patient, "The pharmacist usually likes to spend more time with patients with . . ."—fill in what applies: high blood pressure, diabetes, several medications, etc.

- ☐ Add, "You may want to think about any questions you would like to ask the pharmacist when the two of you are talking."

☐ "If you think of a question later, call us. We will have the pharmacist call back as soon as possible."

☐ "Be sure to read the information the pharmacist gives you with your medication."

While this may take some additional time, it has advantages that may make the time well invested. The patient is given the feeling someone cares and thus it builds rapport and solidifies customer appreciation. It may also reduce the risk of an untoward event caused by the patient's medication. And, in addition, the pharmacist is assisted by putting the patient on notice that the pharmacist may wish to speak to him or her.

Either the technician or the pharmacist may wish to add, "If, while taking the medicine you feel any unexpected effects or just a funny feeling, please call either us or your physician." A patient who has never had a particular drug before will often not know what to expect when first taking it. Some drugs (e.g., drugs to treat cancer) are likely to have very pronounced effects; such a caution could provoke a call. When all best practices have failed, this phone call may be the last opportunity to avoid a medication error.

The Case of the High Blood Pressure Patient and the Cancer Drug

On December 14, 2010, Virgen Diaz Sosa died in Puerto Rico, apparently from an overdose of methotrexate received from her pharmacy.[5] It was reported that Ms. Diaz Sosa had taken 19 doses of methotrexate 2.5 mg. According to the autopsy, she died "of intoxication [caused by methotrexate overdose] and multiple organ failure." According to news reports, her physician had written a prescription for metolazone 2.5 mg for her blood pressure. The Rx was filled at a local pharmacy in the town of Aguadilla, Puerto Rico. Shortly after the death, the local prosecuting attorney said he was investigating whether to charge both the pharmacist and the pharmacy technician with criminal manslaughter.

Methotrexate is used to treat cancer while metolazone is primarily used for high blood pressure. The literature for methotrexate lists its common and serious side effects. The common ones include:

Acne; chills and fever; dizziness; flushing; general body discomfort; hair loss; headache; infertility; irregular periods; itching; loss of appetite; lowered resistance to infection; miscarriage; nausea; sensitivity to sunlight; sore throat; speech impairment; stomach pain; swelling of the breast; unusual tiredness; vaginal discharge; vomiting.

Other side effects are more severe and require medical attention promptly. These include:

Severe allergic reactions (rash; hives; itching; difficulty breathing; tightness in the chest; swelling of the mouth, face, lips, or tongue); black or bloody stools; blood in the urine; bone pain; calf pain/swelling; change in amount of urine; chest pain; confusion; dark urine; diarrhea; dry cough; enlarged glands; fatigue; fever or chills; inflammation of the pancreas (stomach tenderness, nausea, vomiting, fever, increased pulse rate); irregular heartbeat; mental changes; mouth sores; muscle weakness; persistent sore throat; red, swollen, or blistered skin; seizures; serious infection (herpes, hepatitis, blood infection); trouble breathing; unusual bleeding or bruising; unusual pain and discoloration of the skin; vision changes; vomit that looks like coffee grounds; yellowing of skin or eyes.

Both methotrexate and metolazone come in a 2.5 mg tablets. The two do not look alike in either the tablets or the packaging. Because of alphabetical arrangement on the pharmacy shelves, the two products are often situated close or even next to each other. Reaching for the wrong drug is not a new phenomenon; it happens all too often in pharmacies.

There have been other deaths with methotrexate.[6] It is a powerful drug that is used only for a short time and sometimes only intermittently. Often, at the end of a short period of therapy, the patient will be given a "rescue" drug to stop the effects of the methotrexate. This may well be one of those drugs the pharmacy considers for its algorithm.

Ms. Diaz Sosa cannot be blamed for trusting her pharmacist and pharmacy technician, but patients like her can be incorporated into a pharmacy's quality system. Too often patients are the last check to avoid medication errors. If patients like Ms. Diaz Sosa are to be part of the solution, pharmacy staff must educate them. The result in this sad case may have been different had she thought to call when she first became ill, or if she had been asked, "What did your physician tell you this is for?" Some of the things patients should know about their medication are:

- What drug they are taking
- Why they are taking it
- How to take it
- How long they are expected to be taking this drug
- What the drug looks like

OTHER TYPES OF ERRORS

Not all QREs are mechanical errors and not all mistakes are made by the pharmacy. Physicians and patients probably make more errors than do pharmacies. Pharmacists and pharmacy technicians are often in a position to recognize and guard against some, but not all, of these. Preventing all medication errors, including those not caused by the pharmacy, can also be part of the pharmacy's CQI program.

Pharmacists and technicians cannot take full responsibility for all patients or all errors not occurring in the pharmacy. Prescriber errors and patient errors are common and most are beyond what a pharmacy can prevent. Pharmacies can accept fault when they make a mechanical error. In most cases, however, courts have avoided casting blame on pharmacies for tragedies they did not directly cause. While there may not be a legal duty in most of these cases, pharmacies still wish to avoid any injuries that may reasonably be avoidable.

When pharmacists and pharmacy technicians think of reducing medication errors, their vision tends to be myopic, limited to mechanical errors that reach the patient. In this book we have expanded that definition to include drug-review errors such as allergies to drugs and medications that are contraindicated with a patient's condition or other drugs the patient is taking. For pharmacy practice this is a convenient, short-hand, working definition of a medication error. The official definition used by most medical and pharmacy organizations, however, is much broader.

The National Coordinating Council for Medication Error Reporting and Prevention (NCC MERP)[7] is a group of 24 national health care organizations. NCC MERP suggests the following definition be adopted universally:

> *A medication error is any preventable event that may cause or lead to inappropriate medication use or patient harm while the medication is in the control of the health care professional, patient, or consumer. Such events may be related to professional practice, health care products, procedures, and systems, including prescribing; order communication; product labeling, packaging, and nomenclature; compounding; dispensing; distribution; administration; education; monitoring; and use.*

Using this broader definition, pharmacy can expand its definition of CQI.

Physician Mistakes

Pharmacy technicians and even pharmacists often assume that the patient's physician has educated the patient in these matters. That presumption is often not correct. For example, some medications can cause birth defects if taken during pregnancy. Women who may become pregnant should avoid conceiving while taking these drugs and should be made aware of the need for using some form of contraception during and for a time after taking these medications. It is easy to presume that a woman of child-bearing age who is, or will be, taking one of these drugs is at least generally aware of this by the time she arrives at the pharmacy. However, according to a study in the *Annals of Internal Medicine*[8] reported by *Medscape for Pharmacists*, ". . . half of women taking such medications did not receive counseling from their physicians about using contraceptives or birth control measures." The article concludes, "Physicians aren't doing a very good job of warning young women to avoid getting pregnant when taking prescription drugs that can cause birth defects."

There have been cases in which a pharmacy was held liable for failure to warn a patient not to take medication.[9] In Chapter 3 we discussed some of the professional duties of pharmacists, including a duty to counsel patients when drugs should be used with particular caution. Failure to warn a woman not to become pregnant when taking certain drugs could fit within such a duty. Whether it does or not the pharmacy may wish to guard against potential injury to the mother or the unborn child by keeping a list of such drugs. The pharmacy technician filling the prescription or entering data can insert a note directed to the pharmacist who will perform the drug review. Once warned, it becomes the patient's responsibility to take precautions. The pharmacy should maintain some documentation that the patient had been told of the danger. Making patients part of the pharmacy's quality-assurance program means the patient has taken on duties as well.

Prescribers make other errors. A large concern for pharmacy and for society as a whole is the overprescribing of controlled substances. Overuse is often the fault of the patient. Physicians must also accept at least part of the blame. In these cases the pharmacy's best risk-management practice may be to say no and refuse to fill the prescription. A patient may be ignorant of the dangers, so educating patients may be the best way to include them as part of the CQI program.

The Case of Someone Made a Mistake

In 2002 Pauline Deeds[10] had some of her prescriptions filled at her regular pharmacy in Connecticut. In the preceding year she had a lot of prescriptions filled at the same pharmacy. As a matter of fact, she had 149 prescriptions filled in 2001 at the same pharmacy, most written by the same physician. All were filled correctly and all as ordered by Mrs. Deed's physician. She was being treated for "pain relief, muscle tension, anxiety, depression and nausea." Many of Mrs. Deeds's prescriptions were for controlled substances, in particular, oxycodone. She also had several prescriptions for carisoprodol. On January 4, 2002, Mrs. Deeds died. According to the medical examiner, she died of "acute carisoprodol and oxycodone toxicity."

In a subsequent lawsuit against the pharmacy, the court held there was no duty on the pharmacy. The knowledge the pharmacy had was not superior to that of either the physician or Mrs. Deeds. Perhaps the physician was at fault and perhaps Mrs. Deeds was at fault. Deciding that question is beyond the purpose of our study. The question for risk management is: Was the pharmacy in a position to make Mrs. Deeds a part of its quality assurance system? In some similar cases the pharmacist may say, "You are taking too many. I need to discuss this with your physician." In other cases the pharmacist may simply refuse to fill the prescription, at least until the prescriber convinces the pharmacist that he or she has consulted with the patient and the situation is under control.

In some cases of controlled-substance use, there is no question that the physician and probably also the patient are intending to abuse the system. The pharmacy's risk-management system should take these situations into consideration. Interstate 95 runs from Florida through New York. As we saw previously, many pharmacists know this as the "Oxycontin Express." Reportedly, dealers will pay physicians in southern states to write prescriptions for drugs that are in high demand in the North. The dealers, or someone employed by them, will have the prescriptions filled in pharmacies along I95 on the way north. They will then sell the drugs in the northern states. The prescriptions are not for a legitimate medical purpose. They are not written in the regular course of medical practice. Such prescriptions are illegal and are void. While this may not appear to be a risk-management or CQI problem, it is. Filling these prescriptions puts the pharmacists, pharmacy technicians, and pharmacies at risk. It also places some person to whom these drugs will eventually be delivered at risk of death or injury.

> **Quality Note 10-B   Ryan Haight Online Pharmacy Consumer Protection Act of 2008**
>
> Internet prescriptions written by physicians whose only professional relationship with patients is online have been a national problem. Patients, some legitimate and some not, submit answers to a questionnaire, which is reviewed by a physician who has never seen or examined the patient. In response to the patient's request, the physician prescribes the desired medication. The prescription is sent to a mail-order pharmacy that may send it on to a regular pharmacy to be filled and mailed to the patient.
>
> Under the Ryan Haight Online Pharmacy Consumer Protection Act of 2008, and under the laws of several states, the prescription is illegal if it is for a controlled substance. Under Ryan Haight, the prescriber must have conducted at least one in-person medical evaluation of the patient. Prescriptions for drugs other than controlled substances prescribed in a similar manner may also be illegal. The handling of illegal prescriptions should be addressed by the pharmacy's quality program. Not the least concern is the patient, who may only be trying to save time.

Patient Mistakes

Consider a medication error from the perspective of the patient. It would include the wrong drug given or prescribed plus wrong dosage and wrong directions. It would also include medication that did not work, even if, as often is the case, it was the fault of the patient him- or herself. This is particularly true for patients who take medications for chronic conditions. Usually, as with high blood pressure medications, the drug only holds the condition in check and does not cure the underlying disease.

Compliance with a medication's directions for use is important in patients' health. It is estimated that one in three Americans have high blood pressure and spend $20 billion annually on medication. Yet it has been reported that ". . . about 86 percent of hypertensive patients did not properly follow their prescriptions."[11] An article[12] in the *National Medical Association Journal* says, "The morbidity associated with hypertension is high; hypertension is the leading cause of death and the third highest risk factor for disability-adjusted life years in the world. . . . High blood pressure causes half of all heart attacks, strokes, and heart failure cases in the United States."

Education of patients is an important part of quality associated with patient care. In an investigation reported in the *Archives of Internal Medicine*,[13] death among "community-dwelling elderly persons" can be predicted by measuring how well they can read and understand their medical information. This is a type of medication error pharmacists and pharmacy technicians can influence, even if they have no legal duty to do so.

Recall the algorithm used to select vulnerable patients. The purpose is to allow pharmacy staff to selectively target patients who may require more education about their medication. One group of patients suggested for special counseling is people with high blood pressure. Consider Connie (not her real name)[14] and the Case of the Medication That Was Too Expensive. The story takes place before the implementation of Medicare's limited medication coverage under Part D, but it is still relevant in a broader sense.

The Case of the Medication That Was Too Expensive

Connie was in her mid-seventies and suffered from high blood pressure and a heart condition. She had suffered a few "mini strokes." Her physician had prescribed one of the newer medications to treat her high blood pressure, but it was not covered by her insurance. She lived on a fixed income that barely covered her necessities. There was not enough left over for this very expensive medication. She knew she had to take something for her blood pressure, but was embarrassed to talk to her physician or her family about her financial situation. Connie did not know her physician could have prescribed other, less expensive high blood pressure medications that might work as well. Many of these other drugs would have been covered by Connie's insurance plan.

To save money, she began taking her drugs every other day and eventually every third day. Her prescription, designed to last 30 days, was now lasting almost 90 days. No one seemed to notice, neither her physician nor her pharmacy. Connie suffered a full stroke about 6 months later. She was in the hospital for several days and then transferred to a nursing home for rehabilitation. After almost 2 months she returned home. While she was in the hospital and the nursing home, her medication, as well as her treatment, was paid for by her insurance under a different set of rules. When Connie returned home, however, the same problems with finances and coverage were present.

Sometimes medication errors are the fault of the patient, as in the case of Connie. There were people, however, who could have helped Connie manage the risks associated with improper use of her prescriptions. For example, her physician could have tried, had someone talked to him and made him aware of the problem.

When pharmacies institute plans for reducing medication errors, cases like Connie's should be considered so that education and follow-up with intervention, where necessary, is somewhere in the plan. In defense of Connie's physician, he probably did not know the newer medication was not on this particular insurance company's formulary. He also did not know that a 30-day supply was lasting Connie 90 days.

The pharmacy's computer showed that Connie's prescription was lasting three times longer than it should have. The pharmacist was in a position to approach Connie and ask her about her drug use. The pharmacist was also in a position to suggest alternative drugs to the physician. This was a medication error. The pharmacy's CQI plan could have reduced the risks of this error happening.

The Case of the Lumberjack

Patients make other mistakes and unwise choices. Mr. McLaughlin, a lumberjack, was working in the forestry industry in the Northwest.[15] While working, he fell and his back was seriously injured. He was in a lot of pain. He returned to his native Indiana where he was treated by his family physician. Mr. McLaughlin began taking a schedule III pain reliever. At first he took it according to the directions on the bottle, but later began increasing the dose to the point where he was greatly exceeding the prescribed dose. The Indiana Supreme Court later explained the facts of the case:

Over a period of months in 1988, McLaughlin obtained prescriptions for drugs containing propoxyphene from Dr. Edwards. Most of these prescriptions were filled at a Hooks drugstore in South Bend by pharmacists Kathy O'Dell and Craig Merrick. The prescriptions were dispensed either on the basis of written prescriptions from Dr. Edwards brought to Hooks by McLaughlin, telephone calls to the store from the physician's office, or as refills.

McLaughlin consumed these drugs at a rate much faster than prescribed. Hooks' records show that dozens of prescriptions for Darvocet or Darvon were filled for McLaughlin between May 1987 and December 1988. For example, during one sixty-day period in 1988, McLaughlin received twenty-four separate refills of propoxyphene compounds, totalling 1,072 tablets. If consumed according to the prescription, the number of tablets would have lasted a period of 138 days; McLaughlin consumed the tablets in 62 days, almost two and one half times faster than the prescription ordered. In one month alone, propoxyphene prescriptions were filled twelve times, which means that McLaughlin or his wife appeared in the Hooks store once every two or three days.

In late 1988, after Dr. Edwards apparently became aware that McLaughlin was consuming propoxyphene drugs at a rate much faster than prescribed, he refused to furnish any more prescriptions. Shortly thereafter, McLaughlin's wife found her husband holding a shotgun to his head at a time of depression. He did not pull the trigger. Following treatment for drug addiction in early 1989, McLaughlin stopped taking all prescription pain medication.

The legal importance of the case was that it resulted in the Indiana courts, for the first time, recognizing a limited duty of a pharmacist to warn a patient of excessive refills on a prescription. As the court ruled:

Where a pharmacy customer is having a prescription for a dangerous drug refilled at an unreasonably faster rate than the rate prescribed, the pharmacist has a duty to cease refilling the prescription pending direct and explicit directions from the prescribing physician.

The importance in this discussion is that this was a preventable medication error. In the McLaughlin case, it can be said that the pharmacy had special knowledge. That knowledge came from the patient profile that advised the pharmacists how often the patient was receiving this medication.

Unknown at the time of the Indiana Supreme Court's decision, the pharmacists in the McLaughlin case actually did notice the frequency of the refills. As was only later reported, the pharmacists did take action. The case was remanded back to the trial court for a trial based on the supreme court's decision. The full case was never tried. It was settled by agreement of the parties based in part upon the facts that came out only at the time of the settlement. While the amount of the settlement was not disclosed, it was said to be a very low sum. The reason for the lower-than-expected settlement was allegedly because the pharmacists had done what the court had said was their duty. They contacted the physician and counseled the patient and his wife concerning the amount of the drug Mr. McLaughlin was taking. It was reportedly one of the pharmacists' telephone calls to the physician that convinced him to stop authorizing the drug.[16]

Prescription-Monitoring Program

Most states have now adopted a **prescription-monitoring program**. This is a statewide database into which each pharmacy that dispenses controlled substances and each physician who prescribes them must enter the data. The information is then available through a secured online database to all pharmacies and prescribers in the state. They can, by entering the database, see each pharmacy that has filled a controlled-substance prescription for this patient and each physician in the state who has prescribed controlled substances for this patient. It is a tool that needs to be made a part of each pharmacy's CQI program with specific instructions as to when and by whom the database may be viewed. Among other uses, this information could trigger that a counseling algorithm is needed for this patient. It should also set forth when the prescription will not be filled and perhaps when law enforcement may need to be called.

> **RxErcise 10-A**   **Prescription-Monitoring Program**
>
> Use the Internet to research whether your state has a prescription-monitoring program. Discuss:
> The advantages of such a program.
> Why your state has one or why it does not.
> How could a prescription-monitoring program have been used in the lumberjack case and Mrs. Deeds's case?

While counseling patients and use of an algorism, as discussed in Chapter 7, are pharmacist responsibilities, pharmacy technicians can play a major part in a pharmacy's CQI program by recognizing when special problems may exist. The technician at the receiving station may be the first to recognize, by the age of the patient or some other attribute, that the patient is one who meets the criteria for a pharmacist's algorithm.

Education goes beyond individual counseling of a particular patient and need not be completely oral. The pharmacy could be an advocate for those who particularly need an advocate, as in Connie's case, where the family may be unaware of what is happening until it is too late.

Advocacy and education may take several forms. It may be as simple as a pharmacist or a pharmacy technician saying to a patient, "Be sure you read this information, and if you have any questions, call the pharmacist or your physician." A pharmacy may have educational material or videos or websites available for patients to review. The technician who receives the prescription could inform the patient that information is available and suggest that the patient review it while waiting for the prescription to be filled. The patient should be encouraged to ask questions of the pharmacist, rather than just be asked if she or he has questions. Patients may not be in the best position to know whether they need to be counseled.

Summary

Dr. Deming's 14 principles are the basis of his management philosophy upon which his system of total quality management (TQM) is based. Under principle 14, management has an obligation to commit the organization to quality and the obligation to communicate that commitment to all, including employees and customers.

In pharmacy, this translates to having an effective CQI program designed to serve the patient and reduce medication errors, but also to include making the patient a part of that program and admitting that its professionals can make mistakes. Pharmacists and pharmacy technicians have an obligation to use the tools provided to them to reduce medication errors.

In this last chapter we discussed the ultimate extent of a CQI program. Every pharmacy is made up of human beings who can and do make mistakes. Sometimes those mistakes can reach the patient. Sometimes they can cause injury. The message to the patient is that the pharmacy, pharmacists, and pharmacy technicians are dedicated to working with them and helping them care for themselves. Included in the message to patients is: "We do not accept our mistakes, and neither should you."

Review Questions

1. What would first alert the pharmacy technician to the fact that a patient received a different generic on a refill compared to the previous refill?

    A. The NDC number will change when the brand changed.

    B. The patient might say, "This looks different."

    C. The patient will say something when the pharmacist performs "show and tell" counseling.

    D. The pharmacy should post a sign on the shelf next to the generic being used, noting when it changed.

2. What does NCC MERP stand for?

    A. National Coordinating Council for Medication Error Reporting and Prevention

    B. National Centers for Community Medical Electronic Registered Pharmacy

    C. Natural Cause Conditions with Medical Error Reporting in Pharmacy

    D. North Carolina Center for Medication Error among Reporting Pharmacies

3. What name is most commonly applied to state laws that provide immunity for health care professionals who issue an apology when there has been an error?

   A. Sorry laws

   B. Apology laws

   C. Health care Providers' Apology Immunity Act

   D. Pharmacists' Immunity Act

4. What term is usually applied to pharmacy errors: wrong drug, wrong strength, or wrong directions?

   A. Mechanical errors

   B. Intellectual errors

   C. The 3 wrongs

   D. Technician errors

5. What is the best practice rule that covers how pharmacy technicians should respond when a patient says, "This tablet looks different than the one I got last month?"

   A. Obvious-error rule

   B. Pharmacist only question

   C. Apology rule

   D. Triple-check rule

6. Who could be allowed to say to a patient, "If, while taking the medicine you feel any unexpected effects or just a funny feeling, please call either us or the doctor"?

   A. Pharmacy technician

   B. Pharmacist

   C. Clerk

   D. A or B, but not C

7. What should every patient know about their medication?

   A. What drug they are taking

   B. Why they are taking it

   C. How to take it

   D. All of the above

8. For pharmacy practice there is a convenient, shorthand, working definition of a medication error. What is it?

   A. Mistake that reaches a patient

   B. QRE

   C. Adverse medical event

   D. Mechanical error

9. What organization that is a group of 24 national health care organizations developed the official definition of "medication error"?

   A. NCC MERP

   B. APhA

   C. ASHP

   D. NASPA

10. What is the common, slang name given to the illegal traffic of drug dealers who pay physicians in southern states to write prescriptions for drugs that are in high demand in the North? They have the prescriptions filled along the way and sell them in northern states.

    A. "Oxycontin express"

    B. "I95 corridor"

    C. "South-North corridor"

    D. "The super highway"

Endnotes

[1] See http://virtualmentor.ama-assn.org/2001/11/prol1-0111.html accessed March 24, 2010.

[2] Note: Pharmacists Mutual Insurance Company issued a letter to its insureds saying it was not a violation of its policies for them to say they are sorry, if the insured made an obvious error. Before relying on such a statement, the insured should request a copy of the letter from the company.

[3] See http://www.ismp.org

[4] See Pharmacist Only Questions, Chapter 3.

[5] Associated Press, *Miami Herald*, December 10, 2010.

[6] Telephone conversation with Don McGuire, BS Pharm., JD, General Counsel, Pharmacists Mutual Insurance Company.

[7] For more information on NCC MERP, see http://www.nccmerp.org/leadershipMemberOrgs.html accessed March 30, 2011.

[8] See *Medscape for Pharmacists*: www.medscape.com quoting a report by CBS News.

[9] Some of these cases were discussed in Chapter 3, when we examined the role of the pharmacist.

[10] *Deeds v. Walgreen Co.*, 927 A.2d 1001, 50 Conn. Supp. 339 (2007).

[11] McCombs, J. S., Nichol, M. B., Newman, C. M., and Sclar, D. A., The Costs of Interrupting Antihypertensive Drug Therapy in a Medicaid Population. *Med Care*. 1994; 32:214–226.

[12] Shaya, F. T., Gbarayor, C. M., Frech-Tamas, F., Lau, H., Weir, M. R., Predictors of Compliance with Antihypertensive Therapy in a High-Risk Medicaid Population, *National Medical Association*, 2009; 101:34–39.

[13] Baker, D. W., Wolf, M. S., Feinglass, J., et al., Health Literacy and Mortality among Elderly Persons, *Archives of Internal Medicine*, 2007: 167(14); 1503–1509.

[14] Story related by Connie's daughter, who discovered her mother's noncompliance only after her stroke.

[15] *Hooks SuperX, Inc. v. McLaughlin*, 642 N.E. 2d 514 (Ind. 1994).

[16] Conversation with one familiar with the later facts of this case, who asked not to be identified.

Glossary

A

Accreditation Council for Pharmacy Education (ACPE) A national, independent agency for the accreditation of professional degree programs in pharmacy, providers of continuing pharmacy education and certificate programs in pharmacy (Ch. 3).

Adverse drug event Any incident in which the use of a medication (drug or biologic) at any dose, a medical device, or a special nutritional product (for example, dietary supplement, infant formula, medical food) may have resulted in an adverse outcome in a patient. (See http://www.jointcommission.org/sentinelevents/se_glossary.htm) (Ch. 1)

Adverse event An injury related to medical management, in contrast to complications of disease. Medical management includes all aspects of care, including diagnosis and treatment, failure to diagnose or treat, and the systems and equipment used to deliver care. Adverse events may be preventable or nonpreventable. (See http://www.who.int/patientsafety/events/05/Reporting_Guidelines.pdf) (Ch. 1)

Algorithm An algorithm is a list of criteria that form a decision tree. Its use allows a pharmacy to select individual patients or conditions that may most need a particular service such as in-depth counseling. A counseling algorithm may look for certain drugs that would be particularly dangerous because of their method of action or potential interactions. It may also look for disease states such as diabetes, or patient traits such as one who takes more than five drugs (Ch. 7).

Ambulatory A health care facility that services patients who are not in a hospital, nursing home, or otherwise institutionalized. An outpatient pharmacy located in a hospital and retail or community pharmacies are both examples of ambulatory pharmacies (Ch. 1).

American Pharmacists Association (APhA) Formed in 1852, the APhA is the oldest national association representing pharmacists and pharmacy technicians in the United States. See http://www.pharmacist.com (Ch. 2)

American Society of Health-System Pharmacists (ASHP) Originally called the American Society of Hospital Pharmacists, ASHP was formed as a part of the APhA. Today, ASHP is a strong national association representing hospital pharmacists and pharmacy technicians. See http://www.ashp.org (Ch. 2)

Apology laws Laws passed in several states that provide for immunity for health care professionals who issue an apology when there has been an error. Physicians and health care providers can apologize and offer expressions of grief without concern that their words may be used against them in court. Pharmacists and pharmacies are covered only if they are included in the language of the statute or are defined as health care providers in that state (Ch. 10).

B

Benchmark A benchmark is a standard that can be used to measure changes that occur subsequently in a particular area. A benchmark will allow a person to know if improvement has been made. In pharmacy if we measure the number of errors per 1000 prescriptions filled, we can use that figure to compare whether we improved when we filled the next 1000 and each thousand after that. The number we compare each thousand against is the benchmark (Ch. 9).

Best practice A technique or procedure used and developed over time that has been proven to either stop an error before it begins or to catch a mistake before it can reach the patient and become an error (Ch. 4).

Best practice   Best practices are techniques used in the pharmacy profession as a way of stopping or catching mistakes before they reach a patient. They are called "best practices" because they have proven effective in use. An example of a best practice is a **national drug code (NDC)** check during which the number on the manufacturer's bottle is checked against the NDC number printed on the pharmacy receipt (Ch. 1).

Best practices   Techniques that have been proven to be effective. When best practices are used in the dispensing of medications, they help in stopping or catching dispensing mistakes before they reach patients (Ch. 6).

C

Causes of errors   W. Edwards Deming taught that causes of quality-related events can be categorized into five factors. Using these five factors provides a convenient method of identifying the sources of QREs. Once the source is known, it can be eliminated, thereby reducing potential future errors. Deming referred to these five causes as "P, 3 Ms, and E", for:

People: Usually not a specific person, but the position, such as entry technician.

Method: The manner in which a job is being preformed such as the workflow, a process, the "will call" procedure, or the delivery service; it could include software.

Material: All materials used in dispensing a prescription, including shelves, packaging, bottles, caps, and stock bottles.

Machine: Anything electronic or mechanical, including the computer, scanner, cash register, or even the telephone system. It would also include robotics; it could include software.

Environment: Anything that affects what is happening around the pharmacy, including lighting, loud radios, people talking, staff moving through the pharmacy, or any element that could be considered attractive (Ch. 5).

Centers for Medicare and Medicaid Services (CMS)   An agency of the federal government that oversees the rules and regulations associated with federal health care programs, including Medicare and Medicaid (Ch. 6).

Common law   Decisions made by courts can have the effect of setting a rule that other lower courts must follow. The court case thus sets a precedent and has the force of law. Court decisions are referred to as the common law (Ch. 3).

Community pharmacy   Formerly referred to as a *drugstore* or *retail pharmacy*, the community pharmacy is usually located in commercial areas and serves the general public. It may be an independent pharmacy or a unit of a chain pharmacy (Ch. 1).

Continuous Quality Improvement (CQI)   A CQI program is a workflow process designed to reduce the number of errors in any system. CQI is the term most often used in pharmacy practice for systems implemented to reduce the risk of a medication error reaching a patient. Other names often used are total quality management (TQM), quality assurance (QA), and quality improvement (QI). CQI systems should be structured to constantly improve and not remain static. This implies there must be an element of monitoring a system to discover and correct any vulnerabilities in the system (Ch. 8).

Continuous quality improvement (CQI)   Developed from the writings and teachings of Dr. Edwards Deming, CQI is the name often used in pharmacy for a systematic plan to reduce medication errors by identifying the risks, developing a plan, implementing and training staff in the use of the plan, and monitoring the results with the concept of using that information to further improve the workings of the plan (Ch. 1).

Controlled substance While all prescription drugs are controlled by federal and state laws, drugs that have been determined to be addictive have been designated as "controlled substances." Primarily these are narcotics, pain medications, and mood altering drugs such as some stimulants and tranquilizers. They are divided into five schedules, depending on their nature, from Schedule I, considered most addictive with no medical value, to Schedule V, least additive and in some states available without a prescription if sold by a pharmacist to a customer with proper identification. See the Drug Enforcement Administration (DEA) website for drugs in each schedule: http://www.deadiversion.usdoj.gov/schedules/index.html (Ch. 2)

Covered entity A covered entity is an organization or individual that uses electronic means to transmit health care information about its patients. A covered entity and everyone working for it is subject to HIPAA privacy rules (Ch. 5).

CQI station A CQI station is a stage within a series of steps designed as part of a planned workflow. A pharmacy workflow is made up of a series of processes. At each station a person performs tasks leading to the dispensing of medication. Typical stations within a pharmacy workflow are: receiving the prescription, entering information into the computer, filling the prescription, pharmacist final check, DUR, counseling, and delivery (Ch. 4).

Cubic centimeter (cc) A unit of measure often used in medicine. One cc is approximately equivalent to one milliliter (mL). A standard teaspoon is considered to be about 5 cc or 5 mL. A dosage of 5 cc measured in a marked cup or syringe is a more accurate dose than "1 teaspoonful" because teaspoons may vary in size (Ch. 1).

Culture of learning An environment within the pharmacy where all members of staff, including managers and executives of the organization, accept that continuous improvement includes an organized workflow, regular training, quality tools, and an emphasis on the importance of the people who make up the quality team. Everybody is a part of the system and they commit themselves to those goals of quality, service, and continuous improvement (Ch. 7).

D

Drug review, prospective drug review, drug utilization review (DUR) Pharmacists are trained to review prescriptions to ensure patient safety. Medications need to be appropriate for the specific patient, taking into consideration patient age, gender, disease states, drug sensitivities, and allergies. In addition, pharmacists review drug-drug interactions, drug-food interactions, drug–disease state interactions, drug duplications, and patient compliance with prescribed doses and regimens. Also, pharmacists should spend time making sure patients understand their medications. Due to OBRA-90, states are required to have standards for retrospective drug-utilization review and may require prospective drug-utilization review. The Joint Commission standards also mandate prospective drug-utilization review in most settings (Ch. 2).

E

Electronic prescribing (e-prescribing) A method of writing and transmitting a prescription through the use of a computer or handheld personal digital assistant (PDA). The prescriber enters the information into a device and sends it in electronic form directly to the pharmacy. E-prescriptions replace writing, telephoning, or faxing the prescription (Ch. 4).

E-prescribing A method by which a prescriber can electronically send a prescription directly to a pharmacy from the physician's computer or handheld personal digital assistant (PDA) device (Ch. 6).

Errors Also referred to as "preventable adverse drug events." A working definition of

GLOSSARY

errors in pharmacy is mistakes made in the pharmacy that reach a patient. A more complete definition of error from the National Coordinating Council for Medication Error Reporting and Prevention (NCC MERP) is discussed in Chapter 10 (Ch. 2).

Errors   Also referred to as *preventable adverse medical events*, errors are mistakes made anywhere in health care. In pharmacy, an error is usually considered to be a mistake that reaches a patient (Ch. 1).

F

Fishbone diagram   A tool for analyzing the causes of risk-management problems or effects. The fishbone diagram provides a way to examine the effects of Person, Machine, Method, Material, and Environment (Ch. 9).

Food and Drug Administration (FDA)   A consumer protection agency of the federal government, the FDA regulates the safety and quality of drugs, food, cosmetics, and devices. It was created by the 1906 Pure Food and Drugs Act. See http://www.fda.gov (Ch. 2).

H

Health Insurance Portability and Accountability Act of 1996 (HIPAA)   HIPAA is a federal law protecting patient privacy of health care records. Violations can result in fines and even imprisonment. Broadly speaking, release of confidential information is a medical error that should be addressed as part of a pharmacy's CQI program (Ch. 5).

Herbals   Herbals are medicines usually made or derived directly from plant sources. For most purposes, herbals are not regulated by the FDA as are drugs. They can interfere and interact with drugs in the body. For an overview on herbals, visit Wikipedia: http://en.wikipedia.org/wiki/Herbal (Ch. 2).

I

Incident reports   Usually a company-designed report that documents facts and information regarding the events surrounding a QRE that reached a patient. The report summarizes information identifying the patient involved, the medications concerned, and store personnel with information regarding the events. Most pharmacy operations require an incident report to be filed with management. In some states, the law requires such a report to be maintained (Ch. 9).

Indian Health Service counseling   An agency of the federal government charged with health care services for Native Americans and Alaska natives. Its mission statement says: "Our mission . . . to raise the physical, mental, social, and spiritual health of American Indians and Alaska Natives to the highest level." In the 1960s, its officers developed a pharmacy-counseling model using open-ended questions. That model is now taught in all pharmacy colleges in the United States (Ch. 6).

Institute for Safe Medication Practices (ISMP)   ISMP is a not-for-profit organization dedicated to making the delivery of drugs in health care safer. It describes itself as a "nonprofit organization devoted entirely to medication error prevention and safe medication use." See http://www.ismp.org (Ch. 2).

Intellectual error   A name given to claims that are not mechanical in nature, such as placing the wrong drug in the prescription bottle or typing the wrong directions. Intellectual errors may involve an error in judgment or omission of an act requiring judgment. Intellectual errors include release of confidential information, drug review errors, and lack of counseling (Ch. 5).

Interactions   Occasionally, drugs can have an effect when used in combination with other drugs, herbals, or even food in ways that can be dangerous. There can be drug-drug (including herbals) interactions or drug-food interactions or drug–disease state interactions. Many of these drug interactions are known and these interactions are among the items pharmacists will screen for when they perform a drug review or DUR (Ch. 2).

Internal customer   A term used to identify coworkers. The importance of the term is that it emphasizes the need to focus work, at least partly, on other members of the team. Each member of the team serves all others. The importance of customers, discussed in the following chapter, is not diminished by recognizing obligations to internal customers (Ch. 7).

M

Mechanical error   In the Pharmacists Mutual Insurance Company Claims Study, a mechanical error is defined as *wrong drug, wrong strength of drug*, or *wrong directions*. Mechanical errors account for over 80 percent of all claims in the study (Ch. 1).

Mechanical errors   In the Pharmacists Mutual Insurance Company Claims Study, a mechanical error is defined as "wrong drug, wrong strength of drug, or wrong directions." (To look at the study, go to http://www.phmic.com and click on "Services" in the bar at the top and then on "Professional Liability Risk Management" in the menu on the left.) Mechanical errors exceed 80 percent of all claims in the study (click on "Mechanical Errors" in the same menu) (Ch. 2).

Med-guides   Medication guides are described by the FDA as "paper handouts that come with many prescription medicines. The guides address issues that are specific to particular drugs and drug classes, and they contain FDA-approved information that can help patients avoid serious adverse events." The FDA requires that med-guides be given with certain drugs, currently about 100. See http://www.fda.gov/Drugs/DrugSafety/UCM085729 (Ch. 2).

Medical error   Includes all errors throughout the medical professions. The Institute of Medicine, in a summary of its publication, *To Err is Human: Building a Safer Health System*, wrote:

> Medical errors can be defined as the failure of a planned action to be completed as intended or the use of a wrong plan to achieve an aim. Among the problems that commonly occur during the course of providing health care are **adverse drug events** and improper transfusions, surgical injuries and wrong-site surgery, suicides, restraint-related injuries or death, falls, burns, pressure ulcers, and mistaken patient identities. High error rates with serious consequences are most likely to occur in intensive-care units, operating rooms, and emergency departments.

(See http://www.iom.edu/~/media/Files/Report Files/1999/To-Err-is-Human/To Err is Human 1999 report brief.pdf) (Ch. 1)

Medication error   The standard definition provided by the National Coordinating Council for Medication Error Reporting and Prevention is:

> A medication error is any preventable event that may cause or lead to inappropriate medication use or patient harm while the medication is in the control of the health care professional, patient, or consumer. Such events may be related to professional practice, health care products, procedures, and systems (including prescribing; order communication; product labeling, packaging, and nomenclature; compounding; dispensing; distribution; administration; education; monitoring; and use).

(See: http://www.nccmerp.org/aboutMedErrors.html) A medication error is any error occurring in the medication use process. It may be in prescribing, dispensing, or administering a drug. It may also include the overuse or underuse of medication. It includes a mechanical error, a drug review error, or a counseling error (Ch. 1).

Mentoring programs   Mentors are peers who assist new employees in acclimating to the pharmacy. Mentors are particularly helpful in training new hires to understand and use the pharmacy's CQI program. Mentors may not be the trainers, but they function as confidants to whom new employees may go with questions (Ch. 8).

N

National Alliance for State Pharmacy Associations (NASPA)   NASPA is an association representing all state pharmacy associations in the United States. It features a continuous quality improvement program called Pharmacy Quality Commitment®. See http://www.naspa.us (Ch. 2).

National Association of Boards of Pharmacy (NABP)   A national organization that provides services to state boards of pharmacy. NABP administers testing for pharmacists in most states. It provides many other services including the Verified Internet Pharmacy Practice Sites (VIPPS) program that certifies Internet pharmacies (Ch. 3).

National drug code (NDC)   Each drug manufactured in the United States under the authority of the Food and Drug Administration (FDA) is given a unique number code. The code is divided into three segments that identify the manufacturer (four or five digits), the product or drug (three or four digits), and the size of the package (one or two digits). Because the number is also in the pharmacy's computer and printed on each pharmacy receipt, it can be checked against the NDC number on the manufacturer's bottle (Ch. 1).

Near-miss   A pharmacy mistake that does not reach the patient is often called a near-miss. See QRE (Ch. 2).

Near-misses   In pharmacy, a mistake that does not reach the patient, or is caught before it does, is often called a "near-miss." In order to be considered a near-miss, the mistake must have moved from the process or step where it was made to the next step or process. For example, if a mistake is made when typing the information for the label into the computer but is caught before it leaves the computer station, it does not meet the definition of a near-miss (Ch. 1).

Normal variation   A change where none of the factors or causes that work on or influence a system has changed. A normal variation is a change without a cause. It is a change that can be considered as caused by luck only (Ch. 9).

O

OBRA-87 Regulation   The Omnibus Budget Reconciliation Act of 1987 required nursing homes to have all medications for residents who received Medicaid or Medicare reviewed, usually by a pharmacist (Ch. 3).

OBRA-90 Regulation   In 1990 the federal government passed the Omnibus Budget Reconciliation Act of 1990 that required, as a small part of the legislation, states to require pharmacists to perform drug reviews, counsel patients, and maintain a patient profile on some patients. By 1993, the states, through their pharmacy practice acts or board of pharmacy regulations had broadened these requirements (Ch. 3).

Omnibus Budget Reconciliation Act-90 (OBRA-90) Regulation   In 1990 the federal government passed the Omnibus Budget Reconciliation Act that required, as a small part of the legislation, states to require pharmacists to perform drug reviews, counsel patients, and maintain a patient profile on some patients. By 1993, the states, through their pharmacy practice acts or board of pharmacy regulations, had broadened these requirements (Ch. 2).

Over-the-counter medications Medications that do not require a prescription are referred to as over-the-counter drugs (Ch. 2).

Paradigm A common set of patterns or forms that experience has taught us to expect. A paradigm is the lens through which we see the things around us. They help us make quick decisions. A typical paradigm is that high-quality items cost more than low-quality items. While many times paradigms are true and can be useful in helping us recognize patterns, some paradigms are not correct and may lead to mistakes in judgment (Ch. 1).

Patient profile By law or regulations, pharmacies are required to maintain a limited amount of information about each patient. These are referred to as "patient profiles" and may include other drugs the patient is taking in addition to general information such as the address and phone numbers. Disease state may be included in some of these patient profiles (Ch. 2).

Patient Safety and Quality Improvement Act of 2005 A federal law that protects all records collected for the purpose of improving quality in health care, so long as certain conditions are met that are set forth in the regulations. Two primary requirements are (1) the information must be collected for quality purposes, and (2) it must be sent to a patient safety organization (PSO) hired by the health care provider (Ch. 9).

Patient Safety Organization (PSO) A quality organization recognized and certified by the federal department of Health and Human Services to collect and analyze data pursuant to the Patient Safety and Quality Improvement Act of 2005 (Ch. 9).

pH A measurement of acidity, ranging from 1 (most acidic), to 14 (most basic). A pH of 7 is considered neutral, neither acid nor base (Ch. 2).

Prescription drug-monitoring program On-line database for tracking controlled-substance prescriptions filled or prescribed by every pharmacy and physician in the state. Pharmacies and physicians are required to report all controlled-substance prescriptions filled or prescribed by them within a specified period of time. Pharmacists are given a code allowing them to log onto the database and check to see if a patient had any controlled substances filled in another pharmacy in the state. The pharmacist can also see how many physicians are prescribing controlled substances for this patient (Ch. 3).

Prescription-monitoring program A database created by state law of all controlled-substance prescriptions filled or written in the state. All pharmacies and prescribers in the state are required to submit information on all controlled-substance prescriptions dispensed or written. Pharmacies and prescribers who submit information have access only for the purposes allowed under the statute (Ch. 10).

Preventable adverse medical event An adverse medical event is an injury resulting from a medical intervention, not due to the patient's underlying condition. An adverse medical event is preventable if it is attributable to an error. Not all adverse medical events are preventable (Ch. 4).

Preventable adverse medication event Any incident in which the use of a medication (drug or biologic) at any dose, a medical device, or a special nutritional product (e.g., dietary supplement, infant formula, medical food) may have resulted in an adverse outcome in a patient.

Process workflow Just as the pharmacy has a workflow that begins with receiving a prescription and ending with the delivery of the completed order to the nursing floor or the patient, each station or process has its own workflow. An individual station's workflow should be mapped by steps beginning with receiving the order to delivery to the next station (Ch. 7).

Prothrombin time (Pro Time) and international normalized ratio (INR) tests Two tests used to determine the time it takes blood to clot. One of these tests is used for patients on warfarin therapy as a way of determining the amount of this drug in their system and adjusting their dosage from that information. The more common of these two tests used today is the INR. Good INR values are considered as being between 2 and 3 (Ch. 5).

Q

QID (qid) A Latin abbreviation for "four times a day." Prescriptions are often written using such older style of abbreviations. Other common Latin abbreviations are QD (qd) (every day), BID (bid) (twice a day), and TID (tid) (three times a day) (Ch. 1).

Quality-related event (QRE) "Quality-related event" is a name given to a shorthand method used to describe the total of all errors and near-misses. In some instances it is used to describe only errors, but actually it refers to both (Ch. 1).

Quality-related events (QRE) A name given to a shorthand method used to describe the total of all errors and near-misses. In some instances it is used to describe only errors, but originally it referred to both (Ch. 2).

R

Risk-management process A continuous cycle of identification, planning, acting, monitoring, changing and then beginning again with identification of the risks that remain. It may be represented in four or five steps (Ch. 4).

Root-cause analysis An analysis that looks for the one or more causes that, if done differently, would have changed the results. It is not merely one of a number of best practices that would have prevented the error. In a root-cause analysis the cause is looked for, not a solution (Ch. 9).

Rx Only drugs Originally called "prescription" or "legend drugs." *Rx Only* is the new label given to medications that may not be dispensed except upon an order by a prescriber (Ch. 2).

S

Sentinel event A medical or medication error that resulted in serious injury or death. When a sentinel event is reported in a hospital, it must be analyzed by a peer-review committee. The committee will look for what and who caused the error and what measures may be taken to prevent a repeat (Ch. 9).

Shewhart cycle A planning process developed by Dr. Walter Shewhart. It is a way of looking at quality improvement as plan, do check. The Shewhart cycle is sometimes called the "Deming Cycle" or simply PDCA (Ch. 4).

Shift expert A person appointed to act as the quality expert on a shift. There should be at least one person on each shift who knows the quality system and can answer questions. Each shift expert needs to regularly communicate with others to be sure the messages to team members on that shift and throughout the pharmacy are consistent (Ch. 8).

Sig code A sig code is a software-provided shortcut designed to make entering directions into the computer easier and faster. For example, typing "1tqid" causes the directions, "Take one tablet four times a day" to appear (Ch. 7).

Special deviation Unlike a normal variation, a special deviation is a change caused by one of the factors or causes that influence. A special deviation (variation) is a change that was caused to occur. For example, if the pharmacy made a change in its CQI workflow and the number of QREs decreased, the result would be a special variation (Ch. 9).

T

Total quality management (TQM) TQM was the original name given to the systematic process of management and quality improvement by Dr. Edwards Deming (Ch. 1).

Training Training is teaching. It includes guiding, educating, and testing members of the team to be assured that all employees know how the pharmacy's quality systems function, what an individual employee's role is in the CQI program, and why each step in the pharmacy's quality workflow is necessary (Ch. 8).

Verifiers An electronic scanner that uses overlapping systems to verify that the drug in the finished prescription bottle is what was entered into the computer. The primary system is spectrographic analysis of the medication in the prescription bottle and comparison of it with a database of most commonly used drugs (Ch. 6).

Will call A section of the pharmacy department, usually in a community pharmacy, that has been set aside for completed prescriptions that have not yet been picked up (Ch. 7).

Workflow A series of stations designed as a plan for efficiently and correctly filling a prescription order. The workflow begins when a drug order arrives at the pharmacy and ends when the patient receives the correct medication with information for use (Ch. 4).

Workflow Pharmacy-quality systems are arranged as a series of processes that begin at one end of the prescription-dispensing area and move to the other end. They are usually designed as a straight-line flow (Ch. 2).

Workflow Pharmacy quality systems are arranged as a series of processes that begin at one end of the prescription-dispensing area and move to the other end. Workflows are usually designed as a straight-line flow with some deviation for special processes (Ch. 1).

Index

A

Accreditation Council for Pharmacy Education (ACPE), 52, 55
Adderal, 114
Address, 38–39
Adverse drug event, 1, 2, 5
Adverse event, 1
Algorithm
    counseling, 181–183
    definition of, 169
Allergies, 90–91
Ambulatory, 1, 5
American Pharmacists Association (APhA), 25
American Society of Health-System Pharmacists (ASHP), 25, 45
Amitriptyline, 141
Amoxicillin, 141
Anti-diabetic medications, 141
Apology laws, 251, 254
Atenolol, 141
Augmentin, 141

B

Basket system, 85
Benchmark, 220, 227
Best practice, 1, 4, 77, 79, 82–92, 138, 139–153

C

Cause analysis, 231–240
Centers for Medicare and Medicaid Services (CMS), 138, 163
Checklists, 211–212, 214–215
Children, 95–96
Commitment, training and, 195–196
Common law, 52, 60
Community pharmacy, 1, 3
Computer entry, 40–41, 115–116, 173–174
Container, 174–176
Continuous quality improvement (CQI), 1
    definition of, 191
    father of, 6–9
    patient and, 254–255
    risk management and, 77–78
    station, 77

Control, statistical, 14–16
Controlled substance, 25, 33
Conway, William, 6–7
Coumadin, 107–109, 141, 142
Counseling, 42, 68, 99, 129–131, 145–146, 178
Counseling algorithm, 181–183
Covered entity, 104, 126
Cubic centimeter (cc), 1, 11
Culture of learning, 191, 196
Customer
    internal, 169, 186–187
    patient as, 252–255

D

Data collection problems, 245–246
Data recording, 228–230
Data-entry station, 96–97
Delivery, 43, 99, 122–125, 183–185
Deming, W. Edwards, 6–11
DiGiovanni v. Albertson's, 62
Division of labor, 29–30
Documentation, 148–149
Dooley v. Everett, 60–61
Drug review, 25, 40
Drug utilization review (DUR), 25, 34, 42
Duty to warn, 63

E

Economics, 54–55
Education, patient, 68
Efficiency, quality and, 18–19, 64
Electronic prescribing, 77, 163–164
Environment error, 113
E-prescribing, 77, 138, 163–164
Error(s). *See also* Quality-related event (QRE)
    analyzing, 71
    causes of, 104, 112–113
    definition of, 2, 25
    environment, 113
    incidence of, 3, 30–31
    information, 44–45
    intellectual, 104, 126

INDEX

Error(s) (*Continued*)
    mechanical, 2, 5, 17, 112, 223, 255–258
    medical, 2
    medication, 2
    method, 112–113
    physician, 259–260
Expectations, 55–59

F

Fear, 194–195
Filling, 41–42, 97–98, 117–119, 174–176
Final check, 119–122, 176–177
Fishbone diagram, 220, 231
Food and Drug Administration (FDA), 25
Ford Motor Company, 7–9

H

Habits, 92–93, 201
Hand v. Krakowski, 60
Happel, Heidi, 32
Happel v. Wal-Mart Stores, 61
Health Insurance Portability and Accountability Act (HIPAA), 104, 125–129
Herbals, 26, 40

I

Imperfect systems, 222–228
Incident reports, 220, 223
Inderal, 114–115
Indian Health Service counseling, 138
Ingram v. Hooks, 60
Institute for Safe Medication Practices (ISMP), 26, 45, 114
Institute of Medicine (IOM) reports, 4–6
Insulin, 141
Intellectual error, 104, 126
Interactions, 26, 40
Internal customer, 169, 186–187
International normalized ratio (INR) tests, 104, 111

J

Judicial viewpoints, 59–62

L

Label assembly, 174–176
Label preparation, 40–41, 173–174
Labor, division of, 29–30
Law
    apology, 251, 254
    changing, 55–59
    common, 52, 60
    following, 47, 72
Leadership, training and, 196
Learned intermediary doctrine, 61
Learning, culture of, 191, 196
Levesque v. Cluett, 69–71
Levothyroxine, 141
Lifelong training, 196–197
Lipitor, 141
Lisinopril, 141

M

Manual filling, 117–118
Materials, 112
Mechanical error, 2, 5, 17, 112, 223, 255–258
Med-guides, 26
Medical error, 2
Medication error, 2
Method error, 112–113
Monitoring programs, 191

N

National Alliance for State Pharmacy Associations (NASPA), 26, 44–45
National Association of Boards of Pharmacy (NABP), 52, 62
National drug code (NDC), 1, 2, 4
National drug code (NDC) check, 83–85
Near-misses, 2, 10, 19, 26, 44–45, 71
Non-patient, duty to, 68
Non-punitive system, 230–231
Normal variation, 220, 227–228

O

OBRA-87 Regulation, 52, 55
OBRA-90 Regulation, 52, 56
Observation, 110–113, 113–114
Omnibus Budget Reconciliation Act-87 (OBRA-87) Regulation, 55

INDEX

Omnibus Budget Reconciliation Act-90 (OBRA-90) Regulation, 26, 35, 56
Organization, 34–35
Original prescription, 88–89
Outliers, 121
Over-the-counter medications, 26, 40

P

Paradigm, 2, 11
Parata Systems, LLC, 157–160
Pass Rx, 160–162
Patient
    continuous-quality improvement and, 254–255
    as customer, 252–255
    education, 68
    fault, 123–125
    fear of using, 255
    information, 35–36
    mistakes, 262–263
    profile, 34, 40
    in quality system, 252
    vulnerable, 37–38
Patient Safety and Quality Improvement Act, 220, 246
Patient safety organization (PSO), 220, 223, 246
Peer review, 47, 240
People, errors and, 112
pH, 26
Pharmacist
    assisting pharmacy technicians, 65
    evolving role of, 53–59
    expanding legal role of, 59–62
    final check, 119–122, 176–177
    quality check, 42, 65–66
    state statutory duties, 62
Pharmacist-only questions, 31–32, 64–65
Pharmacy technician
    pharmacist role in assisting, 65
    in workflow, 27–28, 35–43
Phone number, 38–39
Physician mistakes, 259–260
Plan, 13
Poison Prevention Packaging Act, 95
Prednisone, 141
Prescription drug-monitoring program, 52, 67, 251, 264–265
Prescription filling, 41–42, 97–98, 117–119, 174–176
Prescription receiving, 35–36
Preventable adverse medical event, 77, 82
Preventable adverse medication event, 77
Privacy, 125–129
Process workflow, 169, 171
Prospective drug review, 25, 35, 66, 90, 146–148, 178
Prothrombin time, 104, 111

Q

QID, 2
Quality and quality systems
    concepts, application of, 13–20
    efficiency and, 18–19
    habits, 92–93, 201
    implementation of, 30–31
    importance of, 16–17
    information, 45–46
    patient in, 252
    from pharmacist end of workflow, 63–64
    pharmacy technician role in, 27–30
Quality check, 42, 65–66
Quality-related event (QRE), 2, 14–16, 151, 238. *See also* Error(s)
Questions, pharmacist-only, 31–32, 64–65

R

Receiving, 35–36, 93, 114–115, 171–173
Recording data, 228–230
Refusal to accept mistakes, 193–194
Results-oriented training, 198–199
Riff v. Morgan, 60
Risk identification, 105–110
Risk management, 19–20
    complete quality workflow and, 77–78
    process, 77
    tools, 139
Robotic filling, 118–119
Robots, 156–160
Root-cause analysis, 220, 240
Rx only drugs, 26, 29, 40

S

Scanners, 154–156
ScriptPro, LLC, 156–157
Sentinel event, 220, 240
Shewhart cycle, 77, 79–81
Shift expert, 191
"Show and tell" counseling, 145–146
Sig code, 169, 174
Sound-alikes, 114–115
Special deviation, 220, 228
Special problems station, 99
State statutory duties, 62

Stations, 82
    continuous quality improvement, 77
    data-entry, 96–97
    final check, 119–122
    observation of, 113–114
    special problems, 99
Statistical analysis, 223–226
Statistical control, 14–16

T

Take 5, 89, 149–151
Teamwork, 186–187
Telephone number, 38–39
Telephone order, 39–40
Testing, 215–216
Toprol, 141
Total quality management (TQM), 2, 7
Tracking mistakes, 233–236
Tracking success, 121–122
Training, 46–47, 72
    beginning, 204–210
    checklists, 214–215
    commitment and, 195–196
    consistency of purpose and, 193
    culture of learning and, 196
    definition of, 191
    effective, 195–204
    fun in, 201–202
    goal of, 192–195
    leadership and, 196
    lifelong, 196–197
    to make quality work, 192
    results-oriented, 198–199
    rewards in, 199
    techniques, 210–215
    testing and, 215–216
    tools, 210–215
    universal, 199–200
Triple check, 87, 151–152
Two-second rule, 85–86

U

Unusual dose, 91–92, 143–144

V

Variation, 226–227, 227–228
Verifiers, 138
Verifying systems, 160–162
Vulnerability, locating, 106
Vulnerable patients, 37–38

W

Warfarin, 107–109, 141, 142
Will call, 169
Workflow
    adding detail to, 171–185
    basket system in, 85
    best practices in, 79, 82–92
    considerations, 185–186
    definition of, 2, 9, 26, 77
    NDC check in, 83–85
    overview of, 170–171
    pharmacist end of, 63–64
    pharmacy technician place in, 27–28, 35–43
    prescription, 81–82
    process, 169, 171
    quality habits in, 92–93
    receiving in, 171–173
    refining, 171–185
    Take 5 in, 89, 149–151
    triple check in, 87
    two-second rule in, 85–86
    unusual dosing in, 91–92